A CULTURAL HISTORY OF THE SENSES

VOLUME 4

A CULTURAL HISTORY OF THE SENSES

IN THE AGE OF ENLIGHTENMENT

Edited by Anne C. Vila

BLOOMSBURY ACADEMIC
LONDON • NEW YORK • OXFORD • NEW DELHI • SYDNEY

BLOOMSBURY ACADEMIC
Bloomsbury Publishing Plc
50 Bedford Square, London, WC1B 3DP, UK

BLOOMSBURY, BLOOMSBURY ACADEMIC and the Diana logo are trademarks of
Bloomsbury Publishing Plc

First published in Great Britain 2014
This edition published 2019

Copyright © Bloomsbury Publishing, 2014, 2019

Anne C. Vila has asserted her right under the Copyright, Designs and Patents Act, 1988,
to be identified as Editor of this work.

For legal purposes the Acknowledgments on p.xii constitute an extension of this copyright page.

Cover image: *The Five Senses*, Gerard de Lairesse, 1668 © CSG CIC
Glasgow Museums Collection.

All rights reserved. No part of this publication may be reproduced or transmitted in any form or
by any means, electronic or mechanical, including photocopying, recording, or any information
storage or retrieval system, without prior permission in writing from the publishers.

Bloomsbury Publishing Plc does not have any control over, or responsibility for, any third-party
websites referred to or in this book. All internet addresses given in this book were correct at the
time of going to press. The author and publisher regret any inconvenience caused if addresses
have changed or sites have ceased to exist, but can accept no responsibility for any such changes.

A catalogue record for this book is available from the British Library.

Library of Congress Cataloging-in-Publication Data.
A cultural history of the senses in the age of Enlightenment, 1650–1800 /
edited by Anne C. Vila.
pages cm
Includes bibliographical references and index.
ISBN 978-0-85785-342-4 (hardback)
1. Senses and sensation—History—18th century. 2. Enlightenment. I. Vila, Anne C., 1961–
BF233.C853 2014
152.1094'09033—dc23

ISBN:	HB:	978-0-8578-5342-4
	PB:	978-1-3500-7791-1
	ePDF:	978-1-4742-3310-1
	eBook:	978-1-4742-3311-8
	HB Set:	978-0-8578-5338-7
	PB Set:	978-1-3500-7783-6

Series: The Cultural Histories Series

Typeset by RefineCatch Limited, Bungay, Suffolk

To find out more about our authors and books visit www.bloomsbury.com
and sign up for our newsletters.

CONTENTS

	LIST OF ILLUSTRATIONS	vii
	SERIES PREFACE	xi
	EDITOR'S ACKNOWLEDGMENTS	xii
	Introduction: Powers, Pleasures, and Perils of the Senses in the Enlightenment Era *Anne C. Vila*	1
1	The Social Life of the Senses: A New Approach to Eighteenth-century Politics and Public Life *Sophia Rosenfeld*	21
2	Urban Sensations: Motion and Commotion in Eighteenth-century Cities *Clare Brant*	41
3	The Senses in the Marketplace: Coffee, Chintz, and Sofas *Joan DeJean*	65
4	The Senses in Religion: Listening to God in the Eighteenth Century *Phyllis Mack*	85
5	The Senses in Philosophy and Science: Blindness and Insight *Lissa Roberts*	109
6	Medicine and the Senses: The Perception of Essences *Patrick Singy*	133

7	The Senses in Literature: Pleasures of Imagining in Poetry and Prose *Rowan Rose Boyson*	155
8	Art and the Senses: Experiencing the Arts in the Age of Sensibility *Sarah Cohen and Downing A. Thomas*	179
9	Sensory Media: Communication and the Enlightenment in the Atlantic World *Richard Cullen Rath*	203
	NOTES	225
	BIBLIOGRAPHY	233
	NOTES ON CONTRIBUTORS	265
	INDEX	268

LIST OF ILLUSTRATIONS

INTRODUCTION

I.1 Claude Nicolas Le Cat, *A Physical Essay on the Senses* (London 1750). Plate X and Plate IX.   5
I.2 Franz Anton Bustelli, *Moor with Sugarbowl*, c. 1760 (cast 1760), porcelain.   8
I.3 Francisco Jose de Goya y Lucientes, *The Chinchillas*, plate 50 of "Los caprichos," (1799 etching and aquatint).   19
I.4 A large gathering of patients and assistants to Mesmer's animal magnetism therapy, showing use of the special tub at his clinic. Wood engraving by H. Thiriat.   20

CHAPTER ONE

1.1 Nicolas Lancret, *A Lady in a Garden Taking Coffee with some Children* (1742).   24
1.2 Engraving, *Feu d'artifice tiré à la place de Louis XV le 30 mai 1770 à l'occasion du mariage de Louis Auguste Dauphin de France avec l'archiduchesse Marie Antoinette, soeur de l'empereur.*   25
1.3 Fresco detail of Sebastiano Taricco, "Saletta del Silenzio" (1706), Palazzo Salmatoris, Cherasco, Italy.   29
1.4 Jacques-Louis David, *Le serment du jeu de Paume, le 20 juin 1789* (1791).   33

CHAPTER TWO

2.1 Michele Marieschi, *L'Entrée du Grand Canal et l'église de la Salute à Venise, c.* 1735–40.   47
2.2 "Buy my fine singing glasses," *Laroon Cryes of London*.   48
2.3 *Life of William Blake* (1880), Volume 2, *Songs of Experience*.   49
2.4 Louis-Léopold Boilly, *L'intérieur d'un café, dit aussi La partie de dames au café Lamblin au Palais-Royal*.   57

CHAPTER THREE

3.1 Anonymous engraving. Frontispiece, Louis de Mailly, *Les Entretiens des cafés de Paris*, 1702.   69
3.2 Painted and dyed cotton produced for the French market. India, Coromandel coast, *c.* 1750.   73
3.3 Jean Dieu de Saint-Jean, "Femme de qualité sur un canapé." Engraving, 1686.   79
3.4 Chiquet, "La Coiffeuse." Engraving, *c.* 1690.   81

CHAPTER FOUR

4.1 William Henry Pyne and William Combe, "Quakers Meeting" (1809).   89
4.2 Electrical machine designed by John Wesley for the treatment of melancholia.   93
4.3 Johann Valentin Haidt (1700–80), "Jesus Showing His Sidewound," n.d.   100
4.4 John Valentine Haidt, "Young Moravian Girl."   101

CHAPTER FIVE

5.1 Thomas Jefferys, *The Russian Discoveries, from the Map Published by the Imperial Academy of St. Petersburg* (1776).   114
5.2 Frontispiece from G.E. Rumphius, *Amboinsche Rariteitkamer* (1705).   117
5.3 *Caroli Linnaei Classes S. Literae*, plate by Georg Dionysius Ehret (1737).   119
5.4 Advertisement for Mr. Cressin and his Chinese automaton, 1796.   130

LIST OF ILLUSTRATIONS   ix

CHAPTER SIX

6.1 Fold-out plate from Fouquet's *Essai sur le pouls* (1767). 140
6.2 Two pages of a consultation letter from Lavergne l'aîné to Tissot, Lyon (France), October 25 [1772]. 142
6.3 Leopold Auenbrugger and his wife. 146
6.4 Title page and frontispiece with portrait of author. Giovanni Battista Morgagni, *De sedibus, et causis morborum* ... (1761). 150

CHAPTER SEVEN

7.1 James Gillray, "The King of Brobdingnag and Gulliver" (1804). 161
7.2 *Laocoön and His Sons*. 167
7.3 Pierre-Paul Prud'hon's "Le premier baiser de l'amour," ink and wash drawing, c. 1792–6. 171
7.4 Silhouette of Goethe in Tieburg, c. 1780. 175

CHAPTER EIGHT

8.1 Antoine Watteau, *La Surprise*, c. 1718–19, oil on canvas. 180
8.2 François Boucher, *Recumbent Female Nude*, c. 1742–3, black, white and red chalk on cream antique laid paper. 184
8.3 Jean-Siméon Chardin, *Still Life with Bottle of Olives*, 1763, oil on canvas. 186
8.4 William Hogarth, *The Enraged Musician*, 1741, engraving. 189
8.5 Angelica Kauffman, *Cornelia, Mother of the Gracchi*, 1785, oil on canvas. 193

CHAPTER NINE

9.1 Edward Collier, *A Trompe l'Oeil of Newspapers, Letters and Writing*, c. 1699. 204
9.2 William Caxton showing specimens of his printing to King Edward IV and his queen. 212
9.3 Post horn. *American Weekly Mercury*, no. 64, March 9, 1721. 217
9.4 William Dickinson (engraver), "The Coffee-House Patriots, or News, from St. Eustatia" (1781). 220

Every effort has been made to trace copyright holders and to obtain their permission for the use of copyright material. The publisher apologizes for any errors or omissions there may be in the credits for the illustrations and would be grateful if notified of any corrections that should be incorporated in future editions of this book.

SERIES PREFACE

GENERAL EDITOR, CONSTANCE CLASSEN

A Cultural History of the Senses is an authoritative six-volume series investigating sensory values and experiences throughout Western history and presenting a vital new way of understanding the past. Each volume follows the same basic structure and begins with an overview of the cultural life of the senses in the period under consideration. Experts examine important aspects of sensory culture under nine major headings: social life, urban sensations, the marketplace, religion, philosophy and science, medicine, literature, art, and media. A single volume can be read to obtain a thorough knowledge of the life of the senses in a given period, or one of the nine themes can be followed through history by reading the relevant chapters of all six volumes, providing a thematic understanding of changes and developments over the long term. The six volumes divide the history of the senses as follows:

Volume 1. A Cultural History of the Senses in Antiquity (500 BCE–500 CE)
Volume 2. A Cultural History of the Senses in the Middle Ages (500–1450)
Volume 3. A Cultural History of the Senses in the Renaissance (1450–1650)
Volume 4. A Cultural History of the Senses in the Age of Enlightenment (1650–1800)
Volume 5. A Cultural History of the Senses in the Age of Empire (1800–1920)
Volume 6. A Cultural History of the Senses in the Modern Age (1920–2000)

EDITOR'S ACKNOWLEDGMENTS

I would like to thank the following people for the roles they played in producing this volume: Constance Classen, who offered incisive comments and sage advice at every stage of the process; Emma Goode and Anna Wright, who replied to technical queries with patience and good cheer; Anne Hajek, who provided timely assistance in standardizing the style and format of the chapters; Donald Kerr, Jon R. Snyder, Micaela Sullivan-Fowler, and Paul Peucker, who greatly simplified the task of obtaining certain illustrations; and most of all, my fellow authors, who brought both enormous scholarly expertise and great professionalism to this collective project.

Introduction: Powers, Pleasures, and Perils of the Senses in the Enlightenment Era[1]

ANNE C. VILA

With light built into its very name, the Enlightenment might seem to be, first and foremost, a culture of sight. The Scientific Revolution unquestionably opened up new visual worlds through advances like microscopes, telescopes, and anatomical dissection; moreover, the eye as physical object and as metaphor preoccupied many of the period's philosophers, physiologists, natural theologians, politicians, and artists.[2] However, just as it was both the Age of Reason and the Age of Sensibility, the Enlightenment had a complex sensory history. Its thinkers and various publics were keenly attuned to all five of the external, physical senses, and to their interdependency: the ways the senses work in concert. They were also fascinated by forms of sensing that were inscribed more mysteriously within the depths of the human being (as we shall see below).

Although the classic hierarchy of the senses that made vision supreme was sometimes upended (or relaxed to allow for multi- and inter-sensorial approaches), it was still commonplace to rank a particular external sense organ as the privileged gateway into the human interior. Theorists of psychology (a term coined in the eighteenth century to refer to the science of mind or mental phenomena—Vidal 2011) often debated which sensory faculty was the most "philosophical," in terms of determining the development of reason or providing reliable information about the world. Whereas some regarded visual perception as the most direct path to knowledge, others—like Denis Diderot (*Lettre sur les aveugles* [*Letter on the Blind*], [1749] 1975), and Johann Gottfried Herder (*Plastik [Sculpture]*, 1778)—championed touch over sight, believing that the haptic sense gives us the surest knowledge of external bodies in their substantial reality (Lichtenstein 2008: 55–72). Smell, too, had its supporters: George-Louis de Buffon hailed the olfactory sense as a key survival tool for animals and "primitive" man; and Jean-Jacques Rousseau called it the "sense of imagination" in *Emile, ou De l'éducation* (Rousseau [1762] 1979: 156; Le Guérer 1992: 164–73). The ear enjoyed special prominence as a conduit for soul-stirring stimuli in secular theories on the origins of language as well as in evangelical Christian notions of spiritual hearing (Schmidt 2000: 50–7). Taste, meanwhile, was central to the definition which many eighteenth-century authors applied to their era. Some prominent figures like Voltaire took pains to expunge taste's corporeal underpinnings when discussing "polite" moral judgment and the discriminating critical faculty of the aesthete; however, David Hume and others were intrigued by the relations between mental and bodily taste (Marshall 2005: 176–96). Partaking in the pleasures of the table was, furthermore, a point of entry into the intellectual pleasures of the Enlightenment: both Voltaire and Hume embodied the "sociable, merry, and moderately gormandizing philosopher of the eighteenth century" (Shapin 1998: 43), and a host of French gastronomes went to great lengths to make the alimentary integral to tasteful connoisseurship (Spary 2012). Taking a more jaundiced approach altogether, the satirist James Beresford invented two fictional characters, Timothy Testy and Samuel Sensitive, who experienced the senses as nothing "but five yawning inlets to hourly and momentarily molestations" (Beresford 1806, quoted in Janković 2010: 56).

Extending the notion of the senses as portals, this chapter considers various points of entry which they offer into the practices and perspectives of those who inhabited the Enlightenment world. This approach will frame the more detailed analyses offered in the nine chapters to come. If we look at dates to anchor the events that did the most to shape the ways in which people understood the world from 1650 to 1800, we are liable to focus on the period's revolutionary bookends: that is, the Scientific Revolution which ushered it in, and the American and French Revolutions at its close. However, developments of a slower sort played an equally critical role in Enlightenment-era beliefs and attitudes about sensory experience. This period introduced new models of matter, the body, and the mind-body connection, which transformed the ways in which sensory perception was held to operate. It also witnessed major changes in living and working habits, including urbanization, travel and exploration, and the rise of comfort and pleasure as values that cut across a range of social classes. Finally, it was marked by some essential tensions: although the Enlightenment is often equated with faith in the expansive powers of human intelligence and creativity, it was equally preoccupied with limits and hierarchies. Similarly, despite our tendency to view it in retrospect as an optimistic period, this was also a time of anxious fretting over the various ills attendant to civilization—not least sensory overstimulation.

Many of those developments were linked to sensibility, a concept that, as Barker-Benfield has put it, lay at the center of a unique "constellation of ideas, feelings, and events" which took hold throughout eighteenth-century Europe and America, albeit with sometimes significant national differences (Barker-Benfield 1992: xix). I will therefore begin with a summary of sensibility's emergence, implications, and influence over this period's thinking about the senses, before shifting into a consideration of the period's mixed attitudes toward intense sensations. Finally, I will sketch some of the ways in which the senses were made useful during the Enlightenment, and the questions and problems which those uses opened up.

SENSIBILITY, SENTIENCE, AND THE MIND/BODY RELATION

Several factors were involved in the rise of the versatile concept that was known as sensibility in eighteenth-century Europe and America: the revalorization of sentiment and the passions in moral philosophy and literature; the emphasis which epistemologists placed on sensations in the formation of knowledge and subjectivity, particularly in the wake of John Locke's *Essay Concerning Human Understanding* (1690); the collapse of mechanism as a philosophical and scientific worldview; and the shift toward a more corporeal conception of the "common sensorium" or seat of the soul. The biomedical sciences also played a key role in the 1740s and 1750s. The Swiss physician Albrecht von Haller conducted ground-breaking investigations on the reactive properties of muscles and nerves which highlighted the inadequacies of dogmatic iatromechanism, a doctrine that used machine-based, hydraulic models to explain the body's physiological processes (Steinke 2005). Drawing on the extensive vivisectionist experiments he was performing on animals, Haller instead proposed the more dynamic notions of irritability, the term he used to refer to contractile shortening in the muscles, and sensibility, which he defined as "signs of painful arousal of the soul" (Figlio 1975: 186).

Not all of the theorists who responded to Haller agreed with his definitions or respected his distinction between irritability and sensibility. For example, the British neuroscientist Robert Whytt refuted Haller by insisting that motions as well as pain responses were dependent on a soul or general sentient principle (Wright 1991: 290–1). On the other end of the ideological spectrum, the physician-philosopher Julien Offray de La Mettrie audaciously seized upon Haller's irritability principle in *L'Homme machine* (1747) to advance a fully materialist theory of thinking and feeling. Another important response came from the vitalist physicians and graduates of the Montpellier medical faculty, who saw sensibility (not irritability) as the key vital power, and elaborated models to explain its operations at all levels in the human being. For example, in the *Recherches anatomiques sur la position des glandes et sur leur action* (1752), Théophile de Bordeu proposed that glands have their own way of "sensing" when it is appropriate to react to a stimulus. Using a metaphor that would soon reappear in other contexts (like Diderot's *Rêve de d'Alembert*, 1769), Bordeu compared the living body to a bee-swarm: that is, a holistic federation of semi-autonomous parts, each of which followed rhythms determined by its particular dose of local sensibility, and which worked in coordination with the rest of the organism in an ongoing process of action and reaction (Williams 2003: 154–60). Opinions differed on how much of that coordination was provided by the brain and nervous apparatus: in contrast to the Montpellier vitalists, life scientists in Scotland and Germany proposed top-down models that located sensibility squarely within the nervous system (Gaukroger 2010: 397–9; Lawrence 1979).

Despite those contrasting opinions, these shifts within biomedical thought had the effect of softening the old mind/body dualism and ushering in a more generalizing vision of vital reactivity that was based upon a simple "impression" model of sensation—often involving fibers (a term taken literally or metaphorically, depending on the theorist). In this view, sensation was "the action of an object upon the property of sensibility" (Figlio 1975: 186), and the presumption of a causal connection between the mind and its underlying physical substrate allowed theorists to use the same vocabulary of impressions or affections to talk about both. The always crucial mind/body relation changed orientation, and the complex involvement of sensory perception in that relation underpinned several of the period's defining medico-philosophical debates. One was Molyneux's Problem, a thought experiment involving the sudden acquisition of sight by a man born blind which was first proposed in 1688 by the Irish scientist and politician William Molyneux in a letter to John Locke, and which surgeons like William Chelseden tested out through cataract operations (Morgan 1977; Riskin 2002). The role of the external sense organs in mediating the mind/

body relation was also a central question for early contributors to the field of sensory physiology, like the Berlin physician Marcus Herz and the Göttingen medical professor Johann Friedrich Blumenbach (Reill 2005: 147–52). Another noteworthy figure in this area was the Rouen surgeon Claude-Nicolas Le Cat, whose *Traité des sens* (1744) included, along with extensive discussion of all five senses (with great focus on Isaac Newton's experiments on color and optics in the chapters on vision), the "extraordinary case" of the monk of Prague, a man endowed with exceptional olfactory acuity:

> He not only knew different Persons by the Smell, but, what is much more singular, could, we are told, distinguish a chaste Woman, married or unmarried, from one that was not so. This Religious had begun to write a new Treatise on Odours, when he died, very much lamented by the Gentlemen who record this Story of Him. For my Part, I do not know whether a Man of such Talents would not have been dangerous to Society.
>
> Le Cat 1750: 32–3

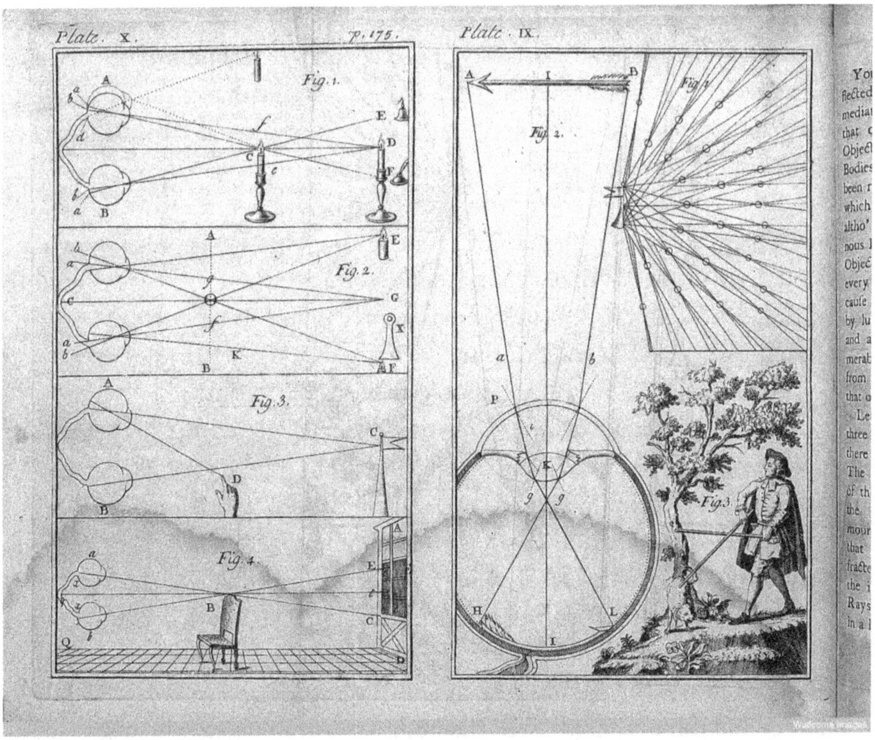

FIGURE I.1: Claude Nicolas Le Cat, *A Physical Essay on the Senses* (London, 1750). Plate X and Plate IX. Wellcome Library, London.

In the context of philosophy, sensibility was the means by which, as David Howes puts it, "aspects of the Aristotelian notion of sentience survived the Cartesian censure of the senses" (Howes 2009: 20). Building on Locke's empirically based, phenomenological approach toward the formation of human knowledge, theorists interested in epistemology largely abandoned the Cartesian notion of "innate ideas" in favor of natural histories of the mind that gave a generative power to sensations. In his 1749 treatise *Observations on Man*, David Hartley argued that sensory perceptions induced vibrations that were represented to the mind as simple ideas, which could then be associated with other ideas; he and his fellow associationists effectively reduced the power of the mind to the ability to receive impressions (Hatfield 1995: 188). Hartley's model helped to make the auditory metaphor of the stringed instrument a commonplace in eighteenth-century discussions of consciousness, memory, and intersubjective passions like sympathy (Jacot Grapa 2009: 267–90; Thomas 2002: 179–200).

The French-speaking reading public also encountered histories of the mind, often in the form of metaphysical "anatomies" designed around the idea of "decomposing a man, so to speak, and consider[ing] what he gets from each of the senses he possesses" (Diderot [1751] 2000: 94). In the *Traité des sensations* (1754), one of the best known works of this sort, Étienne Bonnot de Condillac presented an epistemological fable centered on a statue that acquired all of its intellectual faculties (with the important exception of speech) via the successive activation of the senses, starting with the scent of a rose.

Condillac himself was not a materialist, and he did not draw on physiology or neurology to study the mind's operations. However, his systematic application of the thesis that all ideas come through the senses was central to the so-called sensualist or sensationalist school of philosophy, which culminated with the Idéologues—a group of thinkers who, during the Revolutionary and Bonapartist eras in France, undertook to consolidate all the branches of knowledge into a single "science" of man that articulated the links between physiology, moral character, and intelligence. The physicians Xavier Bichat and Pierre-Jean-Georges Cabanis, two of the most prominent members of this group, endorsed Condillac's emphasis on the impressions the mind received through the external sense organs; however, they gave equal weight to internal sensations originating in the inner organs, which, in their view, were the sources of instincts and passions (Temkin [1946] 2006: 330). Cabanis devoted his major work, the *Rapports du physique et du moral de l'homme* (1802), to examining the forces that affected the bodily substrate from which sensations and ideas arose. He gave special prominence to sex, but also took into account age, temperament, illness, regimen, and climate (Williams 1994: 84–105).

Sensibility thus provided both a dynamic vision of the body's interior, and an equally dynamic way of theorizing the interface between the inner and outer worlds of the human being—the liminal space where the external senses operated. By the second half of the eighteenth century, it was as fundamental to the definition of human nature as was reason. According to philosophical empiricists, sensibility was the root cause of perceptions and mental operations; and, for many contemporary physicians, it was the moving power that drove vital function, the source of both health and illness. Through the interweaving of the moral and the physical so characteristic of this period, sensibility was also made the basis of sociability and sympathic fellow-feeling—an idea vigorously promoted in the sentimental literature and art that flourished during the eighteenth century. Finally, sensibility was often associated with the special energy and affective temperament which were deemed essential to genius, artistic creativity, and aesthetic discernment.

AMBIGUITIES OF THE SENSES: SENSING AND FEELING TOO MUCH

The long Enlightenment invested great powers in sensing and feeling. Vision-enhancing technologies enraptured fashionable audiences and inspired artistic invention from seventeenth-century Dutch art, to British *Georgics*, to Robert Barker's panorama (Alpers 1983; Goodman 2004; Otto 2011; Stafford *et al.* 2001). Grand public fireworks displayed in or near Europe's capitals dazzled the eye while also stunning the ear, especially when accompanied by music by composers like Handel ("Music For The Royal Fireworks," 1749) (see Figure 1.2). As regards architecture, Versailles was constructed to "arrest all of the senses" of its visitors through its brilliant gold, astonishing fountains and grottos, and the outsized proportions of both the chateau and its gardens (Goldstein 2008: 160). Private homes, too, were configured for sensory appeal: fine dining tables enticed the imagination as well as the palates of their guests, through rich and fragrant foodstuffs displayed in exquisitely designed serving pieces. The rooms of wealthy private houses like Keldeston Hall delighted by the "sheen and sparkle of the object, the sparkle of designed space" (De Bolla 2003: 197), and English gardens featured odiferous exotic flowers like jasmine to enhance their multisensorial pleasures (Dugan 2011: 162–7). Shows provided another form of compelling spectacle. Parisian theater audiences wept loudly in response to the striking gestural acting used to depict familial crises in bourgeois dramas (Vincent-Buffault 1991). Opera-goers likewise sobbed upon hearing Gluck's painfully moving music (Johnson 1995: 59–62).

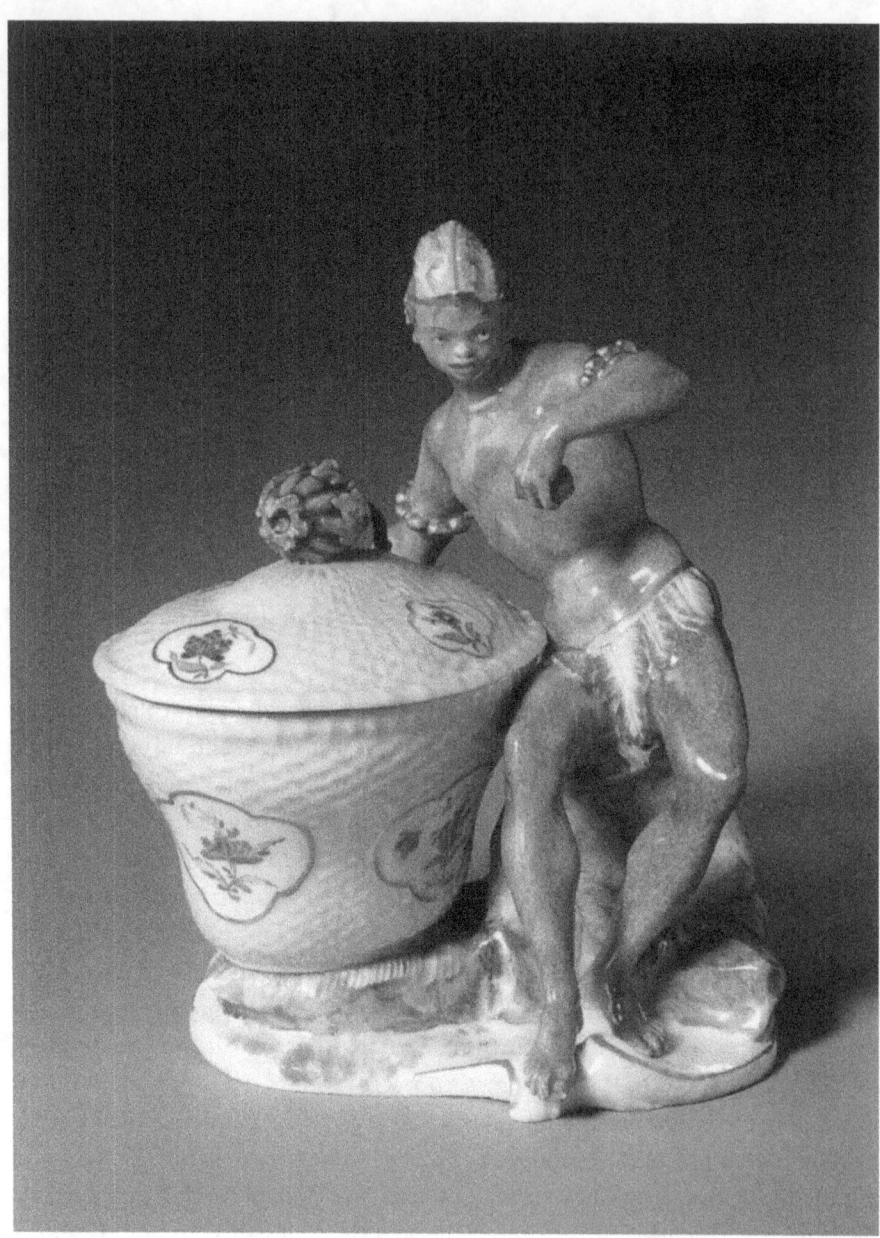

FIGURE I.2: Franz Anton Bustelli, *Moor with Sugarbowl*, c. 1760 (cast 1760), porcelain; from Alfred Ziffer, *Nymphenburger Porzellan Sammlung Bäuml Collection* (Stuttgart: Arnoldsche, 1997), 59, no. 90.

Brave new sensory worlds were opened up by other important threads in this period's cultural tapestry, as well. These included the dramatic surge in the production and consumption of goods, accompanied by the widespread adoption of elite fashions and of physical comfort as an important social value; the growing emphasis on intimacy, familial domesticity, and private life; and the invention or expansion of sensorily inviting public institutions like the restaurant, the coffeeshop or café, the limonadier shop, mineral water spas, and museums. The Enlightenment also saw the discovery of the seaside as a place of invigorating leisure (Corbin 1994); encounters with new parts of the world, like the "howling wilderness" of early America (Rath 2003); ecstatic religious prophecy among Quakers and Jansenist convulsionaries (Mack 1992; Maire 1985); and the elaboration of various voluptuous arts by free-thinking aristocrats and other libertines.

Sensory intensity was not, however, sought or cultivated by everyone. Essayist Joseph Addison pointed out in the *Spectator* (1712) that the mind can take no pleasure if "the Object presses too close upon our Senses, and bears so hard upon us, that it does not give us time or leisure to reflect on our selves" (Addison [1711–14] 1965, iii: 569). The specific context of Addison's remark was aesthetic: writing on the superior pleasures of the imagination, he was intent to underscore the difference between actually witnessing "Torments, Wounds, Deaths, and the like dismal Accidents" versus reading about them in a poem (Addison 1965, iii: 569). However, his emphasis on the mind's need for mastery over immediate sensate experience points to a broader strand of Enlightenment thinking: its insistence on moderation and control, for the purposes of health as well as pleasure and clear-headedness.

Emphasis on moderation was, in fact, paramount among many who undertook to theorize the essential mechanisms of sensibility, a quality that could have either edifying or destructive potentialities, depending on how it was directed. Critiques of sensibility became pronounced in the waning years of the Enlightenment, particularly when it was tied to the terrifying emotional excesses of the French Revolution. However, the double-edged nature of sensibility was already evident in the two articles on the topic which appeared in the fifteenth volume of the *Encyclopédie, ou Dictionnaire raisonné des arts, des sciences, et des métiers* (1751–65). In his short entry "Sensibilité (morale)," Louis de Jaucourt declared that the sensitive were, by nature, more humane, more empathetic, and more intelligent; yet he also remarked that, along with heightened pleasures, they experienced magnified woes (Jaucourt [1765] 2013, xv: 52). Similarly, Henri Fouquet began the long medical article "Sensibilité,

Sentiment" with the lyrical proclamation that sensibility was "the faculty of feeling, the sentient principle, or the feeling of all the parts, the basis and preserver of life, animality par excellence, the most beautiful and the most singular phenomenon of nature" (Fouquet [1765] 2013, xv: 38). However, he devoted a good deal of the article to the pathological disruptions caused when inner sensations became too acute. That negative view was echoed elsewhere in the *Encyclopédie*: in articles like "Digestion" and "Vapeurs," magnified feeling was attributed mainly to people who constantly and fretfully observed their physical sensations, a category that included intellectuals, aristocrats, ecclesiastics, women of leisure "who eat a lot," and the debauched (Venel [1754] 2013, iv: 1002).

Those groups were singled out as vulnerable to chronic nervous susceptibility, a condition which Michel Foucault characterized as "falling ill from feeling too much" (Foucault [1961] 1972: 214). That syndrome was central to this era's sense of its own newness, a modernity that was both exciting and perturbing. For all of the delight that many expressed over the expansion of modern comforts, there was widespread worry that new forms of morbidity were also on the rise, particularly disorders of the nerves—a notion that authors like the Lausanne physician Samuel-Auguste Tissot were very successful in popularizing. The senses were integral to those sorts of maladies. Tissot warned in *De la Santé des gens de lettres* (1768) that excessive study strained the nerves so badly that it could lead to temporary or permanent loss of sight and hearing; he made a similar warning regarding certain forms of "self pollution" in *De l'Onanisme* (1760). In *Dissertation sur les vapeurs* (1756), Dr. Pierre Hunauld maintained that an odiferous sweat as well as impetuous winds emanated from the bodies of those suffering from the vapors (Hunauld [1756] 2009: 124). Overstimulated palates were held to contribute to the dyspepsia and "weak stomach" complaints which seemed rampant among Europe's social elite—yet another condition tied to the nerves. To cure all of these ailments, doctors standardly prescribed bland diets but sometimes proposed more sensorially violent remedies like prolonged ice baths (Vigarello 1988: 114).

Michael Stolberg points out that people suffering from nervous diseases experienced their complaints very differently at the beginning of the century, when humoralism still dominated, versus its end, when virtually everything became a nervous complaint—and nerves were generally seen as overstimulated (Stolberg 2011: 176–7). Physicians commonly blamed civilization for the increasing spread of these complaints, which led them to focus particularly on the lifestyle of affluent, urban patient groups:

Lack of exercise, overly spiced food, fashionable stimulants such as coffee, tea, chocolate, and tobacco, a reversal of the natural succession of sleeping and waking through night-time festivities, constant erotic stimulation due to intensive social contact between the sexes, the excitement of gambling, the artificial stimulation of the imagination through music, novels, and drama, and innumerable other unnatural influences put the nervous system in a state of continual tension and excitement and harmed the entire organism.

Stolberg 2011: 178

We should remember, however, that even morbidity can be made fashionable. For those who lived in the Enlightenment's cultural climate of delicacy—a social context also attuned to climate in the literal, environmental sense—sensitivity taken to the point of infirmity was not just prevalent but chic: it was a marker of rank and refinement, of being up to date (Janković 2010). Thus, just as vaporous complaints were ubiquitous among aristocratic ladies, so too, the true scholar was a sickly fellow; and the bourgeoisie, eager to keep up, also felt vulnerable to nervous disorders and actively sought medical guidance. However much contemporary physicians tried to bring those groups back to nature by evoking the well-entrenched myth of sturdy peasants "free from the ills to which civilization was heir" (Brockliss and Jones 1997: 455), the pleasure-loving urban elite didn't seem inclined to emulate the model. One reason may be that anti-civilization medical discourse tended to depict the simple life of the simple peasant as mind-numbingly boring, devoid of interesting sensations or sentiments (Tissot [1770] 1778: 26–36; Vila 1998: 188–96).

New perspectives on the body, health, and social identity were thus at play in the Enlightenment's mixed attitudes toward sensory experience. Over the course of the eighteenth century, the body became both more private and more susceptible to impressions—or rather, susceptible in new ways, as nervousness supplanted the old humoralist understanding of disease and temperament. The sensibility-inspired conception of the human being as a "reactive" organism, acutely vulnerable to its physical and social surroundings, had a strong effect on both disease theory and the popular perception of sensory stimulants. Among other things, it reoriented the medical quest for the causes of illness toward the environment (interior as well as exterior) and created an almost obsessive concern with things that threatened air quality, including drafts and the "impolite" body odors of which Tobias Smollett's character Matt Bramble complains in *The Adventures of Humphry Clinker* (1771; Janković 2010: 50,

61). This conception also contributed to the rise of hygiene as a distinct branch of medicine, which was closely tied to the growth of the vernacular printing press and the general expansion of the medicable during the Enlightenment (Brockliss and Jones 1997: 459–79). By the end of this era, thorough-going personal hygiene required attending to the air one breathed, the lighting and sound of one's living and work spaces, and the quality of the materials that touched one's person. Sensory hygiene programs were also carried out at the collective level: for example, in the campaigns to purify public space by cleaning streets and cesspools, and transferring cemeteries and their human remains *extra-muros* (Corbin 1986: 111–27; Strauss 2012: 82–102).

THE USES OF THE SENSES

The proper use and management of the senses was a theme sounded in areas other than the medical or hygienic. One was sociopolitical discourse and practice: eighteenth-century English writings on politics were obsessed with the "stink of corruption" in the government (Brant 2004), and Paris police went to great lengths to chase down and arrest anyone "singing or reciting naughty verse about the court" (Darnton 2010a: 22). During the Revolutionary era, the Parisian municipality organized elaborate festivals that carried on the Old Regime fashion for launching hot-air balloons, but festooned the aerostatic objects of the spectacle with a political message in the form of the tricolor, to deepen the impressions made on the huge crowd of spectators gathered on the Champs de Mars (de Baecque 1997: 251–2).

Writings on art were also preoccupied with sensory matters. The German philosopher Alexander Gottlieb Baumgarten first coined the term "aesthetics" in 1735 to refer to "how things are cognized by means of the senses," and he amplified that definition in his groundbreaking *Aesthetica* of 1750, where he redefined beauty as "the perfection of cognition by means of the senses as such" (Guyer 1998, i: 227). Baumgarten's conception of sensitive cognition influenced the esthetics of later German theorists like Moses Mendelssohn, Gotthold Efraim Lessing, and Immanuel Kant. The eighteenth century also introduced notions of aesthetic taste as a sixth sense—within us, as Jean-Baptiste Du Bos put it, "without our seeing its organs" (*Réflexions critiques sur la poésie et sur la peinture*, 1719—Du Bos [1719] 1755, ii: 342). In its final decades, it saw the emergence of new aesthetic categories that stressed strong sensations and emotions rather than pleasing ones, like the sublime, the Gothic, and the fantastic (May 1998, ii: 233–4). The notion of the sublime was a particularly important development in thinking about both sensory experience and the moral/social usefulness of art. As Edmund Burke argued in *Philosophical Enquiry into the Origin of Our Ideas of the Sublime and Beautiful* (1757), the "sublime delight" induced by overpowering works of art was rooted in a radical, somatic stimulation that was painful but therapeutic, in that the mind and its "fine corporeal parts" had to be "shaken and worked to a proper degree" to avoid an indolence that could lead to somber states like "melancholy, dejection, despair" (Burke [1757] 1968: 135–6). Sublime art, as he described it, drew on a unique set of sensory triggers, like obscurity, immensity, and high-intensity contrasts of light and color.

The senses played a particularly important role in Enlightenment-era education reform, a field deeply shaped by the works of Locke, Condillac, and Rousseau (Jütte 2005: 157–79). In *Some Thoughts Concerning Education* (1690), Locke recommended that the physical upbringing of children should promote robust health through a plain diet, loose clothing, playing in the open air, and cold-water bathing; those were, in his view, the best conditions for ensuring that the right impressions of the outside world were made upon the "tabula rasa" which was the human mind (Parry 2007: 217–19). Condillacian sensationalism was applied to education in the controversial works *De L'Esprit* (1758) and *De l'Homme* (1772), where Claude-Adrien Helvétius declared that the human mind was entirely malleable and perfectible—and thus that a program of instruction based on well-controlled exposure to the right sensations could make any pupil a genius. Condillac's more cautious pedagogical tracts, like the *Cours d'études pour l'instruction du Prince du Parme* (1767–73), were followed in the highest circles of European society and remained popular among French educators until the 1830s. Rousseau, who startled some contemporary educational theorists but still attracted many followers, argued in *Emile* that "to exercise the senses is not only to make use of them, it is to learn to judge well with them. It is to learn, so to speak, to sense; for we know how to touch, see, and hear only as we have learned" (Rousseau [1762] 1979: 132).

A basic premise of these works was that enlightened minds could be shaped through the senses to learn how to reason precisely and correctly about the world, and to behave virtuously as moral citizens. Rousseau elaborated his ideas about the latter of those two goals in both his autobiographical *Confessions* (1782–8) and his best-selling sentimental novel *La Nouvelle Héloïse* (1758). In the *Confessions*, he envisioned undertaking a *morale sensitive*, a hybrid brand of moral-physical analysis based on the study of how his own moral behavior was shaped by the impressions made by "the seasons, sounds, color, darkness, light, the elements, food, noise, silence, rest" (Rousseau

1959–95, i: 343), He devoted a good part of *La Nouvelle Héloïse*, in turn, to a detailed plan for the care and maintenance of the exquisitely sensitive heroine Julie in the pristine Swiss countryside. Although Julie is a natural *gourmande* who feels intensely all the pleasures of the senses, she adheres to a regimen of carefully metered doses of enjoyments, starting with her diet, in the belief that her virtue and health depend on it (Rousseau 1959–95, ii: 541–2).

There was, as several commentators have noted, something artificial about the "natural" environment in which some of these programs in sensory education were meant to be carried out. The specific world of Locke's pedagogical scenario was that of an English country gentleman in the making; and Rousseau stuck his fictional child Emile out in the woods—that is, as far away as possible from complicated, denaturing city life ("Cities are the abyss of the human species"—Rousseau [1762] 1979: 59). Isabelle de Charrière pointed up the shortcomings of such a controlled bucolic setting for intellectual and moral development in her melancholic novel *Lettres de Mistriss Henley* (1784), whose heroine is a cultured, urbane woman unsuited for the life she finds herself living at Hollow Park after she marries her own country gentleman. Mistress Henley laments:

> This place is like its master, everything is too perfect, there is nothing to change, nothing that requires my participation or attention . . . the best I can find to do, in this verdant season, is to watch the leaves appear and unfold, the flowers blossom, a cloud of insects fly, creep, run every which way; I don't understand any of it, I apprehend it but superficially . . . I lose myself in this vast whole . . .
>
> Charrière [1784] 1993: 35

Back in the city, pedagogues like the Abbé Charles Michel de l'Epée undertook in the 1760s to educate deaf-mute children by trying to "impart language through their eyes rather than their ears," thereby initiating efforts throughout Europe to develop sign language (Rée 1999: 141–206, quote at 146). Early participants in this campaign, like l'Epée, often expressed the desire to teach the deaf the elements of Christianity, whereas Revolutionary-era educators like the Abbé Roch-Ambroise Sicard tended to emphasize the importance of reclaiming them for society and to promote the education of the deaf "as a model of revolutionary 'regeneration'" (Rosenfeld 2001: 133). Sicard, Epée's successor at the Institution des Sourds-Muets, wrote a dictionary to codify a language of gestural signs and expanded the school's curriculum to include training in artisanal crafts like drawing and printing, creating "a remarkable tradition of deaf painters and sculptors in France" (Rée 1999: 191–2). Sensory education was also of interest to the doctors and philosophers who focused on remedying perceptual deficiencies in wild children in order to socialize them (Douthwaite 2002).

The power to sense in particular ways was central to several fields of professional training, from the emphasis on the artist's physical touch which prevailed in later eighteenth-century artistic practice and theory, to the making of natural historical knowledge at the royal Parisian botanical garden (Cohen 2004; Spary 2000: 196). Equally important, however, was the power to analyze, verbalize, and measure sensory experience accurately. The Philadelphia physician Benjamin Rush told his medical students that "in a sick room, we should endeavor to be all touch, all taste, all smell, all eye, and all ear, in order that we may be all mind; for our minds, as I shall say presently, are the products of impression upon our senses" (Schmidt 2000: 26). Rush's exhortation echoed the idea of the senses as forms of skill which the self-experimenter Sir John Floyer had presented earlier in his *Pharmakos-Basanos, Or, the Touche-Stone of Medicines* (1687–90), a system of medicine based on gustatory practices (Floyer valiantly tasted millipedes and soot to determine their therapeutic value), and in *The Physician's Pulse Watch* (1707–10), where Floyer drew on Chinese as well as European pulse classification systems to offer guidance on what, precisely, should be felt by skilled physicians when taking pulses for diagnosis and prognosis (Jenner 2010). Late eighteenth-century physicians and surgeons taught their students to place as much emphasis on patients' accounts of internal sensations like pain as upon the raw sensory data which the practitioner gathered through physical examination (Lawrence 1993).[3]

A similar distancing from sensory knowledge underpinned the late eighteenth-century chemical revolution: chemical reformers like Antoine Laurent Lavoisier argued that, while sense-based observations like smelling, tasting, and assessing the color of substances were necessary at some points in the experimental process, precise instrumentation and standardized measurement were crucial, and mathematical analysis had to replace sensory analysis "as the final step in chemical determination" (Roberts 1995: 521).

Those developments unquestionably reflect a leaning toward desensualization: that is, a devalorization of human sense, with all of its subjective implications, in favor of reason and objectivity. However, it is important to recognize the fault lines that ran through the separation of sensuous body from discerning mind which occurred in certain arenas of eighteenth-century thought and culture. One was professional hierarchization: as Lissa Roberts, Patrick Singy, and Richard Rath all emphasize in their chapters, the Enlightenment philosophy of observation and manufactures entailed a division of labor which often drew sharp distinctions between keen-sensing workers and their more visionary, reflective managers. Another was gender: the bodily senses were a tool in constructing the theory of sexual dimorphism, or insistence on radical differences between the moral and physical constitutions of men and women, which was advanced by many moralists, philosophers, and speculative life scientists in the final decades of the eighteenth century.

Rousseau was one writer responsible for popularizing sexual dimorphism: he insisted in the *Emile* that there was "no parity between the two sexes in regard to the consequence of sex. The male is male only at certain moments. The female is female her whole life" (Rousseau [1762] 1979: 361). Another was the Montpellier physician Pierre Roussel, author of the widely read *Système physique et moral de la femme* (1775) and its companion piece, the uncompleted *Fragment d'un système physique et moral de l'homme*. Like Rousseau, Roussel saw the consequence of sex spread throughout the entire female constitution, which made it acutely sensitive, impressionable, and "soft" in both body and mind (the same constitution he attributed to children). Women were thus trapped in a state of constant and uncontrollable sensing and feeling, which bound them to hearth and home and made them unfit for serious scholarly endeavor: "The difficulty of shedding the tyranny of her sensations, by constantly binding her [Woman] to the immediate cause which calls them forth, prevents her from rising to the heights which would afford her a view of the whole" (Roussel [1775] 1820: 18). In the male constitution, by contrast, sensibility was selectively channeled to the brain, where it stimulated the soul to rise to "the most sublime operations of intelligence" (Roussel [1775] 1820: 236). Roussel and followers like Cabanis thus masculinized sensibility's most noble, mind-centered qualities while feminizing those that they deemed primitive or less evolved. In essence, they proposed two very different views of human nature: a progressive, meliorist perspective on man's nature, and a biologically deterministic perspective on woman's nature (Rendall 2007; Steinbrügge 1995; Vila 1998).

One might say (adapting Addison) that these theorists believed that the impressions made upon the female mind pressed too close upon it to give women time, leisure, or the proper temperament for sustained, judicious reflection. Similar notions also appeared in debates on taste, going back to the seventeenth century. The Cartesian philosopher and Oratorian Nicolas Malebranche trivialized women's taste by associating it with their soft brain fibers—which, as he argued, produced minds occupied "'to capacity' with misleading sensual information, in constant turmoil due to heightened, ever-changing sensitive reception" (Hamerton 2008: 550).

Clearly, a certain notion of human nature was at stake in Enlighenment-era efforts to draw clear dividing lines between "higher" versus "lower" ways of sensing. Notions of animal nature—and of the difference between animals and humans—also entered into play, especially in the context of the debate over whether animals possessed souls or minds. Buffon answered in the negative in "De la nature de l'homme," a chapter in his *Histoire naturelle, générale et particulière* (1749–88) around which Diderot constructed a lengthy dialogue in the *Encyclopédie* article "Animal." As Buffon contended, animals possess "something similar to our first impressions and our most basic and mechanical sensations" but are incapable of the complex association of ideas that produces reflection, because all they have is the material substrate necessary for thinking, not the divinely granted power of reflection (Diderot [1751a] 1975–, v: 386). Diderot pointed out that the power of human reflection is easily disrupted by activities taking place in the material substrate—like sleep, or deep mental absorption (v: 389–90). His aim was double: he sought both to undermine Buffon's contention that the human mind always acts voluntarily, and to contest Buffon's theory of distinct, identifiable animal species and replace it with a materialist vision in which man and beast were separated only by degrees (Jacot Grapa 2010).

Diderot agreed with Buffon that what truly separated the human from the animal was the intellect—which, as he insisted elsewhere, was far more than the product of mere physical sensibility. However, he viewed human intellect not as a gift from God, but, rather, the result of weaker sense organs and a more complex brain than those possessed by animals. As he put it in his last work, the *Essai sur Sénèque* (1778):

> Man, keep in mind that you owe the quality that distinguishes you from animals to the weakness of your organs. Do you aspire to the piercing view of the eagle? You would be staring endlessly. Do you wish to have a dog's sense of smell? You'd be sniffing around from morning to night. The organ of your judgment has remained predominant and the master; it would have been the slave of one of your senses if it had become too vigorous: that's the source of your perfectibility. If there is a fiber in your brain that is more energetic than the others, you are no longer good for anything but a single thing, you're a man of genius: the animal and the man of genius are alike in that way.
>
> Diderot (1778b) 1975–, xxv: 336

Sensory mediocrity was, in other words, the key to a well-functioning human mind. As for geniuses, Diderot described them as so absorbed by the internal operations of their energetic minds that they tended to go about in a daze, subject to cataleptic moments of utter sensory oblivion.[4]

This brings us to two remaining strands of thought about the senses that bear mentioning, in part because they lead in opposite directions: the universalizing, communitarian strand, evident in the Enlightenment's various theories of common sense as a moral, aesthetic, and political ideal (Boyson 2012: 23–64; Rosenfeld 2011a), and the distrustful strand. One brand of mistrust, pervasive in religious discourse, advocated withdrawal from the world of the senses as the surest path toward happiness and true knowledge. The Catholic apologist Louis-Antoine de Caraccioli expressed such a view in *La Jouissance de soi-même* (1755) while denouncing the relentless pursuit of voluptuous bodily sensations among the "materialists" of his day: "Our soul, victim of an overly credulous ear, or a too curious eye, has succumbed under the effort of the senses, to the point of becoming inseparable from them" (Caraccioli [1755] 1761: xii). A different sort of distrust—but a similar pessimism about the possibility of reconciling the secular Enlightenment faith in reason with uncontrollable somatic desires—marked *Los Caprichos* (1799), where the Spanish artist Don Francisco Goya portrayed the sense organs in monstrous imbalance, with cavernous mouths opposed to "closed eyes and padlocked ears," mouths, anuses, noses, and genitalia conflated, and the line between the human and the animal almost utterly effaced (Schulz 2005: 141).

Ultimately, the Enlightenment's most intriguing contribution to sensory history may be its various visions of a human sensorium expanded beyond the five physical senses. Speculative philosophy provided one framework for that sort of exploration, from Diderot's oniric musings in the *Rêve d'Alembert* over what life would be like for Saturnians endowed with more senses than earthly humans, to Rousseau's reflections on the joy of pure existence—a joy beyond pleasure or pain—in the *Rêveries du promeneur solitaire* (1778). Mysticism as elaborated by Emmanuel Swedenborg provided another framework: as Leigh Eric Schmidt puts it, "no other Christian visionary paid such close, dissecting attention to the bodily and spiritual senses" or strove so intently to find a place in heaven for all the senses (except taste, which was barred; Schmidt 2000: 211, 213). Fascination with expanded ways of sensing was also apparent in public demonstrations on electricity and vital magnetism, which sometimes involved long chains of people holding hands to transmit shocks, or rods and ropes purported to conduct invisible fluids from body to body around a tub

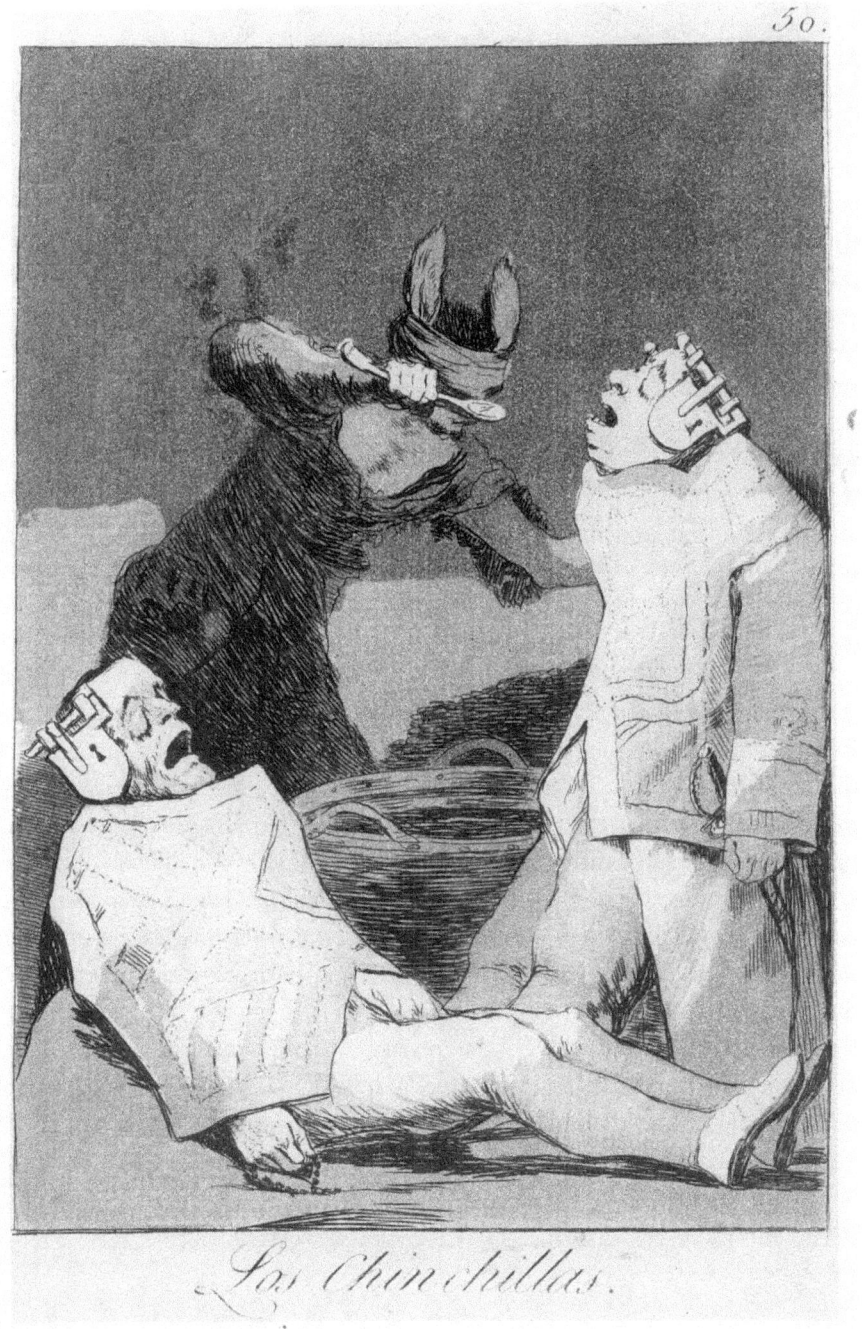

FIGURE I.3: Francisco Jose de Goya y Lucientes, *The Chinchillas*, plate 50 of "Los caprichos," 1799 (etching and aquatint), private collection. Bridgeman Art Library.

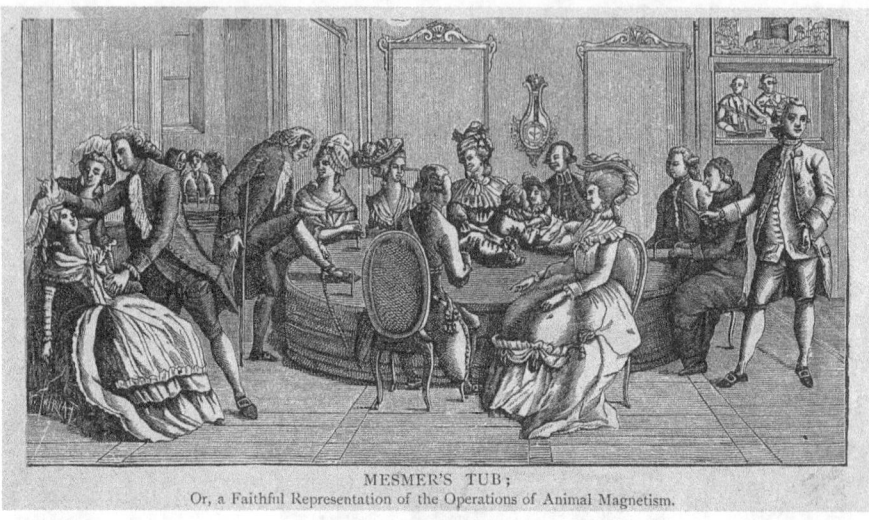

FIGURE I.4: A large gathering of patients and assistants to Mesmer's animal magnetism therapy, showing use of the special tub at his clinic. Wood engraving by H. Thiriat. Wellcome Library, London.

(Darnton 1968; Fara 2002). That fascination was one factor in the late-Enlightenment craze that surrounded Mesmerism, whose practitioners offered the promise of producing an entirely new set of healing sensations through magnetization: sensations deep within the body, guaranteed to cure nervous patients of their most intractable complaints (Azouvi 1991). The Lyon doctor Henri-Désiré Pététin even went so far in his *Mémoire sur la découverte des phénomènes que présentent la catalepsie et le somnabulisme* (1787) as to claim that he had used magnetism to cure cataleptic patients—and that, as he'd discovered, these patients could "see" through their stomachs and "hear" through their fingers through the mysterious phenomenon he called the "transport des sens" (Goldstein 2010: 47–8; Petetin 1787: 69). Along with the philosophers, the aesthetes, and the vaporous, sleep-walking cataleptics have a place in the curious history of the senses during the Enlightenment.

CHAPTER ONE

The Social Life of the Senses: A New Approach to Eighteenth-century Politics and Public Life

SOPHIA ROSENFELD

The senses have, by now, thoroughly infiltrated the study of social life in the eighteenth-century West. *The Foul and the Fragrant, Tastes of Paradise, Intimate Vision*: such book titles suggest that we are now routinely called upon to consider the era of the Enlightenment in sensual terms. The assumption underlying all these works of scholarship is not only that sensory experience was different in the past, but that the senses mattered then in ways that it is sometimes hard to fully feel now. Sensory experience was vital to questions of taste, social distinction, knowledge production, and faith, not to mention the rhythms of everyday life. Indeed, in the view of many scholars, the eighteenth century distinguished itself as an age of sensory excess that it is historians' task to recapture for audiences today.

Except, that is, when it comes to politics. The key story that we continue to tell about public life in the eighteenth century—the coming of revolution and the first experiments with democracy in the modern world—has been noticeably untouched by the flowering of sensory history even as the sensual has saturated other historical domains. Perhaps this is because we still tend to think of politics as a largely abstract business, a matter of ideas and concepts more than bodily sensations. Or perhaps this is an effect of the rapid rate of change we associate with the political, especially in revolutionary eras; sensory experience seems to evolve according to the slower rhythms of custom and social practice. Whichever is the case, what follows is an effort to rethink, from the vantage point of the history of the senses, a key element of the standard narrative of the introduction of popular sovereignty under the aegis of the French Revolution. By rereading the advent of democracy, and especially the act of voting, in light of changing notions of secrecy and exposure, or sensory deprivation versus openness to eyes and ears, we can observe aspects of this moment of rupture that have long remained opaque to us—despite our contemporary commitment to the idea of transparent governance. Ideally, we also gain a model for how the history of the public domain might be fruitfully woven together with the history of the senses.

The initial part of this chapter will sketch the very different roles accorded to the senses in structuring the social life and then the political life of Europe and its principal colonies during the final century of the Old Regime. The latter part will then try to account for two breaks in this political-sensory regime that occurred in France near the eighteenth century's close. The first is the sudden (and well-documented) turn to maximal transparency as political practice between 1789 and 1794. The second is the much less often noted but equally significant turn back to a compromise between sensory openness and desensualized privacy that occurred in 1795: the year of the introduction of that odd phenomenon, the publically administered secret ballot, with which we still live.

*

Any attempt to capture the texture of life in eighteenth-century Paris, London, Amsterdam, Milan, Madrid, or Boston requires attention to smells, noises, vapors, and a kaleidoscopic array of sights that we now only imagine with difficulty. In much of Europe and its overseas outposts, a growing proportion of people left the more open, quiet spaces of farms and villages to move to urban centers. As a result, the already crowded streets of leading cities and towns seemed to contemporaries—and thus to us, reading their words retrospectively—to suddenly teem with human bodies, along with animal bodies and all manner of work, material goods, transport, dirt, and attractions, in very close proximity. For eighteenth-century elites, it became something of a cliché to describe the lives of the urban poor by evoking the myriad sounds of the city (animals braying or being slaughtered, church bells pealing, the shouting in the marketplace of criers and hawkers of goods, the singing of drunks); its strong odors (human excrement, rotting food, horse dung, and the like); its chaotic and often ugly sights; and the feeling of bustle and of restricted movement and space that was thought to be characteristic of the new urban experience (Cockayne 2007; Corfield 1990; Cowan and Steward 2007; Farge 1979, 2007; Garrioch 2003). We read of the sensory pleasures of explicit hedonism: singing, eating, drinking, sex. We read too, especially in the writings of moralists and reformers, of dismay over sewage, smoke, the ailing indigent, and other sensory abominations; such affronts were the starting point for many of the urban reform movements of the later century, such as the rise of new forms of sanitation and lighting (Barles 2005; Corbin 1986; Frey 1997; Koslofsky 2011; Madiment 2007; Melosi 2000). As Emily Cockayne explains in her evocatively titled *Hubbub: Filth, Noise and Stench in England*, the streets of eighteenth-century English cities were rife with "nuisances and irritants" in sensory form (2007: 230). The dwellings of urban workers, moreover, kept out little of this exterior world. For the cramped quarters of city residents too were filled with sound, odor, and close contact with the bodies of others.

But it was not only the world of the urban poor that constituted a veritable sensory bazaar in the eighteenth century. At the other end of the social scale, Europe's nobles and the members of Europe's great courts also distinguished themselves by their sensory trappings, albeit largely ones designed to express maximum distance from the world of their social inferiors. This was, after all, the great age of luxury goods, understood to be sources of both bodily contentment and social prestige for those who owned or consumed them (Berg and Clifford 1999; Berg and Eger 2001; Bremer-David 2011). Consider the design of France's and indeed, continental Europe's greatest eighteenth-century interiors, with their growing differentiation between the spaces of public and private life. Inside these great homes, fine materials—velvet, silk, precious stones—appealed to the touch as well as the eye, covering ceilings, walls, furniture, and selves with conduits for pleasure-producing sensations. Pianos, clavichords, and spectacular clocks that chimed or chirped on the hour made abstract sound—in addition to that generated by animated, polite conversation—a regular feature of daily life. Delicate porcelain services added to the pleasure of imbibing strong, fashionable beverages like coffee, tea, and cocoa, all sweetened with an imported and ever more highly desired complement called sugar. Large fireplaces allowed for warming of the body. Delicate handheld fans and large windows, not to mention sofas for reclining, made possible cooling via comfortable breezes. Perfume masked the smells of bodies or streets, replacing them with strong floral fragrances and musk evocative of the garden instead. And in libraries, sitting rooms, and dining rooms alike, occupants' eyes were tempted to steal a glance in all directions at once: toward elaborate patterned rugs, curtains, and upholsteries; toward large ornamental mirrors, chandeliers holding multiple candles, and gold filigree and metalwork that added light and visual play; toward paintings and tapestries that very often took sensual pleasure as their very theme (Girouard 1993; Whitehead 2009; on specific commodities: Melchoir-Bonnet 2001; Roche 1989; Schivelbusch 1993). Rococo style turned strolling, dancing, swinging, bathing, flirting, and similar pleasures into both its central subject matter and its stylistic inspiration in terms of its evocation of play (Levey 1985). Consider a canvas like Nicolas Lancret's *A Lady in a Garden Taking Coffee with some Children*

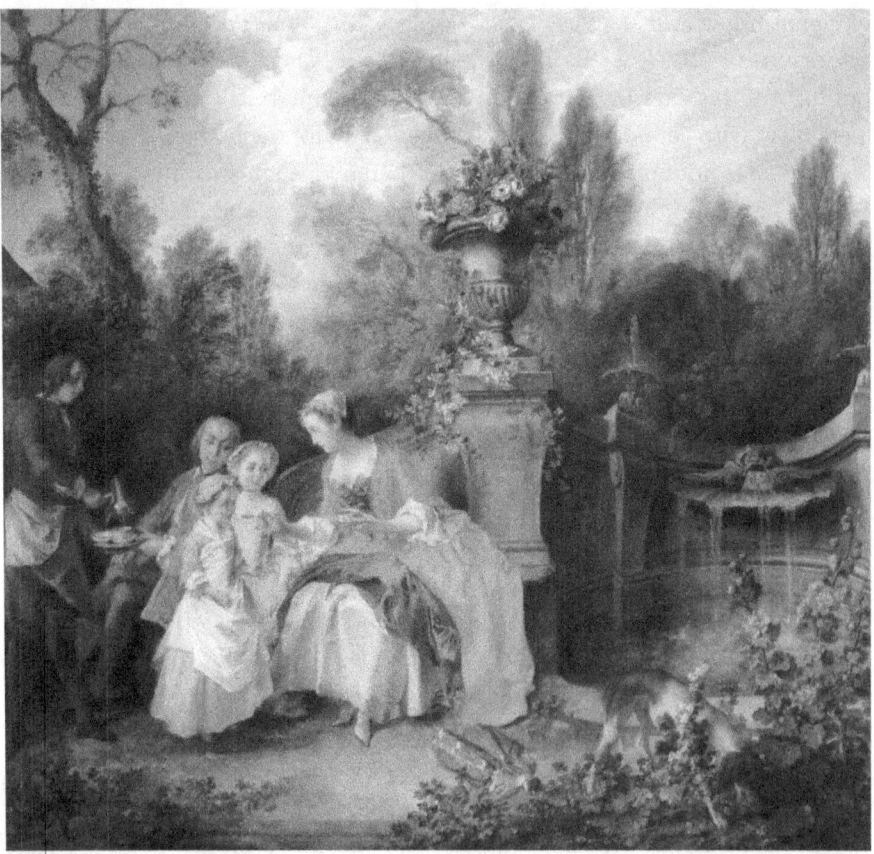

FIGURE 1.1: Nicolas Lancret, *A Lady in a Garden Taking Coffee with some Children* (1742). National Gallery, London.

(1742) in which the central image is the very act of smelling and tasting as a child takes a spoonful of coffee from her mother in an idealized garden filled with flowers, fountains, and other sensual delights. We are a far cry here from the painted warnings of the dangers of gluttony and luxury that pervaded the *vanitas* imagery of the previous century (Jütte 2005: Ch. 4).

It was Louis XIV's Versailles, built at the close of the seventeenth century as a kind of monument to sensation, which set the standard for the great houses of Europe well into the eighteenth century. Louis XIV and his legions of designers were not content simply to turn the statuary, *jets d'eau*, halls of mirrors, and great vistas of his palace and park into feasts for the eyes. They also endeavored to impress French nobles and foreign dignitaries alike by making his home into a setting for spectacles that would have multi-sensory appeal (Burke 1994). From brilliant firework displays, to full-length ballets, to elaborate banquets, classical French taste offered a rival sensory arena to that of Catholic mass (which was also a regular feature of life at Versailles). Such spectacular entertainments were copied all over Europe well into the eighteenth century. In fact, by the last decades of the Old Regime, the appeal

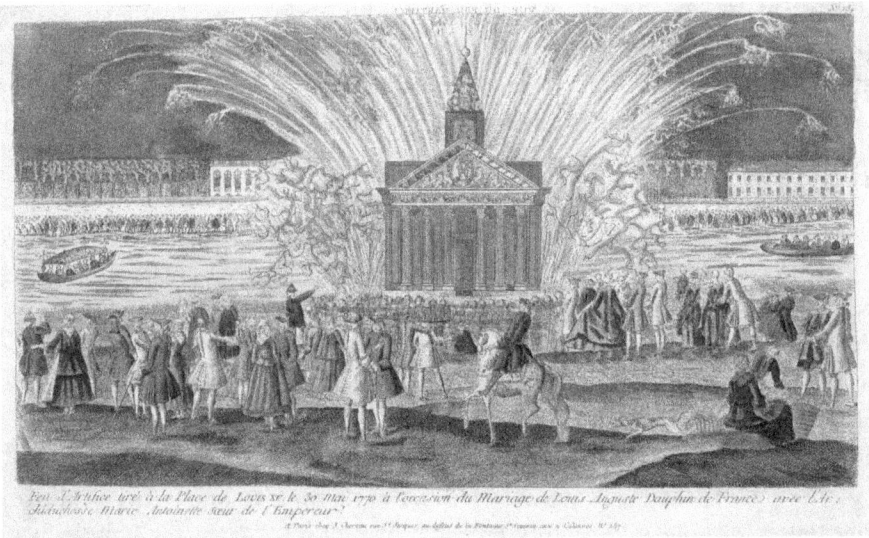

FIGURE 1.2: Engraving, *Feu d'artifice tiré à la place de Louis XV le 30 mai 1770 à l'occasion du mariage de Louis Auguste Dauphin de France avec l'archiduchesse Marie Antoinette, soeur de l'empereur*. Bibliothèque nationale de France.

of such endeavors had begun to spill out from grand private homes into urban settings more generally, as opera and ballet became, from London to Vienna, public, commercial phenomena, at once aesthetic and social, and open to all who could afford the price of a ticket (Hall-Witt 2007; Johnson 1996).

For those in the middle socially, with little chance of creating their own mini-Versailles but eager to distinguish themselves from the urban or rural poor, such novel late eighteenth-century pleasures as opera-going, but also bathing in the sea, visiting coffeehouses or restaurants, and attending public, scientific displays with an emphasis on the experiential, also made sensory pleasure a feature of what was just coming to be called bourgeois life (Brewer 1997; Lowe 1982; Seigel 2012; on specific forms of bourgeois entertainment: Bensaude-Vincent and Blondel 2008; Cowan 2005; Delbourgo 2006b; Ellis 2004; Spang 2000; Walton 1983). So did consumer goods like fine fabrics and spices that were, by the end of the century, no longer beyond the reach of many urban people even when those objects originated in exotic climes or distant colonial outposts (Brewer and Plumb 1982; Crowley 2001). These were items to be used in the home as objects of private sensory pleasure as much as for public display. In northern, Protestant Europe especially, a nascent middle class fostered an ethics of restraint, of not calling too much attention to itself by means of extravagance or libidinal indulgence. But we should hardly imagine asceticism as the dominant value here; Europe's new "middling sorts" distinguished themselves as much by inventing a culture centered on leisure-time entertainment, comfort, and consumption as by establishing a new relationship to the means of production. Sensuality of a very particular sort would soon become a part of bourgeois self-definition.

Indeed, the very idea of "taste" as it emerged in the eighteenth century and eventually became the focus of the new science of aesthetics was closely tied to sensory distinctions among different social classes. At its base, taste was related to the body. What the truly tasteful had in abundance, according to eighteenth-century commentators, was an innate sense of "tact" or a fine touch (Dickie 1996; Ferry 1990; Gigante 2005; Tsien 2012). In the same way, literary works that met with favorable receptions could be described as goûté or savored, just like a fine steak.[1] This was not only a matter of metaphor. For eighteenth-century theorists, to have good taste was, at its root, to know "what pleases our senses," as one mid-century French critic put it.[2] And yet, as Voltaire was to point out in his famous article "Taste" in Diderot and D'Alembert's influential Encyclopédie (1751–65), possessing this perceptual capacity was not always sufficient to mark one as a true person of taste. Taste in art or literature, Voltaire explained, did indeed operate much like the physical sensation one experiences in eating: "It discriminates as quickly as the tongue and palate, and like physical taste it anticipates thought . . . it is sensitive to what is good and reacts to it with a feeling of pleasure, it refuses with disgust what is bad." However, Voltaire went on to point out, taste by itself is liable to make errors, so "it needs practice to develop discrimination," which is to say, cultivation or training. Good taste was the prerogative of the truly tasteful, a social category more than a physiological one. Bad taste, by contrast, signified a lack of refinement in one's person but also in circumstances and breeding.[3]

Increasingly, these sensory distinctions had a gendered dimension as well. Women began to lead the way in the realms of fashion and interior design, linking femininity with heightened sensual pleasure: bright colors, elaborate adornment, refined smells. In this way, a second set of hierarchical oppositions was solidified. The senses, too, were used to establish a growing conceptual chasm between the decorative, bodily sphere that properly belonged to women, on the one hand, and the realm of male reason and disembodied, sober, and immaterial ideas, on the other (Chartier 1993; Classen 2012: 71–92).

*

By this logic, it followed that there remained one central domain of life in Old Regime Europe where this emphasis on sensory pleasure did not hold sway, at least in theory. That was the world of politics and statecraft. This is not to say that the monarchs of eighteenth-century Europe did not keep a close eye on their subjects as well as their competitors. We know that all early modern European states, including Great Britain, were rife with networks of police, spies, and censors of various kinds, listening and peering about for useful information relevant to state security. Michel Foucault, in particular, has drawn our attention to the disciplining gaze of the expanding state apparatus, beginning with what one historian calls the "panoptic monarchy" of the all-seeing Louis XIV (Foucault 1977; Smith 1993: esp. 412). Moreover, elaborate ceremonies, including ceremonies of information designed to convey the majesty and power of the crown, remained a feature of statecraft well into the eighteenth century—even if witnessed by a diminishing few courtiers in close proximity and now largely denuded of bodily contact, including the traditional royal touch (Classen 2012: esp. 158–9, 165–6; Fogel 1989; Giesey 1987). It can hardly be called coincidental that ballet and opera, with their goal of overwhelming the eyes and ears of their audiences, in part by displaying the feats of other human bodies, flourished first as courtly entertainments for an international political and social elite. Yet when it came to the business of governing, we find in the eighteenth century—with the partial exception of England and its colonies—a trans-European culture that largely prized secrecy and closed doors.

From the literal masking of dignitaries in Venice to the ideology of absolutism, with its emphasis on the *secrets du roi*, in France, traditional early modern continental statecraft depended on the idea that affairs of state needed to be hidden from the prying eyes and ears of the public (Kantorowicz 1955; Snyder 2009: esp. Ch. 4; specifically on Venice: Johnson 2011; on France: Schneider 2002). To maintain secrets or to dissimulate and feign, whether about affairs of state or of the heart, was understood to be a vital skill for those in possession of power and eager to maintain it (Elias 1978, 1982). Visibility at the symbolic level was not to be translated into accessibility, or real visibility in the everyday sense, whether for kings or for their closest advisers. Good governance, which was to say, minimizing risk to state or dynastic security, depended upon the opposite: controlling information and shielding the decision-making process from the gaze and audition of the population at large. This was especially true, according to *raison d'état* theorists, when it came to state finances. Even in theories of government far removed from those of Machiavelli, the idea endured that it was important to control what subjects do or do not see since (in Machiavelli's words), "human beings in general judge more with their eyes than with their hands, because everyone may see but few may feel . . ." (Snyder 2009: 112). More than two centuries later, and despite his reformist tendencies, Frederick the Great of Prussia essentially agreed, reiterating the necessity of opacity (except to a king's inner circle) and insisting that private persons had no right to pass judgments on governmental affairs precisely because their knowledge was always, necessarily, incomplete (Van Horn Melton 2001). The Count of Vergennes, foreign minister of France under Louis XVI, concurred, continuing to stress the importance to royal authority of impenetrability and non-disclosure—even as he made public statements about these very matters. Italian statecraft was no different. Another telling eighteenth-century representation of sensory norms can be found in the "Saletta del silenzio," a set of frescoes painted in 1706 by Sebastiano Taricco in an important *palazzo* in the Piedmontese city of Cherasco. For there, perhaps ironically, we see an elaborate visual program constructed precisely to convey the practical value in matters of governance of silence, secrecy, and the hidden (Snyder 2009: esp. 163–76).

Yet, that said, one of the standard stories now told about the coming of the French Revolution highlights the growing antipathy to this mode of conducting state business, a development that dates from well before the emergence of the

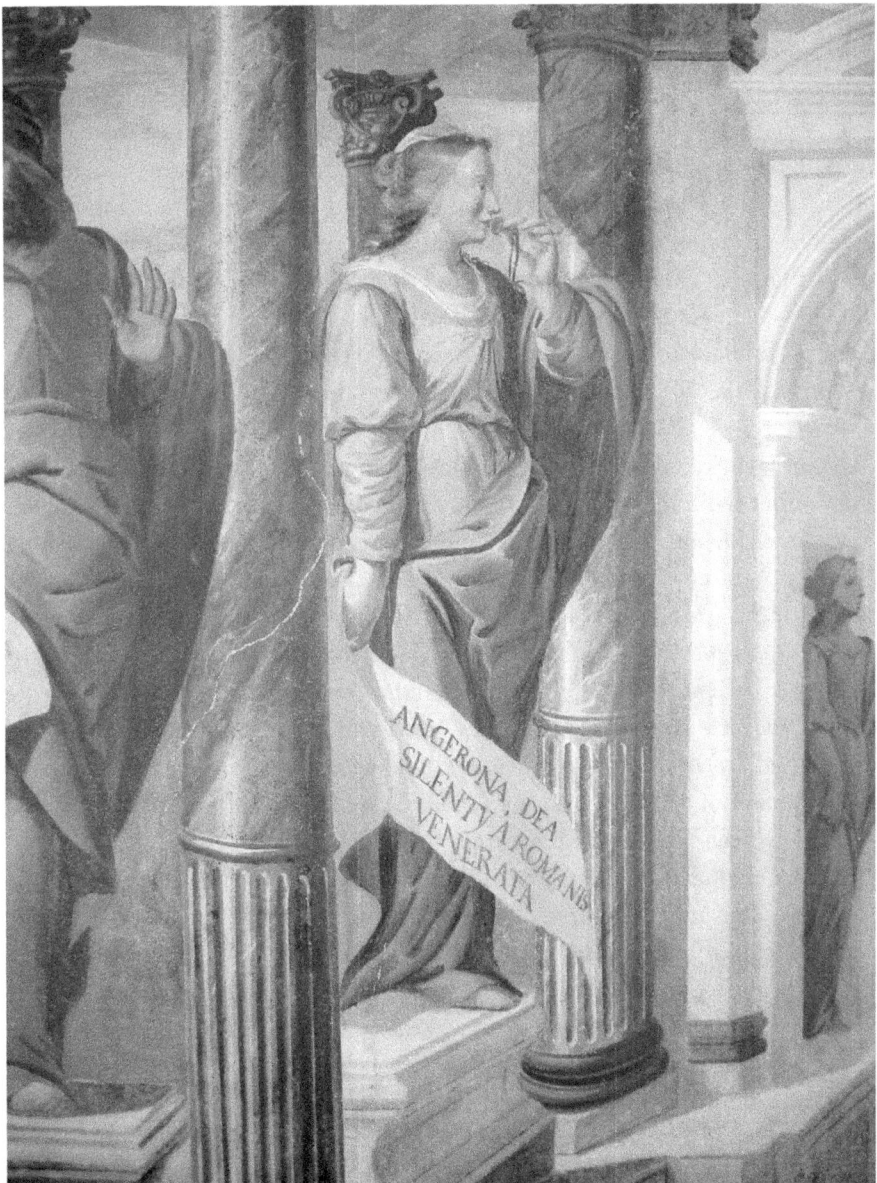

FIGURE 1.3: Fresco detail of Sebastiano Taricco, "Saletta del Silenzio" (1706), Palazzo Salmatoris, Cherasco, Italy. Photograph by Jon R. Snyder.

overt hostility to aristocracy that we associate with the very end of the century. Fifty years ago, the German philosopher Jürgen Habermas introduced readers to a concept that he called the "bourgeois public sphere." By this, he meant an expanding set of spaces, primarily separate from the state or court, that he claimed, were characterized by new kinds of communicative practices that were increasingly rational and egalitarian but also contestatory in nature. In Habermas' telling, this communicative realm emerged alongside the new middle class, first in England and then in France, reaching its apex there on the cusp of the Revolution of 1789. Habermas never attached this story to a history of the senses; "the bourgeois public sphere" was a conceptual innovation designed primarily to describe a changing set of relations between subjects and rulers that was responsible for the growth of the idea of public opinion. He did, however, identify one of its key attributes as a challenge to the politics of secrecy—and a demand for what we now call openness and transparency when it came to the circulation of information, official or otherwise (Habermas 1989).

Habermas' narrative proved compatible in many ways with an even older story about the Enlightenment first formulated by the *philosophes* themselves. One of the chief innovations of the Enlightenment, post-Locke, was the fleshing out of an epistemology, often known as sensationalism, that began from the notion of the senses as the sole paths to true knowledge (O'Neal 1996; Yolton 1984). Ideas were not innate, in this view; they were entirely products of sensory experience on the part of each and every individual. And in the wake of this conception of knowledge, a new, trans-national cohort of self-proclaimed intellectual leaders began to identify its chief function as primarily one of demystification, or full exposure to the eyes and ears of others, of all that had previously been hidden or obfuscated.

On a personal level, partisans of the Enlightenment encouraged a culture of sensibility, meaning alertness to emotions and passions as conveyed by the body itself (Barker-Benfield 1992; Goring 2005; Van Sant 1993; Vila 1998). Fittingly, and concurrently, sincerity and frankness came increasingly to be associated with virtue; it became important in secular terms—much as it long had been according to a Protestant world view—that seeming and being, utterances and actions, be aligned. People would need to become essentially legible to one another (Cavaillé 1998). And on a societal level, this epistemology produced a new pedagogy, to be advanced by the "enlightened," that rested upon the senses as both conduits and receptacles of truths. The very idea of Enlightenment (and its many variants, including *Aufklärung, les Lumières*, and *l'Illuminiso*) depended from the start upon the metaphor of exposure to *light*, of being suddenly able to *see* what had previously been veiled or hidden in shadows (Mortier 1969; Reichardt 1998; on vision more generally in the eighteenth century: Havenlange 1999; Jay 1993: esp. 83–113; Zoberman 1981). In Louis-Sébastien Mercier's 1771 fictional rendering of the distant future, *L'An 2440, rêve s'il en fût jamais*, the glitz of aristocratic experience, as well as the physical misery associated with dire poverty and even the sumptuous spectacle of the Catholic Church, are all gone. But in this Rousseau-inspired fantasy written at the height of the Enlightenment, the whole society has become a "book of morals," completely visually intelligible to all (Darnton 1995: esp. 115–36).

Thus, even as some historians have challenged aspects of Habermas' schema—his insistence that this new "public" sphere rose solely in opposition to the state rather than, just as often, in tandem with it; his desire to yoke this sphere to a specific class, the "bourgeoisie" in Marxist terms, rather than a more heterogeneous elite—other historians have also done much in recent decades to flesh out his central claim. They have also generally agreed that in the course of the eighteenth century the boundaries between the public and private began to shift in ways that at least in part explain the origins of the crisis of 1789 (Van Damme 2007; Van Horn Melton 2001). One might even say that a veritable cottage industry has arisen dedicated to explaining the sources and meaning of this newer impulse toward openness to scrutiny and "publicity" as the motors of public life.

A critique of veiling and secrecy is already abundantly on display in Montesquieu's great novel of 1721, *Les Lettres persanes*. There, degeneracy and corruption—of individuals and of the culture as a whole—flow directly from the structure of the harem, with its locked doors, shaded faces, and thwarted gratifications of the flesh. By the mid-century, the French political economists known as the Physiocrats had translated this message into a demand for exposure, accountability, and greater public knowledge and discussion, especially of state finances (Ives 2003). Even England, where government was already considerably more open to scrutiny from outside, saw radicals in the 1760s demanding the reporting, which is to say illumination, of Parliament's activities as essential to protecting the British people against "dark and dangerous designs" (Van Horn Melton 2001: 26). And as if in response, a whole genre of Francophone publication emerged in the second half of that century that took counter-espionage, or revealing the previously hidden, to be its *raison d'être* (Darnton 2010b: esp. Ch. 21). Consider the revealingly named Milord All'Eye and Milord All'Ear, the fictitious centerpieces of the anonymous serial publication *L'Observateur anglois, ou Correspondance secrete entre Milord All'Eye et Milord All'Ear* (*The English Observer or Secret Correspondence between Lord All Eyes and Lord All Ears*). Typically, the advertisement for the series advances the fiction that what is to be found between its covers is nothing less than an otherwise secret cache of letters, the result of the infidelity of Milord All'Ear's secretary. What is promised is exposure to the public gaze both of the mores of the French people and of the workings of their government—to an extent that all previous travelers' descriptions had failed to match: "I will put before your eyes," one correspondent writes to the other and, by extension, his readers, "the People among whom I live, so to speak, in constant movement." For, he explains, I will be your "observer" (later "spy") and make up for the "total scarcity" of news in London of French doings by "writing day by day what I have seen, read or heard that is memorable."[4] This is a spy whose goal is to turn the tables on the state and subject its greatest secrets to scrutiny. He will reveal all that is generally veiled, from the private lives of celebrated figures to rumors of financial matters generally only whispered in the halls of power.

Such publications derived much of their appeal from the culture of secrecy surrounding the court. But they also, much like the ubiquitous and often pornographic *libelles* of the period, actively contributed to creating a culture of exhibitionism and publicity that would undermine it. Even if much of the news they reported was false, eighteenth-century Parisian newshawkers really did rely on networks of informants and insiders who culled information from taverns, great houses, courts, and the street. Publishers then aimed, as much as possible, to convey the feel and sounds, or "raw materiality," of such spaces back to an abstract public sphere.[5] The proliferation of titles promising "secrets memoirs," "private lives," and all kinds of foreign "spies" suggests a large public for these clandestine works, a readership eager to assume the roles of eavesdropper and voyeur for itself.

In fact, by the 1770s, the French crown, too, had begun to appeal to public opinion, rejecting the old wisdom that politics should be an arena of secrecy. The idea of publicity was most famously taken up (to the horror of Vergennes) by Louis XVI's Genevan finance minister, Jacques Necker, in response to the French crown's ever-growing fiscal crisis. Convinced that public confidence was necessary for credit, itself a crucial question in an age of expensive warfare, Necker took the unprecedented step in 1781 of allowing the state's accounts to be printed and viewed by the public at large. His books may have been cooked. His plan may ultimately have backfired. But with this new form of publicity, Necker made himself a hero of all those who decried the French monarchy's tendency toward despotism, now equated with secrecy in the realm of the political. Even as far afield as Germany, Necker's *Compte rendu du roi* became, temporarily, a best-seller. As one German journalist commented using, once again, a series of metaphors related to sight, "To disclose to public view facts that until now have been counted among the most important state secrets; to brazenly lay bare the wellsprings of government; to reveal with impunity the very secret that has always seemed to be the most jealously guarded: this is indeed a new phenomenon in politics."[6]

We tend now to classify this shift—which can be described as a shift in the sensory dimension of eighteenth-century political life—as a crucial step in the creation of modern democracy. The French Revolution, from this vantage point, can be seen as the logical culmination of the burgeoning politics of publicity, or intense visual and aural scrutiny, as well as a new commitment to the legitimacy of public opinion as a source of law. From the moment of the creation of the National Assembly in 1789, revolutionary leaders promised that the business of making laws would become open to the public's sensory perceptions. All that transpired would be made audible, visible, and, as a last resort, legible, with sound and visual effects recorded alongside words in an effort to recreate the experiential dimension of the proceedings for posterity or those unfortunate enough to have missed the live events. Doors would open, sound barriers and blinders removed. Moreover, the public, too, would make itself heard and seen, from the streets of Versailles and Paris to the balconies of the Assembly's various meeting halls, where spectators immediately took it upon themselves to chant, clap, beat drums, put up placards, shout out threats, and

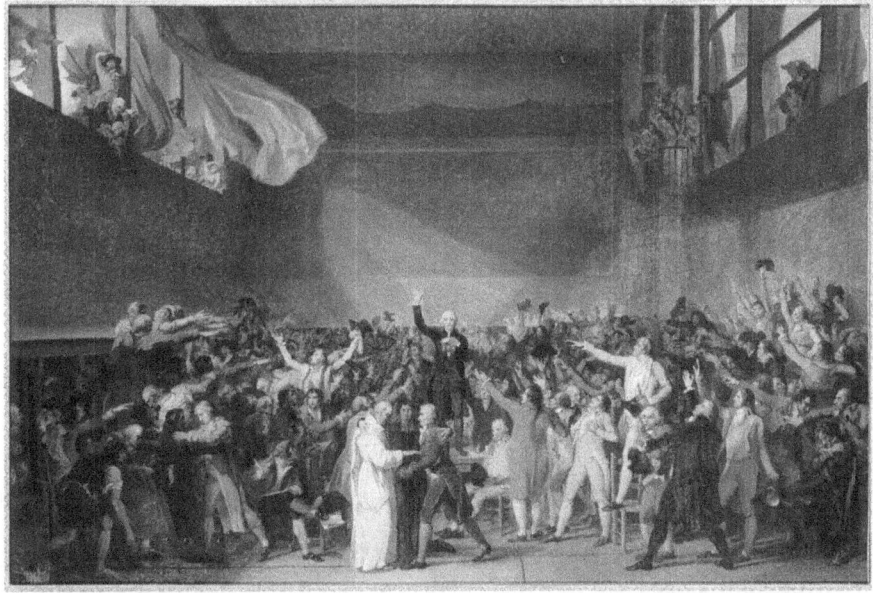

FIGURE 1.4: Jacques-Louis David, *Le serment du jeu de Paume, le 20 juin 1789* (1791). Carnavalet Museum, Paris.

otherwise make their presence perceptible to their representatives and to each other (Rosenfeld 2011b). Rioting became, to borrow from a recent account of the sensory dimension of the American Revolution, a form of "visible and auditory terrorism" on the part of ordinary people (Hoffer 2003: 218). New freedoms of both press and assembly made this possible in entirely novel ways.

Soon the revolutionary state began to harness this idea of maximal sensory exchange for its own purposes, using re-education by means of the senses, most famously through the means of civic festivals. By combining musical interludes and song, speech-making, gesticulation, parading, ritual oaths, communal food and drink, signage, costume, and multi-dimensional scenery, festivals were intended to instill in citizens new tastes, sights, sounds, smells, and physical experiences associated with revolutionary values (Ozouf 1991). As one deputy to the Convention explained in the spring of 1794, the government of the republic had a special obligation to cultivate "all that can speak to the eyes, all that, affecting the senses, can inspire republican morals."[7] The chief precedent here was less the public ceremonies of the Old Regime, with their requirement of passive spectators, than the Catholic Church, whose participatory ethos had long been directed at all ranks in society. The multi-sensory experience of mass would finally find its political corollary.

And as time went by, the very idea of the distinction between the private lives of individuals and the public lives of citizens came to seem obsolete as well. With the advent of republicanism, not just the day-to-day work of representatives but also that of ordinary people, as members of the sovereign body, would, by necessity, have to become open to the scrutiny of all. Transparency, coupled with an anti-aristocratic and masculinist taste for sensory austerity as opposed to the Rococo, became the new ideal, a badge of authenticity, manliness, and deep public-mindedness. As the historian Lynn Hunt explains:

> The ability to conceal one's true emotions, to act one way in public and another in private, was repeatedly denounced as the chief characteristic of court life and aristocratic manners in general. These relied above all on appearances, that is, on the disciplined and self-conscious use of the body as a mask. The republicans, consequently, valued transparency—the unmediated expression of the heart—above all other personal qualities. Transparency was the perfect fit between public and private; transparency was a body that told no lies and kept no secrets. It was the definition of virtue, and as such it was imagined to be critical to the future of the republic.
>
> Hunt 1992: 96–7

Thus began a novel sensory regime.

Starting in 1792 and accelerating through Year II (1793–4), this impulse extended to French social life, where, for example, communal meals (albeit not luxurious ones) were staged for public benefit, creating a newly shared sensory realm. It also extended to that activity deemed most essential to the realization of popular sovereignty: voting. Many French people had certainly voted prior to the Revolution; despite France's relative lack of representative assemblies prior to 1789, a strong popular tradition of collective deliberation and suffrage had long held sway, especially in guilds and village assemblies. They had done so (and continued to do so after the formation of the new National Assembly) by employing a wide range of techniques, ranging from standing in a show of support to paper balloting. But in the course of the Revolution, enthusiasm grew, especially among radicals in the Paris sections, for the idea of voting in ways that were public enough to be open to the scrutiny of all (as was the standard in eighteenth-century England and many of its colonies, where voting had, since the seventeenth century, acquired many of the qualities of a raucous popular festival—see Dinkin 1977; O'Gorman 1989, 1992). It was already widely agreed that citizens were, in the aggregate, up to the task of choosing representatives precisely because, as Montesquieu had pointed out at midcentury, "They have only to base their decisions . . . on facts that are evident to the senses."[8] That meant, in an age before party politics, electoral campaigns, or even stated candidates, simply the virtue and personal merit of possible representatives of the people. But radical republicans began pushing circa 1792–3 for the act of voting to become public in every sense: occurring under the watchful eyes of the community and with the community's best (collective) interest in mind. In practical terms, that meant voting in public spaces, by means of signs, whether visual, gestural, or acoustic, that could be observed or heard by every other voter and by the wider community as well.

At the time of the choosing of delegates for the Estates-General in 1788, the first round of voting had already taken place in the open—both for the sake of determining the vote of illiterates and because the initial decision had less to do with competition among varied positions or factions than with the expression of a shared ethos. But the second round of voting had been conducted by written ballot, or *scrutin*, in an effort to eliminate excessive communal pressure on individuals making important choices. At the height of the Terror, in contrast, many revolutionaries insisted that all voting become a matter of standing up, doffing one's hat, raising one's hand, moving to one side of the room or, most often, declaring one's preference *à haute voix*: ritual enactments that gained meaning precisely because they could be witnessed by the eyes or ears of all present (see Crook 1996; Gueniffey 1993; Tanchoux 2004; specifically on the question of the secret ballot: Crook and Crook 2007, 2011). In many instances, these acts were to be accompanied by ceremonial oaths and fraternal embraces similarly intended to substantiate the sovereignty of the people and its unified general will. Such displays were thought to be effective means to this end. Secrecy, in contrast, signaled selfishness or, even worse, the need for disguise.

But as we well know, the republican push for full disclosure came at a price. Many historians have noted the centrality of plots and conspiracies in the French revolutionary imagination (Campbell *et al.* 2007; Tackett 2000; and for comparison: Wood 1982). What has been less remarked upon is the animating fear behind this tendency, a fear that began at the level of epistemology and grew in tandem with the impulse towards full publicity. Excessive worry focused on the hunch that what was visible or audible was never the whole truth, that revolutionary images and utterances always hid behind them some other truth—generally, disloyalty or bad intentions—that remained inaccessible to the ears and eyes of others (Hunt 1984; Maslan 2005; Rosenfeld 2001). Such anxiety was at the root of the punitive culture of the Terror, with its efforts to root out unseen and unheard impurities and to criminalize the harboring of deviant interior intentions (i.e. the Law of Suspects). It also produced the eventual fall of Robespierre on 9 Thermidor Year II.

And ultimately, fear of the limits of sensual perception as the path to utopia constitutes the source of another twist in our story of the advent of democracy at the end of the eighteenth century. The final stage of our well-rehearsed tale of the expansion of publicity to a central value of the new, revolutionary state was a *second* sensory shift that was equally important for the long history of politics. But it is also one that has been much less well documented—in part because we tend not to think of questions of senses and questions of political practice together. That was a reaction following the death of Robespierre against the culture of total transparency and sensory openness and a turn to the limited, strategic re-introduction of secrecy and veiling in decision making, albeit this time within the new public sphere.

This shift becomes concrete once again when we look to the (neglected) history of voting practices. Specifically, we need to consider the new appeal of an ancient idea known as the secret ballot. For in reaction against the Terror, the Thermidoreans now concluded that it was efficacious to make voting in secrecy, shielded from full exposure to the senses of others, the standard means by which to determine the public's preferences and, more generally, enact the rule of the sovereign people.

In England, in the late eighteenth century, the secret ballot had its advocates as well. But it remained the exclusive pipedream of radicals like Major John Cartwright, who attached themselves to the often related goals of expanding the franchise and championing the downtrodden as political actors. Secrecy promised to break the enormous role of patronage and obligation to one's social betters in the determination of how to vote. Precisely for this very reason, it also took decades more for the idea to gain any real traction in England or certain of its colonies, where collective voting long remained the norm (Kinzer 1982).

In France, by contrast, the move at the close of the eighteenth century towards mandating the use of secret or hidden ballots stemmed from a very different set of impulses. On the one hand, it indicated a new desire on the part of the post-Thermidorean Revolution's leaders to try to thwart organization or pressure on voters, in this case, from below. On the other, it marked the beginnings of a shift toward a more individuated notion of voting that took suffrage to be a matter of expressing a distinctive—and largely interior—choice.

This change in law came into being with the new anti-Jacobin Constitution of Year III (1795). This third revolutionary constitution is usually taken to be significant only insofar as it marked the formal end of the Terror and the rejection of its most radical innovations in favor of a more moderate strand of republicanism (Bart 1998; Conac and Machelon 1999; Jainchill 2003; for comparison: Dinkin 1982: esp. 101–6). However, from the perspective of a sensory history of eighteenth-century politics or, indeed, of modern politics as a whole, this document carries considerably more weight. It marks the first time that secret ballots were constitutionally mandated for all kinds of elections. As such it also marks a significant step toward the kind of semi-privatized democracy with which we remain familiar today.

Article 31 of the Constitution of Year III required that ballots (typically papers to be filled out, folded, and placed in an *urne*) be free from sensory scrutiny, even if they continued to be cast in public spaces and aimed at determining the public good. The sentence announcing this change read simply "All elections will be conducted by *scrutin secret*."[9] A new electoral law determined shortly thereafter required stated choices for voters to ponder. This was on top of new constitutional restrictions on the franchise itself, not to mention new limits on freedom of assembly and press and restrictions on the number of spectators who could observe the new government's representatives at work. Such was the backlash in the years following the Terror. By the time of the Consulate (1799), the Senate—much like Louis XIV's ministers—met once again behind closed doors.

The logic behind this second revolutionary turn in sensory regimes can be discerned from a contemporaneous pamphlet that went even further than the new constitution, suggesting the use not only of secret, written ballots but also of compartments within assembly halls that would further shield the act of voting from prying eyes or ears and cordon off distinct bodies from one another. The author was a lawyer and political moderate named Jacques-Vincent Delacroix. Eager to find a way to safeguard popular sovereignty but also determined to reattach the revolution to the property-owning classes, Delacroix published in 1795 a dialogue on the perennially sticky question of how, exactly, to determine the public's will. One of the text's two conversationalists, standing in for the author, worries, yet again, that one cannot be sure about citizens' true feelings about the republic from what one perceives with one's senses: "I rest neither on exterior signs [visual cues] nor on applause [auditory clues] inspired by fear or by the desire to imitate." The only solution, he continues, is to hold new elections. But for them to be legitimate yet also effective in maintaining the republic, he insists, it will be necessary, first, to restrict who constitutes the legitimate "people." Then, it will be equally essential to change the means by which those legitimate voters vote so that they are not, this time, intimidated by "anarchists" and "agitators." To learn the true people's true wishes, what will be needed is a "divided" space in which citizens will be asked to fill out a paper "without being seen" and put the results in a "closed box." Then, the results could be formally analyzed, by a small set of expert eyes, and announced at a later date.[10]

This plan was never adopted into law. It is, however, suggestive of the new kind of thinking that would gain traction in the years to come. For the practice of democracy was—starting circa 1795—partially re-secretized just as Delacroix imagined in a slower, yet equally revolutionary transformation to the one that produced the beginning of political-sensory openness. What Thermidorean moderates like our lawyer successfully proposed in 1794–5 was a turn back towards the Old Regime's culture of secrecy in decision making but now rendered a mass phenomenon. In the future, the major means of enacting the sovereignty of the people would involve even less outward display than the political decision-making of the Old Regime court. Voting was to become a dry exercise with little sensual appeal. For the suffrage was just starting to be reimagined—in France as in England, and even as other techniques like election nullification were sporadically employed as well—as about the expression of interior sentiments and opinions on an individual basis, not an expression of communal will. Once, to be seen or heard to vote in a particular fashion had been a way of being accountable for one's choice, not to mention a way to demonstrate one's public-spiritedness and integrity. Now voting began to take on the contours of a private right, one that would be compromised if individuals were subject to the influence or surveillance of others, whether local notables (as English reformers initially worried) or Jacobins (as French ones initially did).

Today, of course, the *totally* secret ballot has become the norm, enshrined as a key tenet of human rights. It is perceived to be both essential to individual liberty and fundamental to the workings of a healthy democracy. Candidates may be officially announced, usually with formal parties behind them. Collective results of elections must be publicized almost immediately and in all kinds of previously unimaginable media. Ditto for representatives' voting in various political bodies. But individual decisions at the polls—whether about matters of policy in the case of referenda or about choices in representatives—are understood to be private, not to be revealed to the eyes and ears of one's fellow citizens. This is the process that we now unthinkingly equate with freedom, the way we believe most suited to guarantee the expression of interior inclinations and private determinations.

We do not, however, often examine how this state of affairs came to be. The full story takes us all the way to the twentieth century. But only by tracing the sensory dimension of the origins, nature, and outcome of the revolutions that paved the way for modern democracy are we any closer to perceiving—or dare I say, sensing—this for ourselves. The American and Haitian Revolutions are no less deserving of this kind of analysis than is the French one. It is time that the great body of political history written about the eighteenth century opened itself up to sensory history as well. We are steeped now in considerations of the role of the senses in structuring both public and private social life in the eighteenth century, from the interiors of boudoirs to the taverns and markets of big cities. But the very nature and significance of those terms—public and private—take on new meaning when we stop to consider political behavior as also intimately related to the history of the senses.

CHAPTER TWO

Urban Sensations: Motion and Commotion in Eighteenth-century Cities

CLARE BRANT

One would think there's no end of the streets, but the land's end.
   Then there's such a power of people, going hurry skurry! Such a racket of coxes! Such a noise, and haliballoo! So many strange sites to be seen!
— Smollett [1771] 1982: 60

The astonished reaction of a Welsh *ingénue* to London in a satirical novel which delights in exaggerating sensual discomfort gives a nonetheless typical Enlightenment idea of urban life as a shock to the senses. A language of violence runs through eighteenth-century representations of towns and cities: senses are assaulted, overpowered, assailed. Yet the energy of urban life, characteristic of *activity*, was accompanied by a commensurate *reactivity*, in which senses were the more intently alert. Stimulation raised questions: what stimuli were good—for health, for society? What forms of order should be cultivated in new behaviors between people and new locations of pleasure? What Penny Corfield has called the "kaleidoscopic appeal" of city life (Corfield 1990: 174) may be applied to the varied ways in which the senses were perceived afresh in the bustle, throng, and hurry of eighteenth-century cities. In that kaleidoscope, there emerge strong contrasts: between positive and negative experiences; between rich and poor; between delight and disgust; between immersion and alienation. Each of these has their own history, but one may collate them through a common history of the body and movement. And one may particularize them through places, each with different flavors and textures which nonetheless contributed to a general concept of urban life as one of motion and commotion.

The long eighteenth century, stretching from the late seventeenth to the early nineteenth century, could be said to be the period in which cities transformed from early modern to modern. That claim supposes an evolution, in which growth—of population, housing, trade, and civic amenities—sees cities grow physically and change culturally. An index of growth through numbers is an established way of defining and measuring urban locations— more people, more density of buildings, more material and cultural networks characterize and hence define urban life. Although this model holds good for many Enlightenment-era towns and cities, and its use of data makes it appealing to many historians, it can be a blunt instrument, masking both particular changes in cities and how urban life accommodated space in new ways even as it enveloped more of it. In London, for instance, the Great Fire of 1666 burnt down a large part of the city, and in both rebuilding and new building, more consideration was given to spacing buildings so there would be less risk of fire spreading fast through densely built areas. The Enlightenment era also saw urban centers spring up in new countries like America, with growth so fast it barely had time for evolution. Philadelphia, for instance, had begun as a settlement on wooded ground; within one lifetime it had transformed to a city rivaling many cities in the Old World. According to Edward Dunker, who died in 1782 aged 103, there were now regular streets where he had hunted hares; churches rising on marsh where he had often heard frogs croaking; wharves and warehouses where Indians used to fish; ships, where there used to be only canoes, and grand legislative buildings on the site of Indian council-fires (*The Universal Magazine* 1783: 420). Conversely, some Old World cities were falling apart. Thus Cracow, where houses were pockmarked with shot after a siege by Charles XII and depredation by the Russians: "Cracow exhibits the remains of ancient magnificence, and looks like a great capital in ruins: from the number of fallen and falling houses one would imagine it had lately been sacked, and that the enemy had left it only yesterday" (Coxe 1784, I: 171). Decline and poverty made some cities melancholy places: "the suburbs chiefly consisting of the same wooden hovels which compose the villages, we had no suspicion of being near the capital of Poland until we arrived at its gates"

(Coxe 1784, I: 203). So a grand narrative of growth needs to acknowledge there were counter-currents too.

New cities in the eighteenth century had layouts that were grid-like and rational—notably in America but also in European towns, especially those devastated by natural events. A great earthquake in Sicily in 1693 reduced several flourishing towns to rubble: Ragusa, Modica, Noto, and others were rebuilt on a new baroque style of grand plan, in which imposing cathedrals, open vistas, and widened approaches gave urban life a distinctly progressive feel, a three-dimensional form of Enlightenment. In 1669, lava from Mount Etna's most powerful eruption reached the town of Catania ten miles away: the townspeople engaged digging channels to divert it (said to be a world-first tactic), but to no avail; about 20,000 died. After another earthquake in 1693, Catanians inventively rebuilt their city using lava as a building material. The great earthquake that leveled much of Lisbon in 1755 was followed by a tidal wave and a terrible fire, again leading to the deaths of thousands. It too ushered in new and grander design. The contrast, sufficiently interesting to be the subject of a panorama on show in London in 1800, had a profound effect on the imagination:

> It is not to be expressed by human tongue how dreadful and awful it was to enter the city after the fire was abated; and looking upwards one was struck with terror in beholding the frightful pyramids of ruined fronts, some inclining one way, some another: then, on the contrary, you beheld with horror dead bodies six or seven in a heap, half buried and half burnt, in the streets and squares.
>
> *An Account of the Earthquake* 1800: 6

These actual catastrophes provided materials for necropolitan visions of hell as a city of burning souls; they also swept away medieval towns to enable broad streets and open squares to replace meandering mazes. What distinguishes cities from towns in this evolution of urban environment is that in cities, especially those with royalty in residence, building aspired to magnificence. But a common aesthetic of durability, elegance, and airiness could be found too in the assembly rooms, theaters, pump-rooms, opera houses, and other public buildings of provincial towns across Europe. Observations on the density of build and height were a common part of urban sense-impressions. So one admirer of Genoa wrote, "The City itself makes the noblest Show of any in the World. The Houses are most of them painted on the Outside; so that they look extreamly gay and lively, besides that they are esteemed the highest in *Europe*, and stand very thick together" (Addison 1718: 18). Light and space were indicators of good use and health: thus Smollett, entering Montpellier, observed "The town is reckoned well built, and what the French call *bien percée*; yet the streets are in general narrow and the houses dark" (Smollet [1766] 1981: 85). The senses commonly have evaluation attached to them, or an affect—sensations are causal, emotive, productive of pleasure, pain, numbness, stimulation, or overstimulation. Visual evaluation of attractive and unattractive density in urban environments points to a balancing act akin to that decorum valued in Enlightenment models of social emotion.

Enlightenment urban life was shaped both by evolution from existing conurbations and by idealism occasionally put into practice. The architect of St. Paul's Cathedral, Sir Christopher Wren, turned his attention to designing the whole of London anew following disasters of plague (in 1665) and fire (in 1666). However distinctive the character of different Enlightenment-era cities, comparison was a common practice amongst their architects. In 1665 Wren visited Paris, whose buildings concentrated his mind through his senses:

> the Antique Mass of the Castle of St *Germains*, and the hanging-gardens are delightfully surprising, (I mean to any Man of Judgment) for the Pleasures below vanish away in the Breath that is spent ascending. The Palace, or if you please, the Cabinet of *Versailles* call'd me twice to view it; the Mixtures of Brick, Stone, blue Tile and Gold make it look like a rich Livery: Not an Inch within but is crouded with little Curiosities of Ornament; the Women, as they make here the Language and Fashions, and meddle with Politicks and Philosophy, so they sway also in Architecture; Works of Filgrand and little Knacks are in great Vogue; but Building ought certainly to have the Attribute of eternal, and therefore the only Thing uncapable of new Fashions
>
> Wren 1750: 261

The heroic simplicity of Wren's baroque was thus deliberately masculine. Yet gender influenced the idea of the city: London should be beautified, wrote Wren, to reflect her own wealth and grandeur "and in respect also of the Rank she bore with all other trading Cities of the World, of which tho' she was before one of the richest in Estate and Dowry, yet unquestionably the least beautiful" (Wren 1750: 267). Other travelers used the template of femininity to evaluate foreign cities: it provided a shorthand for sensual response. So Lady Mary Wortley Montagu, traveling across the continent to Constantinople in 1716, surveyed a number of cities. Pleased by the neatness and cleanliness of

Rotterdam, she saw it reflected in women: "the common servants and little shopwomen, here, are more nicely clean, than most of our ladies, and the great variety of neat dresses (every woman dressing her head after her own fashion) is an additional pleasure of seeing the town" (Wortley Montagu 1763, I: 4). Vienna's smartness in white stone was offset by dirt, cramped streets, and overcrowding: a town clapped on a town, she wrote, without social zoning "so that the apartments of the greatest ladies, and even of the ministers of state, are divided, but by a partition, from that of a taylor or shoemaker" (Wortley Montagu 1763, I: 29). Commodiousness and cleanliness were pleasures for eighteenth-century travelers, who sought them in domestic space, in the rooms and houses they occupied, and also in the streets and districts of those houses. For all the rich lexicon of dirt, malodor, and filth in the eighteenth century, there was also a vocabulary for positive sensual experience.

William Cowper's assertion that "God made the country and man made the town" (in *The Task*, 1785, Book 1) was orthodox in its emphasis that urban experience was man-made. Hence there was interest in how it might be made better, by reducing its moral shortcomings of crime and dishonesty and by opening up its literally dark ways. Different cities followed different trajectories—Amsterdam, hub of world trade in the seventeenth century, focused on enabling institutions of global capitalism, in the form of joint stock companies, banks, a magnificent town hall, chambers of insurance, merchants' homes, elegant new canals, and "a proliferating array of civic and religious institutions" (Blumin 2008: 2), whereas Rome, home of kings and popes, counts and cardinals, primary center of Catholic pilgrimage and an emergent secular tourism, fits what Paul Hohenberg and Lynn Lees identify as a model of "cities of surplus" whose economy turns on exaction of rents and in which relative decline paradoxically produces architectural brilliance (Blumin 2008: 4–5). Amsterdam was modernized by its citizens, Rome by Pope Alexander VII, who obsessively straightened streets, built *piazze* and lined streets and squares with impressive new buildings eloquent of cultural magnificence (Blumin 2008: 85). Yet, if the burghers were developing civic community and the pope was modernizing the Eternal City, the cities of both were re-envisioned through a new form of visual representation in art, what Stuart Blumin terms "streetscapes":

> Artists of this era did, in fact, multiply images of cities, and expanded the modes by which cities were represented—in maps, "map views", and other more or less acutely angled panoramas; in city profiles limned from across harbours and approaching plains; and, most notably, as a fresh

departure of the seventeenth and eighteenth centuries, in closer views of the city's streets, squares, waterways, buildings and daily life.

Blumin 2008: 1

Streetscapes were promoted and circulated around Europe thanks to crisscrossing artist networks, the growth of Grand Tourism and the proliferation of print shops everywhere. These urban views or *vedute* organized perspectives, recorded improvements, and promoted understanding of cities through rationalizations of their sites, sights, and occupants. Stuart Blumin makes a convincing case for seeing them as part of a common, modernizing culture which is emphatically secular and characteristically Enlightenment (Blumin 2008: 12–18).

The evolution of urban depiction may suggest an increase in the importance of sight, solidified by the growth in souvenir images of cities for tourists. Yet other senses are evoked too, making the streetscape an urban scene in which sounds, smell, and touch are active. In Michele Marieschi's series of twenty-one etchings of Venice published as *Magnificentiores Selectioreque Urbis Venetiarum Prospectus* in 1741, there are evocations of movement in clouds, flapping flags, fluttering pennants, and curving smoke (Blumin 2008: 138). As in Canaletto's paintings of similar scenes, there is often rippling on the surface of the water which manifests a light wind's touch. Almost every principal city in this period was on a river or a coast: many—Amsterdam, Venice, Lisbon, Constantinople, London, Copenhagen, Stockholm to name a few—had harborage or docks as an important part of their urban landscape. Sounds of loading and unloading, masts and timbers creaking in the wind, clatter of anchor, ruffle of sails, oaths and songs of watermen, smells of wood and tar, rope and salty tackle—all may have been liberated rather than repressed by a visual frame. Sound was curiously pictorialized in popular engravings: a seventeenth-century series by Abraham Bosse, *Les Cris de Paris* (c. 1630) was given new life in Marcellus Laroon's very popular series *The Cryes of the City of London drawne after the life*, originally published in 1687 and much reprinted. Using models from life they show a wide selection of street hawkers who sold all sorts of goods including fish, fruit, matches, pins, vinegar, oysters, and spectacles. Writers, who also minded watchmen calling the hours, noted their intrusion: "I never could be poetical in this Town, if my imagination was preparing to rise on the wings of the Eagle in that moment perhaps a wretch under the window cryd oysters, and I have been immediately awakend from the vision".[1]

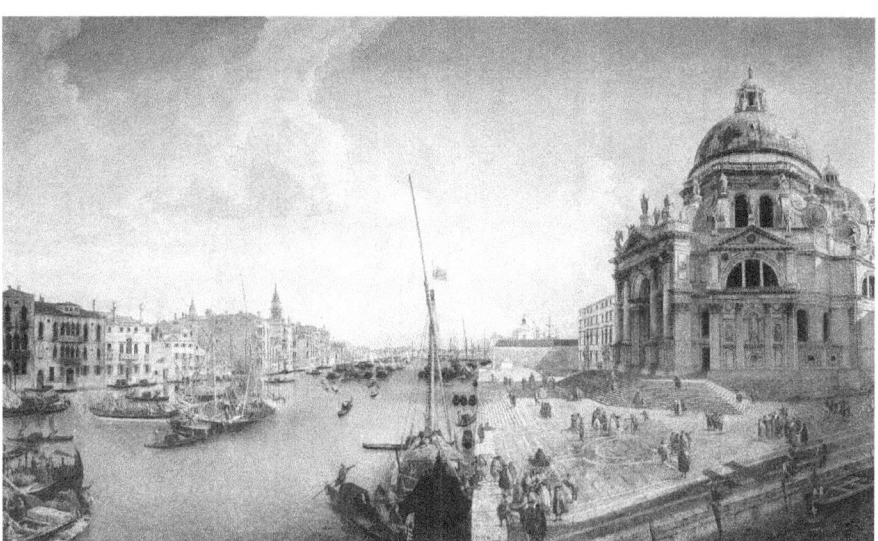

FIGURE 2.1: Michele Marieschi, *L'Entrée du Grand Canal et l'église de la Salute à Venise*, c. 1735–40. Louvre Museum, Paris

On the page you can't hear these distinctive cries, but their inscriptions evoke an aural world in which the urban poor literally made themselves heard. "When I first entered the city of London, I was almost stunned, while my curiosity was not a little excited by what is termed the 'cries of London'—the streets were thronged by persons of both sexes and of every age, crying each the various articles which they were exposing for sale, or for jobs of work at their various occupations." The writer of this, an escaped American prisoner of war, joined them of necessity, crying "Old Chairs to Mend" for thirty years. He recorded he needed strong lungs to compete, suggesting elite clichés of urban noise (and smell) had a real basis (Potter 1824: 68–9). Some Laroon prints show refined goods in rough hands, like the hawker who sells short-stemmed "singing glasses" and longer "glass trumpets" or "glass horns," and although the extreme poverty of such sellers is tidied up in the prints, there is a suggestive contrast between the delicate goods on sale and the ragged, emaciated state of their sellers. In these prints sight doesn't replace sound but frames it as a key urban sense. Blake's London is dominated by hearing:

In every cry of every Man,
In every Infants cry of fear,
In every voice: in every ban,
The mind-forg'd manacles I hear.

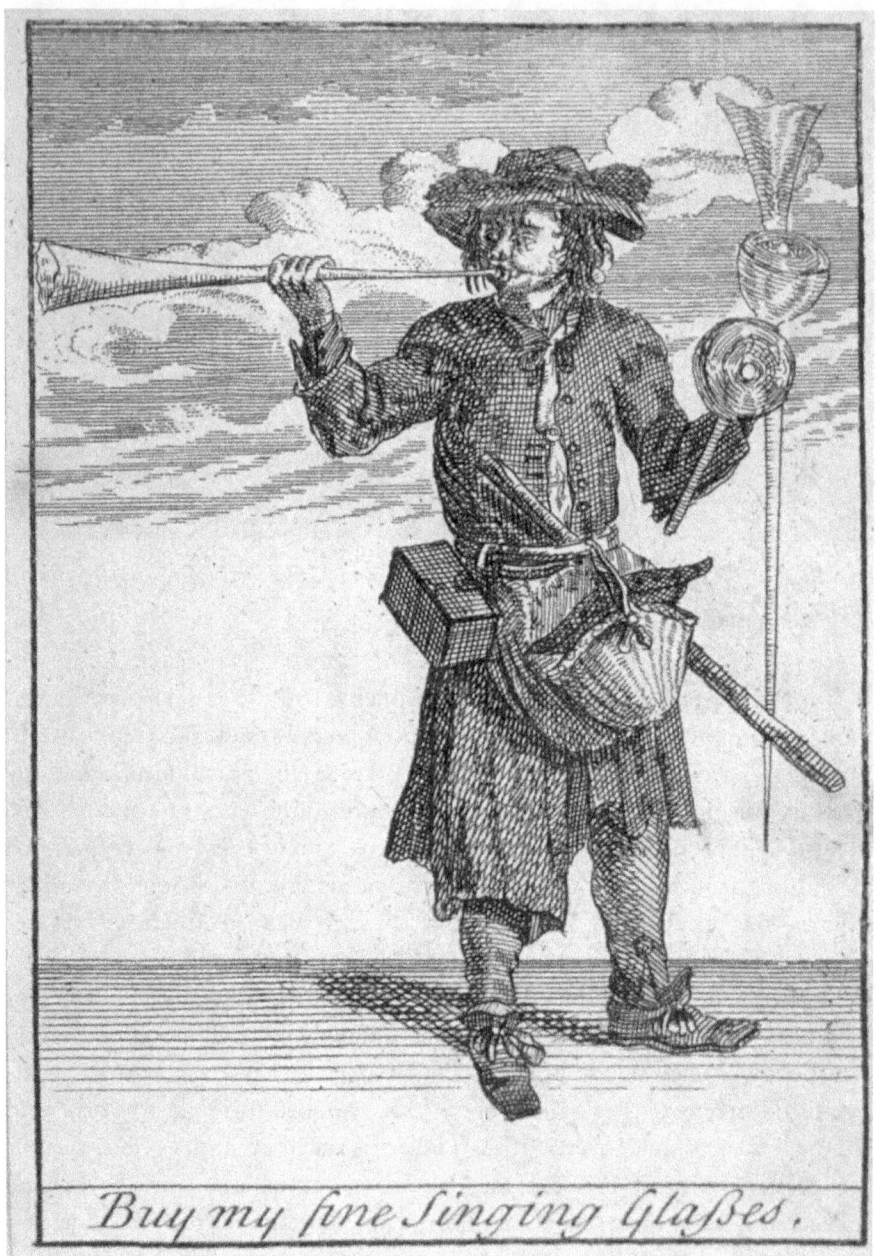

FIGURE 2.2: "Buy my fine singing glasses," *Laroon Cryes of London*. City of London, London Metropolitan Archives.

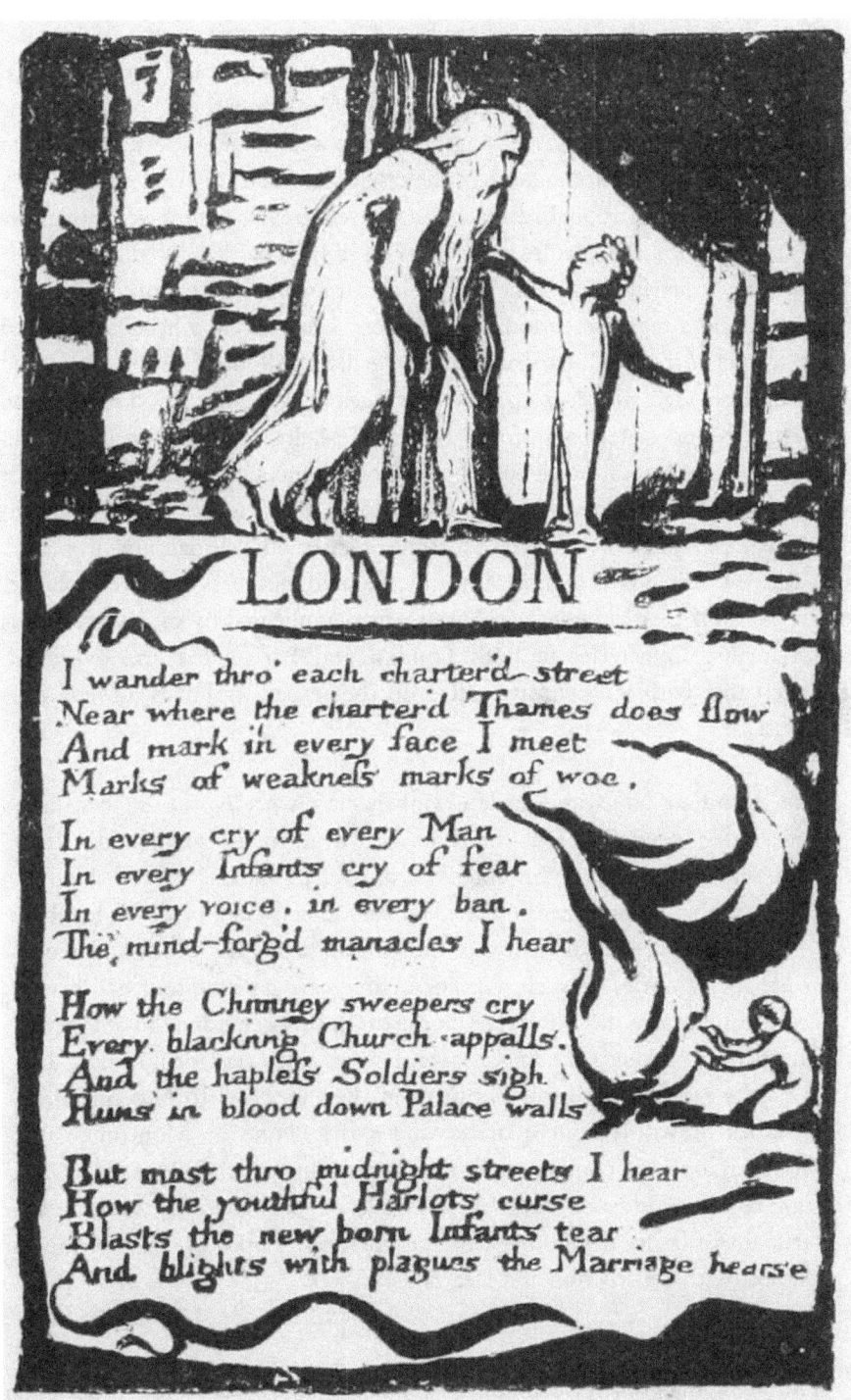

FIGURE 2.3: *Life of William Blake* (1880), Volume 2, *Songs of Experience*.

The chair mender, Isaac Potter, found London magnificent, noisy and unwholesome, a sense-based bewilderment that paradoxically clarified social difference: "There is not perhaps another city of its size in the whole world, the streets of which display a greater contrast in the wealth and misery, the honesty and knavery, of its inhabitants, than the city of London" (Potter 1824: 61–2). One English traveler thought Moscow had even greater contrasts. Though he was a devotee of the picturesque, he was simply baffled by the churches: "Something so irregular, so uncommon, so extraordinary, so contrasted, never before fell under my observation." Some streets were paved; others "are formed of the trunks of trees, or boarded with planks like the floor of a room; wretched hovels are blended with large palaces, cottages of one story stand next to the most superb and stately mansions" (Coxe 1784, I: 361). A sense of the gap between rich and poor, heightened by sensibility, encouraged denunciations of luxury. "Golden girls and boys all must / Like Chimney sweepers, come to dust": Blake's version of antithetical fortunes is sorrowful, elegiac, and prophetic.

Cities published bills of mortality and operated measures to prevent plague. In the wake of Death the leveler, burial was complicated by divisive religious requirements. Cemeteries in both London and Paris filled and overfilled. Change came with a convulsive effect on the senses, as James Stevens Curl explains:

> The Arcadian landscape-garden, embellished with *fabriques*, became a desirable exemplar for burial of the dead when compared with unsavoury, even vile, urban churchyards. Yet politicians moved slowly, and it was some time before the idea was officially adopted. Under the *Ancien Régime* the Churchyard of the Innocents in Paris which had been in use for centuries, was closed. For many years its condition had been scandalous, and in the 1780s the Church of the Innocents and the *charniers* (charnel-houses) surrounding the putrid ground were demolished. In 1785 the transfer of bones began from the Innocents to underground ossuaries in worked-out quarries under the Plaine de Montrouge in Montparnasse, but contemporary descriptions suggest they were places of nightmares, worlds of darkness and silence broken only when new cartloads of bones from other closed crypts were tipped in. There Chaos reigned, with Destruction and Death.
>
> Curl 2012: 195

Following the French Revolution, Arcadian designs modulated into Elysian Fields "which would be dramatically contrasted with Church-controlled burial grounds where skulls, bones, foetor, horror, and loathsomeness were to be found in plenty. Agreeable philanthropic ideals and sweet reason were to replace despair, terror, hellfire, superstition, and disgusting sights and smells" (Curl 2012: 196). City authorities did organize new places for burying the city dead, assuming a physical closeness between living city and necropolis. The sensual offensiveness of urban burial was replaced by cemeteries devoted to restfulness, in which the senses were to be soothed by peace and silent mourning.

One other kind of city needs to be included in an Enlightenment urban sensorium: the heavenly city. Though the Bible provided tropes for heaven from both nature and culture, city imagery suited visions of the sociability of heaven. Charles Wesley imagines such a city in his hymn "Away with Our Sorrow and Fear" (ironically often sung to a tune called "Green Fields"):

> We see the new city descend,
> Adorned as a bride for her Lord;
> The city so holy and clean,
> No sorrow can breathe in the air;
> No gloom of affliction or sin,
> No shadow of evil is there.
> By faith we already behold
> That lovely Jerusalem here;
> Her walls are of jasper and gold,
> As crystal her buildings are clear;
> Immovably founded in grace,
> She stands as she ever hath stood,
> And brightly her Builder displays,
> And flames with the glory of God.
>
> Wesley 1746: vii

Wesley takes streets of gold and a crystal river from the Bible (Revelations 21:21; 22:1) and supposes the contemporary city to be a place of filth and suffering, yet his version of transcendence also mirrors actual cities like London in using magnificent materials and rhetorics of antiquity and power to give ideological purpose. Vision is purified—bright, crystalline—and so too is touch—unshakeable. The most unusual transmogrification is Blake's Golgonooza, a city of Art and Imagination which stands between earth and heaven. It has four gates and intricate layers of cosmology within; its enfolded meanings depend on symmetry, like a mandala, including, in a typically Blakean way, an asymmetry between actual London and a spiritually translucent city in which dirt, noise, and suspicion have been transformed into sensually perfect cleanness, peace, and trust. Negative sense impressions have to be included in these visions in order to be cast away; Blake foretells the ideal by passage through and beyond the real. Urban dirt—an expansive category which here includes literal filth and the figurative stain of sin—dissolves in the radiance of celestial redemption, made possible by holiness inherent in humans: "I write in South Molton Street what I both see and hear, / In regions of Humanity, London's opening streets" (Blake, *Jerusalem* 38). Golgonooza introduced a kinder, compassionating city. "The stones are pity and the bricks well-wrought affections / Enamel'd with love and kindness, & the tiles graven gold,/ Labour of merciful hands: the beams and rafters are forgiveness" (*Jerusalem* 12). "It is the Spiritual Fourfold London" declared Blake. Though it is a singular vision, it contributed to a common perception of urban life as sensorily negative because social difference was great. The sensual pleasures of luxury were for some less pleasurable, and for some contemptible, because only the rich could afford them and because they circulated at the expense of the poor. Others argued that luxury benefited the poor by increasing demand for fine goods and the trades associated with them.

Social distinctions were especially evident in relation to food and its accompanying senses. In urban settings, the sensory world of eating was one shared by all, in that urban people by definition were not generally food producers, but also a world striated by class distinctions. What the rich consumed was often conspicuously sumptuous. In 1727, George II's coronation banquet took place in Westminster Hall. It lasted for three days, featured seventy-five different dishes, "thirty of which were replaced as the repast continued, so that 105 different taste sensations were available in one place" (Varey 1996: 36). Guests were tempted by piled-high platters of jellies, veal, geese, crabs, cheesecakes, pasties, fruit, and wet and dry sweetmeats in grand pyramids. Generally, Britons were carnivores; Londoners of all classes were keen on pies. The chair mender's London is full of instances of the starving. He reports one such case where a baker furiously followed home a woman who had stolen a loaf of bread. In her wretched dwelling was a platter with some roasted meat. It proved to be dog, all they had eaten for three days. Roast meat had symbolic importance in the roast beef of Old England, held by the English to be superior to French ragouts and stews where inferior meat was disguised by sauces. In 1762, Boswell, fresh from Scotland, spent a whimsical day in London acting English, in eating a big beefsteak and going to see a cockfight. He recorded:

> A beefsteak house is a most excellent place to dine at. You come in there to a warm, comfortable, large room, where a number of people are sitting

at a table. You take whatever place you find empty; call for what you like, which you get well and cleverly dressed. You may either chat or not as you like. Nobody minds you, and you pay very reasonably. My dinner (beef, bread, beer and waiter) was only a shilling.

Boswell [1762–3] 1950: 86

Eating at chophouses, taverns, and inns gave more substantial refreshment than coffeehouses; the popularity of clubs and societies also involved food, though often in second place to prodigious quantities of drink. The sandwich, slices of meat between bread, is said to have been devised in 1762 by John Montagu, fourth Earl of Sandwich, so he could continue gambling without leaving the table for food. In their cities the English promoted fast food; the French encouraged restaurants.

The London Tavern, which opened in 1768, gives us a flavor. Situated just inside the City of London, it was patronized by East India Company directors from their nearby premises; it was also popular with the radical John Wilkes and his supporters. It came to be associated with revolutionaries—in 1791 at a dinner to celebrate the anniversary of the French Revolution, Thomas Paine proposed a toast to "The Revolution of the World" (Farley [1783] 1998: 5), an association between radical politics and good dining (anticipating champagne socialism!) which carried over to Paris, where in 1782 the great chef Beauvilliers opened a restaurant called La Grande Taverne de Londres. Bills of fare for each month show the presence but not dominance of French culinary taste. January, for instance: first course Soup a la reine, Harrico of Beef, leg of lamb Boil'd, Rabbits florendine [sic], Almond soup, boiled chickens, oyster patties and pork cutlets circled two fish dishes and a raised French pie. The second course features hen turkey, asparagus, larded fowls, wild duck and larks, a wonderfully-named amulet of oysters, roast hare and sausages arranged around crayfish flanked by dishes of orange jelly and blancmange. The few puddings morph into barely-edible ornaments: Moonshine, Rocky Island, Snow and Cream, Silver Web (Farley [1783] 1998: 219–30, 325–8). The Tavern's principal cook uses a fascinatingly specialized vocabulary for the carving of cooked small fowls: to wing, allay, lift, display, rear, unbrace, unlace, designated precise and different procedures, a new repertoire of touch. When choosing provisions, feel, look and smell determined freshness:

> If you squeeze young mutton with your fingers, it will feel very tender; but if it be old, it will feel hard and continue wrinkled, and the fat will be fibrous and clammy. The grain of ram mutton is close, the flesh is of a

deep red, and the fat is spongy. The flesh of ewe mutton is paler than that of the wether, and the grain is closer. Most people give the preference to short-shanked mutton.

Farley [1783] 1998: 22–3

This egalitarianism—everyone is an eater—was partnered by comparativism, in noticing sense differences between cultures: "A porter of London quenches his thirst with a draught of strong beer; a porter of Rome, or Naples, refreshes himself with a slice of water-melon, or a glass of iced-water" (Smollett [1766] 1981: 161).

The eighteenth century saw French cuisine become the touchstone of culinary taste, universally and sometimes grudgingly acknowledged. It had a philosopher in Jean-Anthelme Brillat-Savarin (1755–1825; the richly creamy cheese named for him was invented in the 1930s). He thought there were six senses, the sixth being physical desire. "I am also tempted to believe that smell and taste are in fact but a single sense, whose laboratory is the mouth and whose chimney is the nose" (Brillat-Savarin [1825] 1994: 41). The aetiology of the senses was, however, much less important to him than analyzing their operations and effects and developing a richer language for them. On taste, for example, which he thought operated through humidity, he lamented the fewness of terms of description, limited to sweet, sugary, acrid, and bitter. But he argued those were always contained in "agreeable or disagreeable," and it is in the whisking together of pleasure and the senses that Brillat-Savarin became an exemplary and influential Enlightenment gourmet.

Unlike other philosophers, Brillat-Savarin was not looking to reason to advance enlightenment, but to an understanding of the body that was also bodily understanding. Food is an intelligent pleasure, he demonstrated, in which the mind is enriched by being attentive to senses. The gastronomic equivalent was *osmazome*, "that highly sapid part of meat which is soluble in cold water" (Brillat-Savarin [1825] 1994: 64) that gives soups, caramelized meat, and game their savor. Brillat-Savarin was not a simple epicure—he liked Welsh rarebit and *potage*—but he brought senses together in amity that could be shared with others. He also united urban and rural space through a common appreciation of food: categories of raw and cooked were connected through people's care with ingredients. And he was amusing: "it would be fair to say that it is gravy that distinguishes feasting from fasting." Brillat-Savarin is attentive to a sequence of senses—how wine is only fully tasted once it has been swallowed, for instance—and to the sensuality of gastronomic language, sharing orality with sexual pleasure. He celebrated aphrodisiac foods for the sensuality of language they encouraged: "Whoever says 'truffles' utters a great word, which arouses erotic and gastronomic memories among the skirted sex, and memories gastronomic and erotic among the bearded sex" (Brillat-Savarin [1825] 1994: 90). He adventurously explored new flavors, tasting an extraction of hemerocallis (*hemerocallis fulva*, the orange daylily, is edible; later cultivars are dubiously so): it might flavor pastilles, liqueurs, or ice cream, he thought (Brillat-Savarin [1825] 1994: 313). Like many Enlightenment philosophers wrestling with the relationship between ancient and modern, he paid tribute to classical models. Roman gourmands could distinguish between the flavor of a fish caught upriver and one caught downriver, but moderns could match them. "Have we not men among us today who have discovered the peculiar savour of the leg on which a partridge rests its weight while it sleeps?" (Brillat-Savarin [1825] 1994: 47). Such skills were not only for urban sophisticates.

Fasting laws had relaxed as the authority of the Church weakened, Brillat-Savarin noted, changing calendar eating patterns. Diurnal eating patterns also changed. "More than a third of Paris is content, in the morning, with the lightest of meals" (Brillat-Savarin [1825] 1994: 235)—thus began the continental breakfast. Trades related to food had increased: new professions included that of *petit-four* pastrycook. "A wide variety of vessels, utensils, and other accessories has been invented, so that foreigners coming to Paris find many objects on the table, the names of which they do no know and the purpose of which they often do not dare ask." Conviviality invented new forms in breakfast parties, tea parties, political banquets, and restaurants—"the effect of which is that any man with three or four pistoles in his pocket can immediately, infallibly, and simply for the asking, procure all the pleasures of which taste is susceptible." Among restaurateurs, he singled out Beauvilliers (who set up in 1782, and died in 1820), "the first to combine an elegant dining-room, smart waiters, and a choice cellar with superior cooking" (Brillat-Savarin [1825] 1994: 263–73). Two particular innovations helped spread gastronomic pleasures: the fixed-price menu and the inclusion of imported foods—from Asia, for instance, rice, sago, curry, soy, shiraz wine, and coffee—so that a meal in Paris became an experience of world products. In the sociability of urban space, pleasurable eating became a desirable part of entertainments both private and public. Brillat-Savarin ended his disquisitions with a mythological vision in which "the great city is now just one immense refectory" (291), as if the heavenly city turned out to be a giant restaurant.

Accompanying the development of relatively democratic sensual space in the form of the restaurant (Spang 2000; Spary 2012), eighteenth-century cities also provided sensual space for a wider demographic in the form of green space. Many Enlightenment cities had significant green space. Royal parks, monastic orchards, and open fields survived variously; tree-lined avenues, like Unter den Linden in Berlin, were partially stratified for mixed use by aristocratic hunters, middling classes, and laborers. Most important was the development of pleasure gardens. London's Vauxhall Gardens was perhaps the most influential: it inspired imitations as far afield as Russia (Coxe 1784: 344). The Tivoli gardens too became a model, though the grand Renaissance gardens of Villa D'Este itself fell into decline. Pleasure gardens, like spas and wells, promoted health, selling bottled source water where they had no well of their own. Materially, they temporized to accommodate fashion, an increasingly important part of urban life. Ornamental buildings were run up at speed, alcoves and arbors were rapidly replaced. "Water, of course, played its part, either for the supposed medicinal properties, or as decorative elements such as fountains, ponds, or canals. There were more substantial ponds too, used for bathing" (Curl 2010: 243). They displayed a scene of *rus in urbis* and gave cities smaller versions of royal parks and gardens, where sex the leveler was free to stroll.

> As Peter Borsay and others have pointed out, Georgian men and women enjoyed outdoor entertainments, and the whole business of seeing and being seen, dressing up, and promenading, was an essential part of eighteenth-century urban life, requiring suitable tree-lined walks, flower-beds, seating areas, and facilities for refreshments to be laid on. Even quite small Gardens had provision for walks, secluded seating where conversation could be enjoyed and refreshments consumed, and games such as bowls or skittles played. Some large part of such places of popular resort, of course, was dalliance.
>
> Curl 2010: 243

Pleasure gardens promoted optical intensity and ease, and combined them in ease of looking, especially for men looking at women, that was newly sensual.

In Paris, the Palais Royal "turned into the most spectacular spot for pleasure and politics in Europe" (Allen 2006: 45). In 1782 the Duc de Chartres (from 1785, Duc d'Orleans) invested in "an extravagant plan to turn what had been gardens into an arcaded resort, combining shops, cafes, theatres, and places of more doubtful recreation." The works took six years and "succeeded in bringing a raw and Rabelaisian popular culture right into the heart of aristocratic Paris" (Allen 2006: 46). Among the attractions were marionettes, farces, and melodramas in the packed-out theaters; genteel and risqué cafes; "grocers, bookshops, jewellers, haberdashers, silk merchants, fan makers, tobacconists," and makers of wigs and lace. Visitors could read political satires; hear bawdy songs; sip lemonade; play chess or billiards; watch magic-lantern shows, dancers and acrobats. Mercier wrote admiringly: "this enchanted little spot is in itself a little town of luxury . . . it is the very temple of pleasure, where vice is so bright that the very shadow of shame is chased away" (Allen 2006: 46–7). In describing the allure of pleasure gardens, witnesses often use the word "enchantment." Why? A holiday from the moral effort of politeness was part of the attraction: promenading slid into voyeurism, and conversation into intrigue and sex. Like Vauxhall Gardens, the Palais Royal offered a rational version of carnivalesque pleasures, a Bakhtinian playground in which reason took second place to the senses. Like the cinema in the twentieth century, pleasure gardens were a place in which social encounter was also sensual encounter. Carrying on some of the populist enterprises of fairs, pleasure gardens refined them, with the added attraction of class mingling: "all the orders of citizens are joined together, from the lady of rank to the dissolute, from the soldier of distinction to the humblest official in the Farms" (Schama 1989: 136). Entrance to the Palais Royal was controlled by Swiss guards and there was a dress code, but participants remarked often on the diversity of crowds and the magic of their circulation. Enchantment

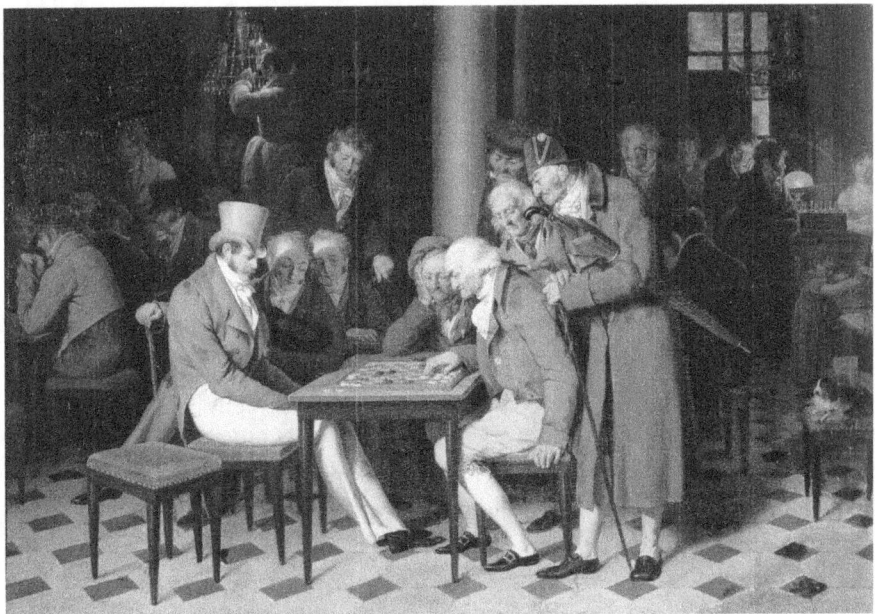

FIGURE 2.4: Louis-Léopold Boilly, *L'intérieur d'un café, dit aussi La partie de dames au café Lamblin au Palais-Royal* (1824). Wikimedia Commons.

invites surrender to performance cast by something or someone else: in pleasure gardens, like theaters and masquerades, people could polish, adjust, experiment with and abandon personae. "Every body is talked of as having some *Ton*; and many People that are walking about Paris *keep up a Character*, as if they were at a Masquerade for Life" (Allen 2006: 101). Keeping up could partner letting go. Enchanted bodies move differently, impelled and slowed by astonishment, wonder and delight. Enchanted minds need think nothing. So pleasure gardens reconciled the energy and entropy of urban space into animation, organizing procession and riot into dialogue.

Tourists in classical and holy cities watched religious processions that went back centuries: as Thomas Gray reported from Rome, "Mr. Walpole says, our memory sees more than our eyes in this country" (Letter 119, Thomas Gray Archive, 350, May 1740). Traditions of carnival were celebrated, most famously in Venice. "It is an *Omnia Bene* for Peccadillo's. No *Where have you been? Who have you passed the Night with*? To wife or daughter" (*Amours* 1795: 8). Carnival continued the tradition of Saturnalia valued by the early modern period as "the world turned upside down"; it was "a confused Scene of intermixt Pleasure, jumbled together without any Regularity" (*Amours* 1795: 10). Frost fairs sprung up on frozen rivers:

> Booths sudden hide the Thames, long Streets appear,
> And num'rous Games proclaim the crouded Fair.
> So when a Gen'ral bids the martial Train
> Spread their Encampment o'er the spatious Plain;
> Thick-rising Tents a Canvas City build,
> And the loud Dice resound thro' all the Field.
>
> Gay 1716, II: 369–74

Old fairs like St. Bartholomew's near London remained, though their very traditionality helped inspire an Enlightenment version of sense-impressionism: "the quick dance / Of colours, lights, and forms; the Babel din; / The endless stream of men, and moving things" as Wordsworth put it in "Residence in London," the seventh book of *The Prelude* (1805, VII: 156–8). "The more efficient ... city dwellers," William C. Sharpe maintains, "screen out the adverse stimuli that buffet them—what Wordsworth himself alludes to as the city's 'shock/For eyes and ears'" (1805, VII: 685–6). Quoting this, Michael Meyer argues "the uncertainty engendered by the pervasive theatricality of life may induce a desire to avoid any involvement with individuals" (Meyer 2003). Getting away from the crowds became a Romantic preoccupation, along with finding space: "To one who has been long in city pent, / 'Tis very sweet to look into the fair / And open face of heaven,— to breathe a prayer/ Full in the smile of the blue firmament" (Keats [1817] 1884). City and sky acquired new Enlightenment sensual pleasure with the appearance of balloons, which from 1783 brought out great crowds to view aerial ascents. The first accounts of cities viewed from above by aeronauts gave those crowds a new sense of their urbanity and teeming humanity. An Italian ascending over London struggled to describe his downward view: "I saw the streets as lines, all animated with beings, whom I knew to be men and women, but which I should otherwise have had a difficulty in describing. It was an enormous beehive, but the industry of it was suspended" (Lunardi 1785: 32; on ballooning: Brant 2011; Lynn 2010; Thébaud-Sorger 2009).

Enlightenment city iconography favored cornucopia, and no wonder: on the ground, the great hive produced astonishing goods and variety of experiences. Yet abundance could cause sensual fatigue, even sensory overload. The pursuit of pleasure was frequently manifested through social codes which entailed etiquette, obligation, a culture of *comme il faut* which could be hard to learn and tiring to practice. *A la mode* came into English in the 1640s: it appeared first as an adverb, associated with doing. Fashionable amusements kept up that compulsive energy. As Frances Anne Crewe sojourning in Paris wrote on March 4, 1786,

> Miss Carter said the other Day that there was so much trouble about every Sort of Amusement at Paris, and so much to be done about every other thing, that She thought what we often all Complained of here ought to be called the *Day Mare*. I protest it is so apposite to what I have forever felt in Paris, that I was quite charmed with the Idea
> Allen 2006: 183

Six years later, the husband of Crewe's friend the Duchesse de Brissac was guillotined, and his severed head thrown in at the window of Mme du Barry, his mistress (Allen 2006: 108). Revolution gave a violent jolt to any ennui.

Home to violence, riot, and crime as well as pleasure, urban space was for the laboring classes and distressed poor a sensual world only partly shared with the prosperous. The poor went hungry and cold; many curled up on hard floors or ash heaps to sleep. Yet there were sensual pleasures common to all: drinking and sex were common appetites. For the richer classes, provisioned with the best in town and country, an ideal of rural retirement was powerful not simply as a binary divide between town and country but as a withdrawal into a microcosm whose value is defined in part by the urban experience from which it retires. Town was communicative: in Britain, the popular format of letters from A Gentleman in Town to a Friend in the Country endorsed dialogue. Mr. Urban, the persona of *The Gentleman's Magazine*, gave the middling classes an urban figurehead.

Enlightenment opinion was not uniform about whether urbanity had a civilizing effect on the senses, or whether increasing sophistication tended to corrupt the senses. Rousseau argued at length in *Emile* that "The further we are from a state of nature, the more we lose our natural tastes; or rather, habit becomes a second nature, and so completely replaces our real nature, that we have lost all knowledge of it" (Rousseau [1762] 1921). Conversely, Mary Wollstonecraft reflected that civilization "produces a variety which enables us to retain the primitive delicacy of our sensations" (Wollstonecraft [1796] 1987: 72). She recorded instances of that in herself and others, like a prisoner at Lisbon: "A wretch who had been imprisoned several years, during which period lamps had been put up, was at last condemned to a cruel death; yet, in his way to execution, he only wished for one night's respite, to see the city lighted" (Wollstonecraft [1796] 1987: 113). Urban life could feel attractive and annoying simultaneously: as Frances Anne Crewe wrote, "my Life has been, what, I think, every Paris one may be called, a regular Confusion—indeed most Lives in Capitals are such when they are formed upon a large Scale, and not closely linked with a small, regular Society." Regular confusion put strain on fellow feeling and produced prejudice, often sense-based. One view in Paris was that the English language "was a Combination of Sounds *scarcely human*! And that it might be compared to the *Hissing Noise of Animals* more than any other" (Allen 2006: 155).

The senses gave people a cultural spectrum in common, but the pressure of urban life produced and aggravated social divisions. In such contexts a language of low senses lurked, ready to color insults. In Philadelphia, Benjamin Franklin organized street lighting, street paving, a newspaper, and a subscription library—"the Mother of all the N American Subscription Libraries now so numerous" (Franklin 1986: 71). Nonetheless, this active citizen resented improvements benefiting immigrants:

> Why should the *Palatine Boors* be suffered to swarm into our Settlements, and by herding together establish their Language and Manners to the Exclusion of ours? Why should *Pennsylvania*, founded by the English, become a Colony of *Aliens*, who will shortly be so numerous as to Germanize us instead of our Anglifying them, and who will never

adopt our Language or Customs, any more than they can acquire our Complexion.

Franklin 1986: 259

Complexity of urban idiolects and behaviors could also be read as a Babel, overpowering, divisive, and threatening.

Social mixing gave a sensual disorderliness to Enlightenment literature of the city. Tom Brown makes the most of this in a piece about London. He imagines showing the city to an Indian who has dropped from the clouds. The two of them will ramble about, once the Indian has got over the shock of traffic:

> At first Dash the confused Clamours *near Temple Bar*, Stun him, Fright him, make him Giddy. He sees an infinite Number of different *Machines*, all in violent Motion. Some Riding on the Top, some Within, others Behind, and *Jehu* on the Coach-Box before, whirling some Dignify'd Villain towards the *Devil*, who has got an Estate by Cheating the Publick.
>
> Brown 1702: 11

Brown's hectic prose stresses the variety of people in a city of heteroglossia, of different kinds of language and sounds on the street. Jostling is physical and linguistic:

> Here a Sooty Chimney-Sweeper takes the Wall of a Grave *Alderman*, and a *Broom-Man* jostles the *Parson* of the Parish. There a Fat Greasie *Porter* runs a Trunk full Butt upon you, while another Salutes your Antlers with a Flasket of *Eggs* and *Butter. Turn out there, you Country Put*, says a *Bully*, with a Sword two Yards long jarring at his Heels, and throws him into the Channel [ditch]. By and by comes a *Christning*, with the *Reader*, screwing up his mouth to deliver the Service *alamode dè Paris*, and afterwards talk immoderately nice and dull with the Gossips, and the *Midwife* strutting in the Front, and Young Original Sin as fine as fippence, follow'd with the Vocal Musick of *Kitchen stuff ha' you Maids*; and a damn'd *Trumpeter* calling in the Rabble to see a Calf with Six Legs and a Top-knot. There goes a Funeral with Men of Rosemary after it, licking there [sic] Lips after three Hits of White, Sack and Claret, at the House of Mourning, and the Sexton walking before, as Big and Bluff as a *Beef-Eater* at a Coronation. Here a Poet scampers for't as fast as his

Legs will carry him, and at his Heels a Brace of *Bandog Bayliffs*, with open mouths ready to Devour him, and all the Nine Muses; and there an *Evidence* [an informer] ready to spew up his *false Oaths* at the sight of the Executioner.

Brown 1702: 12

Even allowing for poetic licence, the energy of Brown's urban world turns on oral and aural intensity. Urban space becomes a place of idiolect, different kinds of speech understood to express occupation, age, class, and character.

Brown and many other writers of the period represent intensity and density of urban movements with reference to touch, and more specifically to *avoidance* of touch. Rousseau, interested in active touch, proposed it as a powerful sense:

> Although touch is the sense oftenest used, its discrimination remains, as I have already pointed out, coarser and more imperfect than that of any other sense, because we always use sight along with it; the eye perceives the thing first, and the mind almost always judges without the hand. On the other hand, discrimination by touch is the surest just because of its limitations; for extending only as far as our hands can reach, it corrects the hasty judgments of the other senses, which pounce upon objects scarcely perceived, while what we learn by touch is learnt thoroughly.

Rousseau [1762] 1911: 125

In *Crowds and Power* (1960 1962) Elias Canetti argued that urban experience is unpleasant because it imposes involuntary touch. He writes: "The repugnance of being touched remains with us when we go about among people; the way we move in a busy street . . . is governed by it" (Canetti [1960] 1962: 15). Ava Arndt argues that touch replaces sight as the primary sense of urban space, and that it does so in the eighteenth century. She also proposes that "An obsession with motion, financial, fictive, and corporeal, is arguably one of the major effects of a move into capitalism" and it manifests in a modernity overwhelmingly tactile (Arndt 2007: 104). There's good evidence for this approach to underpin a case for a composite history of the senses. Consider this confession by a Londoner in 1763:

> Somehow or another, I was very low-spirited and melancholy, and could not relish that gay entertainment [of Vauxhall Gardens] and was very

discontent. I left my company, and mounting on the back of a hackney-coach rattled away to town in the attitude of a footman. The whimsical oddity of this, the jolting of the machine, and the soft breeze of the evening made me very well again.

Boswell [1762–3] 1950: 286

Here movement is sensual. Moreover, the three forms of movement all relate to air, to which eighteenth-century people were sensitive, and which helped make movement sensual. Air and movement are important terms in music of the period, a parallel suggestive of how eighteenth-century perceptions of the senses were often related to a sense of the body, which incorporated the senses.

It has been argued (Jancović 2010: 3–5) that eighteenth-century urban residents spent more time indoors to pursue new entertainments and forms of sociability, which created a new sensitivity to the passage of air, for instance between indoors and outdoors. The boundaries between urban home and street were newly and often noisily emphasized by the rattle of sash windows. One of Montesquieu's Persians writes of Paris as "a town built in the air, with six or seven houses all on top of each other . . . exceedingly full of people, and when everyone comes out into the street it makes a splendid muddle" (Montesquieu [1721] 1973: 72). Satire involves exaggeration, of course, but Montesquieu's refrain about the hurry, noise, and press of street life may be taken as symptomatic. His character Rica, like Brown's Indian, is unused to rush, speed, and jostle:

No people in the world make their bodies work harder for them than Frenchmen: they run; they fly . . . I sometimes get as cross as a Christian: for, not to mention getting covered in mud from head to foot, I cannot forgive being regularly and systematically elbowed. A man coming up behind me turns me right round as he overtakes me; another, passing in the opposite direction, abruptly puts me back where the first one got me; and before I have gone a hundred yards I am in a worse state than if I had done ten leagues.

Montesquieu [1721] 1973: 168

Always in a hurry, these citizens create noise: "Front doors suffer more from the way they bang the knocker than from winds and storms." Energy in urban life could appear perilously close to entropy; the phenomenon was expressed through movement and sound in combination. The duplication involved helps explain the invention of a new word in English, *hurry-scurry*. Its multiple functions—verb, adjective, adverb, and noun—and its compound rhyme evoke a need to catch something more than mere hurry. The urban world was represented as social whirl, understood through the senses. It is this pressing sense of urban motion—frenetic and creative motion—that the Enlightenment passes on to us.

CHAPTER THREE

The Senses in the Marketplace: Coffee, Chintz, and Sofas

JOAN DEJEAN

The age that began in the 1660s was the first key moment in the development of a modern luxury goods industry worthy of that name. Over the course of the next century (1660–1760), many items in categories ranging from clothing and fashion accessories, to exotic new foods and beverages, to furniture and decorative objects for the home were invented. In addition, luxury goods were made available in new ways and marketed far more actively and widely than ever before. The modern shopping experience traces its origins to this period: the shop itself was redesigned; advertising techniques such as the flyer and the poster came into broad use for the first time. As a result, luxury goods gradually began to reach an ever broader public, in both geographic and social terms.[1]

Numerous sensory experiences first became part of daily life for Europeans during this period. Many of them were exotic, brought to Europe from distant lands, and no foreign import was more successfully implanted than coffee. The taste of and the taste for coffee spread through European society so quickly that coffee can be thought of as one of the greatest success stories in culinary history and the history of taste.

During these decades, the way Europeans dressed was just as spectacularly transformed as the way they ate. In this domain, a second foreign import knew a commercial success as striking as coffee's: cotton fabrics imported from India. These textiles, previously virtually unknown in Europe, came into ever more widespread use—in table linen and bed linen, in interior decoration, and above all in clothing. The soft, easily washable fabric brought both comfort and convenience into the lives of those who used it; the foreign import's exotic colors and patterns made cotton the darling of fashion trendsetters.

At the same moment, another market was created, for various kinds of items used to furnish and decorate the home. Types of furniture then invented—capacious armchairs and the sofa in particular—transformed both the look of most rooms in the home and the experience of sitting down. They made experiences ranging from entertaining to reading more comfortable and inviting than ever before.

Each of these developments began in a different country: coffee, for example, seems to have first been publicly consumed in either England or Italy, while cotton was originally marketed in the Dutch Republic, and new models of furniture first went on sale in France. Each of them, however, quickly became a pan-European phenomenon. Thus, within decades of its entry into the European marketplace, coffee was being drunk in public in every major capital, and it was not long before cotton was made available to consumers all over the continent. Foreign visitors to Paris saw recently invented furniture models on display in shops there and placed orders so that their homes in Germany, Spain, and Sweden could feature the latest designs. Trends that began in Europe also quickly made their way to much more distant markets, to European colonies in North America for example (see Crowley 2000).

In the course of the decades during which novel kinds of luxury goods such as these touched more and more lives, a new body language was created, and the developing art of portraiture recorded it for posterity. People stretched out and reclined; they draped their arms casually over nearby surfaces. Rigidity and formality were replaced by casual poses and a far greater ease of movement. As artists made clear, the new sensory experiences and sensations had transformed the way individuals thought about and interacted with personal space and furniture (see DeJean 2009).

A MAGICAL NEW DRINK: COFFEE

Europe experienced one of the most significant culinary revolutions in modern times during the period when consumerism was on the rise. New foods, new seasonings, new ways of preparing food, and even of eating it were introduced. This was, for example, the age when the fork was first widely used, the moment when many fruits and vegetables—from baby peas to strawberries—became widely cultivated and made their original appearances in cookbooks, as well as the period when the concept of the sauce was codified (see DeJean 2005). It was also at this time that foods and beverages were first widely consumed in public places, as well as the moment when the original upscale eating establishments began to be established. Of all the new taste experiences that then went public, none was a bigger, a faster, or a more widespread success than the consumption of coffee.

Europeans were introduced to coffee in private homes early in the seventeenth century when travelers to the Orient brought beans back and prepared coffee for their friends. Then, during the second half of the century, public establishments in which the exotic beverage could be purchased and consumed began to be established all over the continent, as well as in European colonies in the New World.

The first coffeehouse whose history can truly be documented was founded in 1650 or 1652 in Oxford by someone identified as "Jacob, one Jew" in a rented room in the Angel Inn on High Street. In 1652, Bowman's coffeehouse opened in Saint Michael's Alley in London. By the 1660s, coffee was being publicly consumed in Paris. A coffeehouse opened in Vienna in 1683, but the first was established in Berlin only in 1721. The original coffeehouse in North America was founded in Boston in 1689; coffee was first drunk in public in New York City in 1696, and in Philadelphia in 1700.

A distinctive coffee culture developed in each country in which the new beverage was introduced. The contrast could not have been clearer, for example, between the two types of establishments that can be most extensively documented—the English coffeehouse and the French café.

In England, the coffeehouse was almost exclusively a male preserve (see Cowan 2005; Ellis 2004). A Dutch engraving of a late-seventeenth-century English coffeehouse depicts a group of men, most of them seated at long communal tables. They are drinking from what appear to be small, handleless bowls. When someone wanted a second cup, their bowl was passed down to the end of the table, where it was filled by a young man who poured the beverage from a large, rather rustic pot. A woman is stationed behind a counter to serve their beverages, but not a single woman is at the tables drinking. Many of the men are smoking pipes; English coffeehouses were known as smoke-filled places. The décor is minimal, and the room was surely rather dark: a few candles are lit on the tables and a fire burns in the back of the room. The space is reminiscent of what would today be called a tavern or a pub: it is the setting for a scene of male camaraderie, a camaraderie founded on the still novel experience of purchasing and drinking a popular beverage in a public establishment.

We know little about the decade during which public coffee consumption began in Paris. When Englishman Edward Browne visited the city in 1664, he frequented "the Coffee House which one Wilson, an Englishman, keeps in the rue du Boucheries" (near Saint-Germain des Prés). Wilson provided "beere and Tobacco and Ale" as well as coffee and thus ran a true English establishment (Brown 1923, 7: 14). Wilson's English coffeehouse may have been short-lived, for no other mention of it survives.

Then, on December 2, 1666, a periodical announced that a beverage already popular in England, Italy, and Holland was now coming to Paris. This second attempt to introduce the French to the experience of drinking coffee in public was, the periodical explained, to be masterminded by Armenians (Subligny [1666] 1882, 2: 196). Once again, however, the experiment does not seem to have been a success, for this announcement is the sole record of coffee's second arrival in Paris.

It was only in the mid-1670s that coffee was successfully implanted in the French capital. From then on, its Parisian history began to be extensively recorded. At first, the establishments where one went to drink the new beverage were referred to by names translated from the English: *maisons* or *cabarets de café*.[2] Within about a decade, however, they were being referred to as *cafés*, a new name for a new kind of establishment.[3] Foreign visitors frequently remarked that cafés were completely different from the English coffeehouse model popular elsewhere in Europe.[4]

The café that launched the new tradition of coffee consumption opened its doors on the Rue de Tournon near Saint-Germain des Prés in 1675 or 1676. It was the brainchild of an Italian, Francesco Procopio dei Coltelli, whose name was Gallicized as Procope. Procope's establishment set the tone for the cafés of Paris, a model still being carefully followed at the turn of the eighteenth century, as the engraving shown in Figure 3.1, the earliest depiction of a Parisian café, demonstrates.[5] This image makes plain both the qualities that set the café apart from the coffeehouse and the reasons for the new model's success.

The tables at which customers are seated are small and individual rather than communal. The waiter, who appears in the rear doorway holding a rather elegant pot (Procope used silver ones in his café), will come to their tables first to take their order and then to serve them—a practice unique to cafés and one that, even in the early eighteenth century, still astounded German visitors to

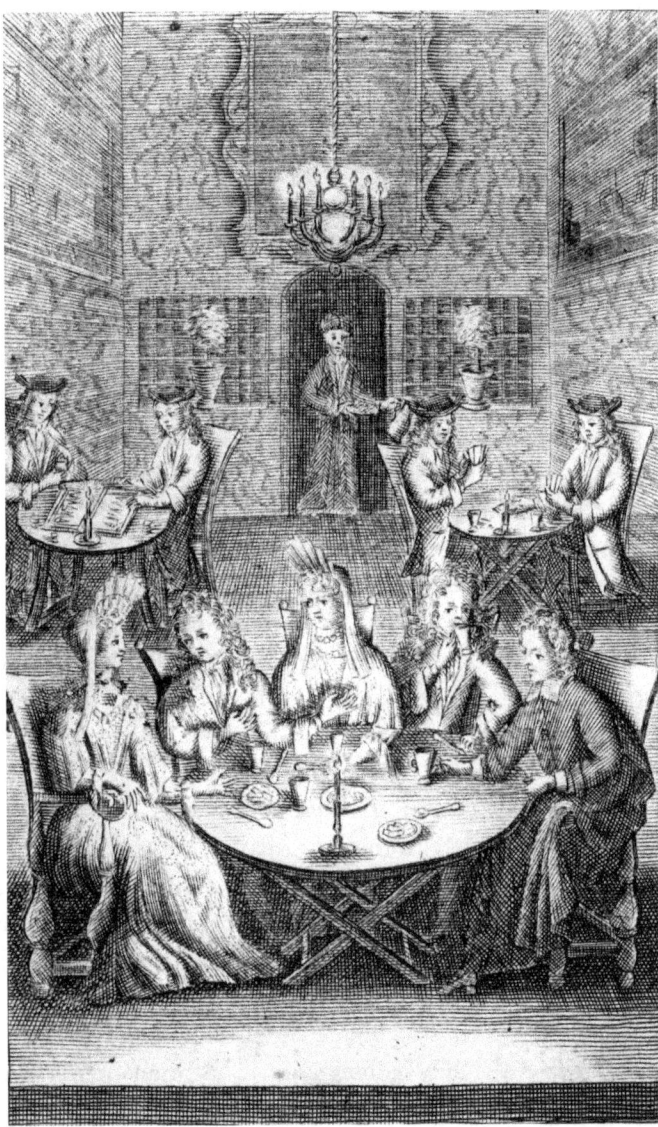

FIGURE 3.1: Anonymous engraving. Frontispiece, Louis de Mailly, *Les Entretiens des cafés de Paris*, 1702. Photograph: Gérard Leyris for Joan DeJean.

Paris.[6] The waiter is also garbed in a very distinctive uniform—a fur-trimmed hat and an exotic, flowing caftan, exactly the outfit worn by waiters in Procope's establishment. The style was described as "en Arménien," the Armenian style. (The Armenians who arrived in December 1666 surely started this fashion.)

The customers drink their coffee out of elaborate, large cups with handles. There are candles on every table, as well as a grand, central chandelier hanging from the ceiling. Overall, the café's décor is elaborate and elegant, a perfect reflection of the standards set by Procope, who used marble-topped tables and hung large mirrors on the walls.

The tables shown here are set with cutlery—spoons in particular, which indicates that clients had adopted the still recent practice of using individual spoons and also that some clients are following the new custom of sugaring their coffee. (When English physician Martin Lister visited Paris in 1698, he found the use of sugar far more prevalent there and warned that "these sugar'd Liquors add considerably to their Corpulency"—Lister 1699: 168.) There are also small plates, some of which appear to contain food. All over Europe, establishments that served coffee also offered a limited menu. But in this respect as well, national traditions were worlds apart.

In England, patrons of the coffeehouse were also able to drink beer there and to eat sausage and other simple fare. Beer was not served in cafés—nor was smoking allowed there. The cafés' offerings were more up-scale—champagne and pastry in particular. Both champagne's bubbles and pastry's buttery flakiness were sensory experiences that Parisians discovered at the same moment when they were introduced to coffee's bitterness. Champagne was invented in the early 1670s, just as coffee was first publicly commercialized in France. In 1653, *Le Pâtissier français*, *The French Pastry Chef*, the first cookbook devoted exclusively to the art of pastry, was published. It included the original recipes for everything from *pâte feuilletée* to *chaussons aux pommes*. By the late seventeenth century, the pairing of coffee and pastry, and flutes (a type of glass only recently invented) of champagne had both become associated with Parisian cafés.

The Parisian café was thus a completely distinct model for the marketing of coffee. With what the best contemporary historian of the marketplace called their "magnificent decoration," they seem quite like what we would now call a restaurant—and a quite up-market restaurant at that.[7] Coffee was widely advertised both as a stimulant and as "a sovereign antidote to sadness" (Marana 1714: 46). Cafés were thus promoted as key to the excitement of Paris: as consumers stirred their coffee, cafés were stirring up Parisian society.

Cafés were also seen as an integral part of the city's sensorial experience. At the turn of the eighteenth century, a guidebook for foreign visitors introduced them to a Parisian custom: "almost everyone" goes out for coffee after lunch in one of the "endless number of cafés in Paris." Its author advised foreigners that because of institutions like its cafés, more than any other European capital Paris "charms and contents your senses" (Nemeitz 1719, 2: 582, 1: 41).

Their elegant setting surely explains what may be the most basic difference between the coffeehouse and the café, the fact that women were not only able to frequent cafés but constituted an important part of their clientele. In fact, the women featured in the engraving from 1702 are not mere generic women but noblewomen: their clothing and hairstyles are markers of their social status. Every early account of Parisian cafés makes it clear that they were the first public establishments in which the sexes mixed freely and in which people of the highest rank came to eat and drink.

A true coffee culture took shape in these different settings in which coffee was consumed. In 1690, François Laurent opened the Café Laurent in the Rue Dauphine, also near Saint-Germain des Prés. This was the first of what became a Parisian institution, the literary café, a place where writers came to discuss their works. Other cafés, both in Paris and London, became known as places where current events were discussed and political ideas debated.[8]

This public success story naturally influenced behavior in private homes. By 1690, the Marquise de Sévigné was drinking coffee in the morning on a regular basis (Sévigné [1646–96] 1972, 3: 952). In May 1696, the *Mercure galant*, the most widely read Parisian periodical of the day, published a lengthy "Eulogy of coffee" by someone who identified himself only as "a frequent coffee drinker." It proves that barely three decades after coffee was first consumed in public, it was no longer an exotic rarity but had been completely integrated into French culinary habits. The author, obviously a true coffee aficionado, explains to the newspaper's readers every step on the road to obtaining a perfect cup: how to choose the freshest beans, the best manner of torrefaction or roasting, which model of coffee grinder and which coffee maker to use, even the best water (see Anon 1696).

In his memoirs, the Duc de Saint-Simon reports that, also in 1696, Louis XIV first drank coffee with his breakfast; a decade later, he was having it served on a daily basis at Versailles. By 1734, in a scene in Marivaux's novel *Le Paysan parvenu*, *The Upstart Peasant*, when the hero Jacob, a peasant newly arrived in Paris, appears for breakfast on his first morning in a new apartment, he is stunned by the whiteness and the quality of Parisian bread but is in no way surprised by the choice of coffee as a beverage and even knows how to drink it (Marivaux [1734] 1965: 101). Louis XV was so fond of coffee that he would personally prepare it for the guests he entertained at small dinners in his private dining room. Less than a century after coffee was first drunk in public in Paris, it had become the breakfast drink of choice for the French in general.

THE TOUCH OF COTTON

Only one other new commodity introduced to European markets in the seventeenth and eighteenth centuries was marketed on a similarly broad scale: cotton.[9] First in Portugal, then in Holland, and next in England, small amounts of cotton arrived in Europe as a byproduct of the spice trade. Some cotton also reached Europe via overland trade from the Levant. Until the second half of the seventeenth century, however, only very few Europeans had ever seen the new textile. At that moment, the Dutch and the English began marketing cotton in a serious way, and France first became a player worth noticing in the Indies trade. In the 1670s, the volume of cotton being imported exploded: by 1684, the East Indies Company was exporting to England over a million pieces of Indian cotton annually (Lemire 2003: 68). Already in 1680, the Comtesse de La Fayette wrote to a friend that "in France, we love everything that comes from India"—which is just what the directors of the East India Company in London kept repeating about the English in their letters to their Indian agents (La Fayette 1942, 2: 99–100).

Europeans' enthusiasm for the foreign textile is easy to understand. Prior to this time, they had known only far heavier native fabrics, wool and linen. For women whose gowns required many, many, yards of fabric, the light foreign import must have been an extraordinary liberation after the weight of outfits in textiles such as wool velvet.

The new cloth, hand-dyed and painted by Indian craftsmen, was also far more colorful than anything Europeans had ever seen. Cottons appeared in previously unimaginable shades. And since several brilliant shades were often juxtaposed in any pattern, an Indian cotton fabric could be a positive riot of color. No European cloth had been nearly so bold.

Because of the new cottons, colors earlier found only infrequently became common. Red in particular, which had been expensive for Europeans to make and was therefore considered a color that signified prestige, became a common accent and background color because it was used so widely in Indian textiles, which were produced using different dyes and techniques (see Gittinger 1982). Designs common in Indian textiles destined for the European market featured a bright red background and a foreground composed of bouquets and sprigs of flowers in a variety of colors. The Indians quickly learned that the French were wild for these red-field cottons, but that the English were much less taken with them and preferred a tamer white ground.

In addition, European textiles had never had patterns like these. The techniques used by Indian craftsmen (a combination of printing and hand-painting) produced designs that made European woven fabrics with their more uniform patterns seem in comparison overly symmetrical and tightly controlled.

Indian fabrics often featured in particular something never seen in European textiles, figures of all kinds—humans, animals, strange birds and beasts, some imaginary, others real. The detail from a cotton textile shown in Figure 3.2, produced for the French market in the mid-eighteenth century, for example, depicts kinds of flora and fauna that would have been exotic to European eyes and in ways that serve to emphasize that exoticism—the elephants and the bird seem huge in relation to the rather tiny flowering trees; the elephants are in

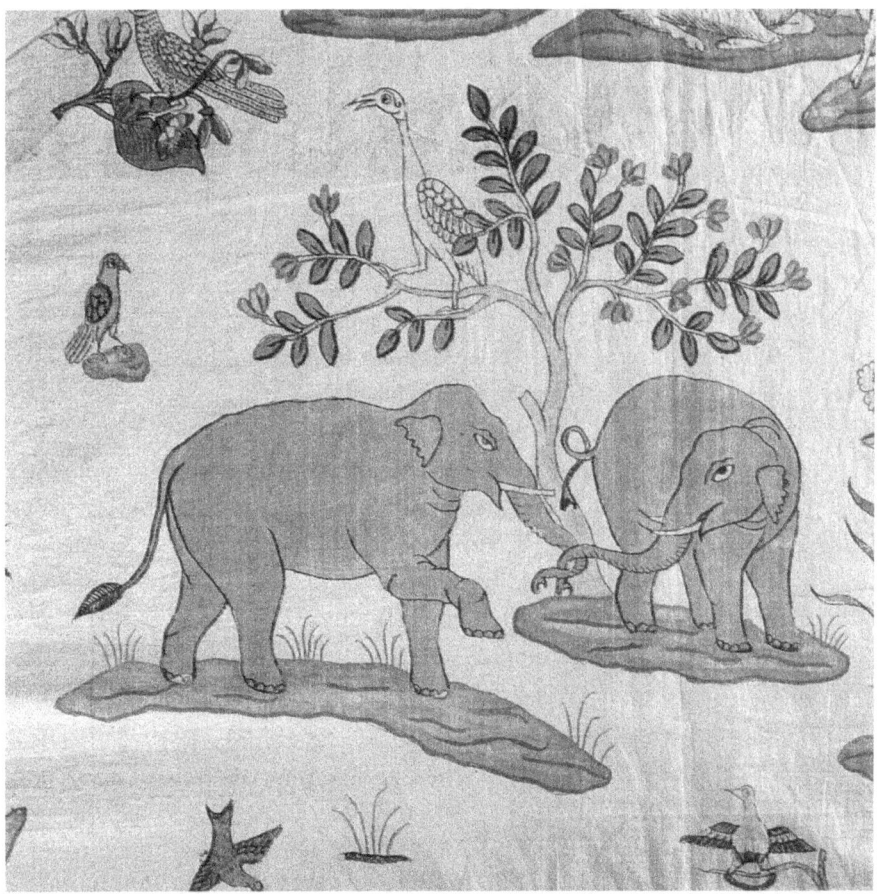

FIGURE 3.2: Painted and dyed cotton produced for the French market. India, Coromandel coast, *c.* 1750. Collection Maison Georges Le Manach. Photograph: Alain Damlamian for Joan DeJean.

addition a dazzlingly bright blue, and they are frolicking on what appear to be shocking pink carpets.

The French in particular always begged for shipments of fabrics with what their East India Company's directors described as "petits personnages," "little people." Other panels of this same chintz depict Indians dressed in wildly patterned painted cloth and turbans, smoking hookahs, and shooting with bows and arrows at fantastic beasts.

Then, there were the flowers. There had been floral designs in earlier European cloth, but for the most part depictions remained too heavily stylized and formal to be confused with real blooms. Asian textiles introduced Europeans both to more graphic ways of depicting flowers in cloth and to many varieties such as magnolias and camellias not then found in Europe. (Europeans soon began importing the actual plants.) As a result, European dress became for the first time floral in a dramatic fashion. Women wore entire outfits made of brightly flowering cottons. Men had vests, handkerchiefs, and neck scarves with similar motifs.

Indian textiles also inspired the first great age of floral interior decoration in the West. This was particularly evident in the new kinds of more private rooms then beginning to appear in domestic architecture all over Europe, in particular in bedrooms. Beds were completely decked out in floral prints. Their coverlets, the canopies of tester beds, the curtains that closed beds off to provide privacy and warmth—all were made from matching cloth. Window curtains were also done up in the same fabric—and many even completely upholstered their bedrooms' walls in matching floral prints.

Once again, national usage varied: the Dutch, for example, were apparently the first to cover entire walls with hangings of Indian cotton, while the French made extensive use of cotton as an upholstery fabric for furniture such as folding stools and chairs, decades before the Dutch, and continued to make far more extensive use of cotton as an upholstery fabric (Deville 1878–80, 1: 196, 471). (Cotton was naturally more fragile than traditional upholstery fabrics; by choosing it, the French were privileging fashion over durability.) In short, in a matter of just a few decades, bright cottons must have seemed to be cropping up everywhere Europeans looked.

Europeans had many names to refer to Indian cottons. Most originated in an attempt to reproduce a Hindi word: *chint* (singular), *chintes* (plural), from *chitta*, "spotted cloth." Beginning in 1614, the English said everything from *chint*, to *chites*, to *chinke* (Samuel Pepys' choice in 1663), to *chints*, and finally *chintz*. The French used mainly *chitte*. More often, however, they preferred simple generic terms, *toile peinte*, "painted cloth," or just *indienne*, "Indian (cloth)."

Indian designers cornered a vast new market and held onto it for decades because their products were so innovative, providing a radically new visual and tactile experience. In addition, they worked hard at predicting European consumers' desires—and even at shaping those desires. In this, they had the collaboration of the directors of the various East Indies companies. English directors, for instance, sent them engravings by French artists that were then popular in England and asked the Indians to copy them in cotton, with requests that they do so "in the Indian manner." The product that was then shipped back to English shores after this collaborative effort was naturally a hodgepodge: Indian designers' vision of a French artist's concept popular in England (Irwin and Brett 1970: 4, 9). That cultural jumble, however, seems to have been just what Europeans were after.

During the period when coffee achieved dominance at breakfast tables all over France, "painted cloth" took over the same market, first with a trickle-down effect as it spread through the social ranks. Cotton textiles made early, high-profile appearances at the French court. In 1675, two bedrooms in the new château being built at Versailles were completely decorated in Indian cotton, a floral pattern on a red background. In 1687, Louis XIV's son and heir was seen wearing a vest made from painted cotton. In 1699, ladies of the court, including the wife of the king's grandson, danced at carnival balls wearing Indian cotton.[10] In the early eighteenth century, employees in aristocratic homes in Paris were being spotted in the city's streets in garments made from Indian cotton textiles.[11] By the 1750s, less expensive textiles made up a sizeable share of Indian imports; the least expensive of all became the new "everyday dress of the common folk," in the words of one of the period's most noted economists, François de Forbonnais.[12]

At the same time, Indian textiles came to represent an ever greater proportion of all wardrobes. In 1743, when one of Louis XIV's daughters by his long-time mistress the Marquise de Montespan died, her probate inventory indicated that thirty-seven of her thirty-nine casual dresses were made of cotton, in patterns ranging from a floral that mixed various shades of violet to a multi-colored medley of trees, fruit, and flowers on a white background. In the mid-1780s, a young Frenchwoman, Henriette-Lucy Dillon, proudly remarked of her vast trousseau that all her dresses were made of cotton and that "there wasn't a single silk dress." And by that time, over half the clothing owned by female servants working in Paris was made from cotton (DeJean 2009: 216; see also Styles 2010).

The rage for Indian cotton even caused important changes in the design of fabrics made in Europe. In a number of countries all over the continent, local textile manufacturers tried, with varying degrees of success, to produce cotton fabrics that imitated Indian methods and styles—manufactories established in Switzerland were among the first to create imitations that garnered praise from consumers. Silk patterns imagined by English, French, and Italian textile designers soon showed the influence of exotic imports. Silks now known as "bizarre," for example, were produced at a number of centers all over Europe, from Venice to Lyon, beginning at the turn of the eighteenth century. They featured fantastical elements, such as stylized leaves and flowers, all clearly borrowed from Asian textiles. In the 1730s, designers of so-called "naturalistic" silks experimented with a bolder use of color to achieve more realistic images of flowers and fruits. They developed new weaving techniques that, for example, used shading and blending to make their patterns more three-dimensional in appearance. These designers thus created new looks in silk patterns in an attempt to lure European consumers back to European-manufactured textiles.

The take-over of the European market realized by Asian textile designers was responsible for one of the biggest revolutions in color and pattern of all time. Painted cloth transformed the look of Europeans and their interiors. In the 1660s and 1670s, both dress and décor were overwhelmingly monochromatic, and even elite consumers had a quite limited exposure to color in their daily lives. Everyday dress was dominated by the beiges and pale earth tones of linen; interiors by the brown of wood. By the 1770s, bright colors and bold patterns were found everywhere and at all times—on people's backs, on their beds and their tables, and on their chairs.

A REVOLUTION IN FURNITURE

At the moment when the Indian invasion began, European interiors were lacking in more than color. They were also missing many of what are now seen as the most basic kinds of furniture, in particular, anything we would consider an adequate form of seating.

Until about the mid-seventeenth century, chairs were never numerous. In addition, the sole models were primitive and utilitarian, with low, straight backs, no arms, and at the most only minimal upholstery (perhaps a bit of leather stretched across the back or a cushion placed on the seat). People perched on trunks; they sat on backless, unpadded benches, as the patrons of the English coffeehouse are shown to do in that Dutch engraving referred to earlier in the chapter—a form of seating convivial but hardly plush. The only seating in the house that could be considered in any way comfortable was the bed, and seventeenth-century engravings frequently depict scenes in which family members and guests are sitting side-by-side on a bed. A new age for seat furniture began in the 1670s, the same decade when coffee and cotton were first seriously marketed in Europe.[13]

At that moment, armchairs finally became a standard option. Seats were made wider and deeper, backs wider and taller. Modern upholstery techniques began to be invented, and fixed upholstery came into increasingly widespread use. Within about fifteen years, almost all modern upholstery techniques had been invented, and French furniture makers were beginning to produce the earliest furniture with fixed padding on all surfaces, front, sides, and back—as well as on the trickiest surface to pad, the armrest. Thus reinvented, the chair became more and more frequently encountered in many settings. The patrons portrayed sitting in a French café in the 1702 engraving, for example, all occupy chairs with ample, upholstered backs; a number rest their arms on armrests (see Figure 3.1). In this respect, too, the café was a far cry from the coffeehouse.

The English were never as fond of well-padded upholstery as the French: even later in the eighteenth century, when French upholsterers were cushioning all surfaces in an extremely plush manner, across the Channel padding remained firm and shallow, intended to provide no more than a bit of support. An English armchair considered well-cushioned had upholstered surfaces that were at the most barely rounded.

The contrast between French and English tastes in seating became especially evident with the invention of what quickly became the quintessential piece of furniture in Parisian homes: the sofa, the first form of comfortable seating designed for more than one person.

Earlier in the seventeenth century, in both England and France, daybeds began to appear in elite residences. Then, in the 1670s, some of the earliest pieces of seat furniture produced for the French court at the new château at Versailles were a new kind of daybed with fixed upholstery. These hybrid pieces soon morphed into the original prototypes for the modern sofa.

The earliest known representation of a sofa is an engraving dated 1686; the earliest known purchase of a sofa by a private individual was recorded in 1688, when the Prince de Conti ordered one from a craftsman named Grémont in Paris, who described himself as "a specialist in armchairs and sofas," a phrase that proves how quickly the new seating had become a sought-after item in the French capital (Havard 1890, 4: 1038). A mere seven years after that, Daniel Cronström, a Swede posted to his country's embassy in Paris, described the French as "sofa-mad" and claimed that "there is hardly a room in Paris without one." In 1695, when he wrote to a Swedish friend about the new craze,

Cronström was himself on a self-described "sofa campaign" to find a matched pair. It took him six months to locate a pair that he promptly had shipped back to Stockholm (Tessin 1964: 67, 79, 81, 106).

It's impossible to know what either the Prince de Conti's or Daniel Cronström's sofas looked like because none of the earliest sofas have survived. French designers realized, however, how popular the new furniture could be with buyers outside of Paris who could not easily visit their shops. They thus began the first known advertising campaign for a piece of furniture.

The 1686 engraving shown in Figure 3.3, based on a drawing by Jean Dieu de Saint-Jean, seems to have been the image that launched that campaign. The model depicted in this image and in other plates from the late 1680s was clearly inspired by the humble bench. It is, however, a bench with back support as well as clearly defined armrests. And in a very early display of modern upholstery techniques, all its surfaces are nicely padded with rounded, fixed padding.

As has been the case ever since, a variety of very different types of sofa existed from the start. Engravings from the 1690s depict, for example, a model with a very high and straight back that looks rather like a double-wide version of the already wide armchairs then in fashion. This model continued to be produced in France until about 1720; in England, however, where it became known as a "double Windsor chair without a division," it remained perhaps the most popular kind of sofa through much of the eighteenth century.[14] Other models of sofa advertised in Paris by the mid-1690s are quite close to styles available today. A sofa depicted in a 1696 print, for instance, has a nicely carved wooden frame, higher in the middle and curving down to join carved armrests. It features both ample padding and matching throw pillows.

The English may have preferred the "double Windsor chair" style precisely because it was so lightly padded. All through the eighteenth century, they remained wary of sofas, which they saw as a form of furniture both somehow morally dangerous and typically French. In 1745, the English man of letters Horace Walpole, writing from Paris, joked about the sofa's bad reputation and said of the experience of sitting on a French sofa that it was rather like "lolling in a *péché-mortel*"—a mortal sin (Walpole 1954, 18: 315). His correspondent and fellow countryman, Horace Mann, answered that he couldn't imagine such a sofa and added that "we [the English] are always some years behindhand." And still in 1770, an Englishwoman wrote to one of her friends to describe how, when guests were expected, sofas "were banished for the day" (Delany 1900: 205). It was as if simply owning a sofa might be enough to imperil a family's reputation. It's hard to imagine the reaction if someone had happened upon family members "lolling about" in a French sofa's curves.

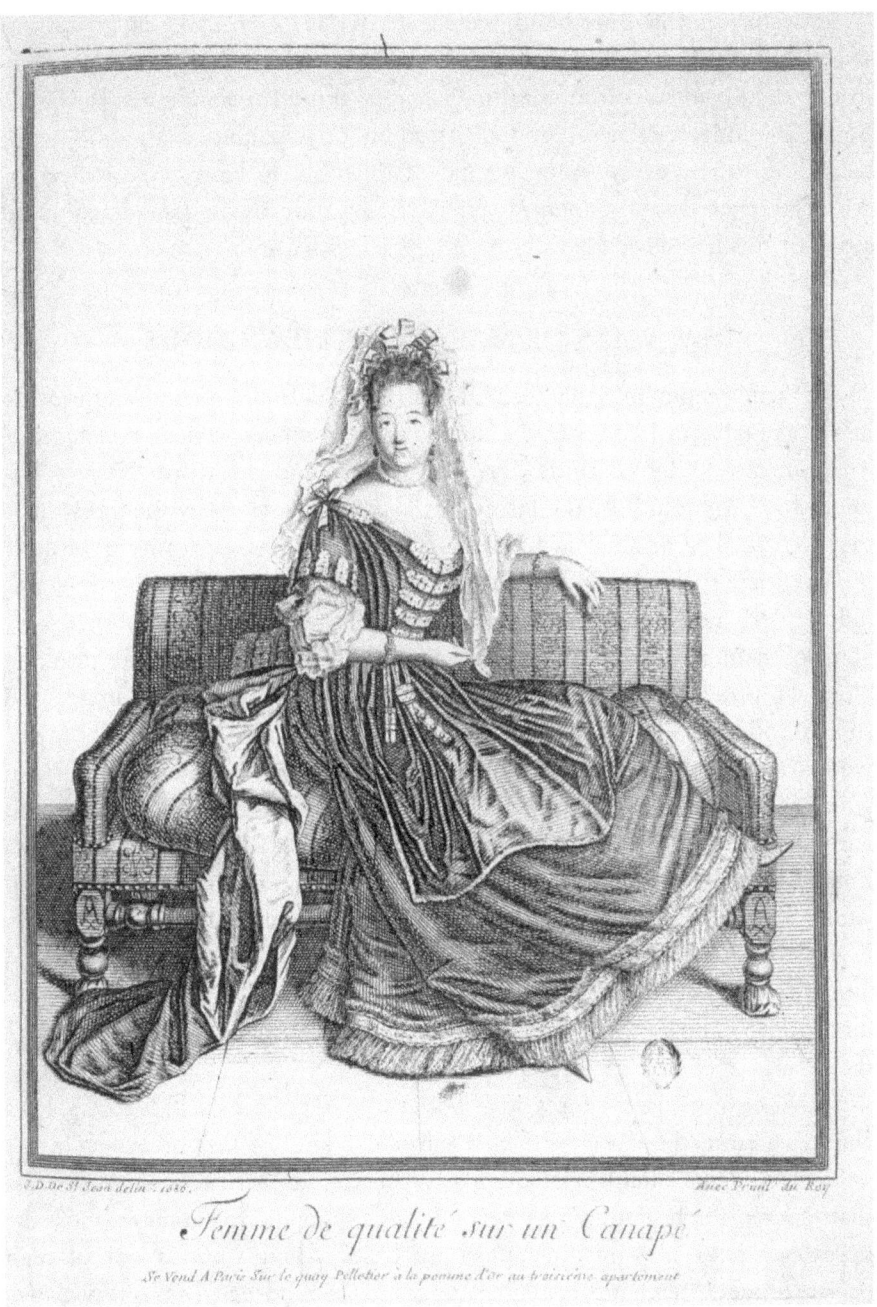

FIGURE 3.3: Jean Dieu de Saint-Jean, "Femme de qualité sur un canapé." Engraving, 1686. Photograph: Patrick Lorette for Joan DeJean.

Parisians, on the other hand, were every bit as "sofa-mad" as Cronström said. Louis XIV's daughter, the very one who owned thirty-seven outfits made from Indian painted cotton, outfitted her very grand Parisian home, the Palais Bourbon—today's French National Assembly or Assemblée Nationale—with sofas in virtually every room, a total of thirty-six to be exact. Eighteenth-century French design manuals depicted dining rooms with sofas lined up all along the wall, and even bathrooms equipped with a sofa or two.

NEW WAYS OF MARKETING NEW GOODS

Those French engravings that, beginning in the mid-1680s, advertised furniture newly available in Paris soon became known as *modes*, styles or fashions.[15] They are now referred to as "fashion plates," and the word "fashion" is understood to mean only the fashions, the garments, worn by the individuals they depict. The original fashion plates, however, had in reality a broader mission: they showed off all the latest inventions of the Parisian luxury goods industry, the range of stylish novelties available in the Parisian marketplace. Some of them, for example, portrayed aspects of the new art of coffee drinking along with the fashionable outfits of those shown drinking it. The image of a sofa introduced in 1686 promoted, along with the new furniture, both the woman's garments and above all textiles—in particular, the striped fabric in which the sofa is upholstered. In 1686, the king of Siam sent a delegation to Paris as part of his project of opening his country to the West. The French followed every move of those they called "the Siamese ambassadors," who were often seen wearing striped textiles. Parisian fabric merchants immediately began marketing all striped cloth with great success. This could be seen as an attempt by upholsterers (who sold both cloth and furniture) to promote two innovations in tandem—striped fabric and a newly invented piece of furniture: the sofa.

Other fashion plates simply advertised the marketplace itself. Figure 3.4, an engraving from the late 1680s, is a particular kind of fashion plate. In the 1680s and 1690s a number of engravers depicted another new institution, one that marked the beginning of a revolution in shopping for luxury goods: the upscale shop. Prior to this time, most purchases of luxury goods took place in private homes. Merchants brought samples to the residences of wealthy clients for their selection, and a merchant's shop was mainly a storehouse for his inventory. In the final decades of the seventeenth century, the shop was reinvented as a place where consumers could find a wide selection of the latest and most desirable merchandise in an elegant setting. This transformation

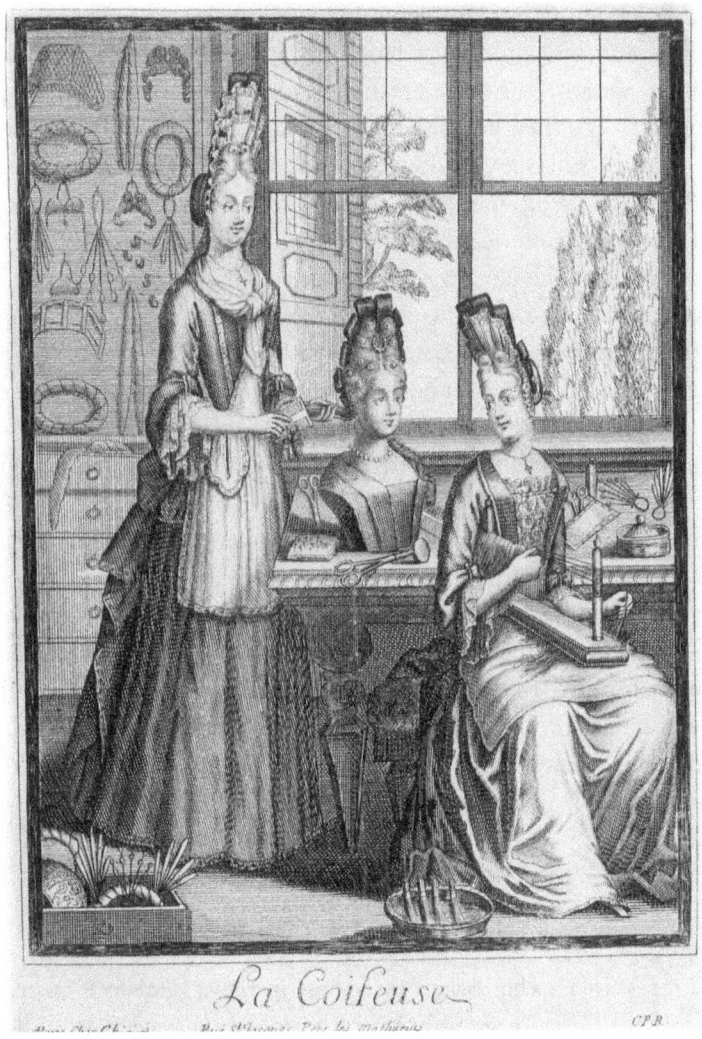

FIGURE 3.4: Chiquet, "La Coiffeuse." Engraving, c. 1690. Private collection.

took place in both Paris and London, though it seems likely that Parisian shops led the way.[16]

This *mode* depicts the shop that two *coiffeuses* or hairdressers have organized in the latest fashion. Instead of the simple counter on which most of the merchants who opened the original modern shops relied as their principal display space, they use an elegantly carved table, an example of the fine furniture for sale in Paris. They have added another very recent innovation of French designers, built-in drawer based storage and, above it, arranged in an eye-catching pattern, various implements for adorning or propping up the elaborate hairstyles then in fashion. The image highlights still another recent development, extra-large windows fitted out with something that French glass-making technology had only recently made possible: large panes. Such windows made shop interiors far brighter, and they also opened them up to the city outside. As for the hairdressers themselves, they are fashionably dressed, much as their elite customers would have been.

The image advertises the new kind of shops and the new experience of shopping as offering both an appealing setting and a wider range of goods than ever before. And it was in a setting much like this that the newly available luxury goods—from painted cloth to sofas—were displayed for potential customers such as Daniel Cronström.

By the turn of the eighteenth century, European consumers thus had access to novel products of many different kinds. They also had access to a variety of innovative settings in which new kinds of public life developed—from cafés in which more and a wider range of people ate and drank in public than ever before, to the original modern shops in which individuals who had previously seldom if ever shopped in public had their initial experiences with modern techniques for selling desire. Those who sought to attract consumers for newly available commodities can thus be said to have reinvented the marketplace.

THE SENSES IN THE HOME

The new marketplace that began to emerge in the seventeenth century's final decades provided previously unheard of sensory experiences, from the feel of cotton next to the skin to the sensation of comfortable seating. And all these experiences combined to create in turn, as many fashion plates seemed designed to prove, a new way of experiencing furniture.

Earlier depictions of individuals using seat furniture always portray them sitting bolt upright, their backs straight up against the chair's back, their legs and arms carefully and formally positioned. In contrast, the lady of quality posed on the original sofa (see Figure 3.3) seems to have been introducing, along with the new seat furniture, a new way of using such furniture. She doesn't so much sit as stretches out, taking full advantage of the sofa's new expansiveness. She's kicked up one foot on the sofa; one arm is draped across its back, making her the picture of relaxed informality.

Many of the earliest images of sofas illustrated related poses: a lady deep in thought, leaning back into a sofa's curves with her arm supported by a soft cushion; a gentleman reading with his back against the armrest, both legs extended out on the sofa and a book propped up in front of him. They depicted individuals obviously quite content with themselves and their surroundings. And in all cases, these men and women were portrayed in poses that could never have been possible before the invention of the new kinds of seating. And this behavior was no mere fantasy of the artists who created these images. As soon as there were sofas, people began to lounge on them or to deploy themselves in other non-traditional fashions. We know this because many contemporary observers were completely taken aback by the new ways of using furniture.

Louis XIV's German-born sister-in-law, the Princesse Palatine, complained to her cousins at home that, because men could frequently be spotted "stretched out full-length on sofas," Versailles "no longer looks at all like a court." The worst offender was the king's first-born and heir, the dauphin, who, she claimed, "was capable of spending an entire day lying down on a sofa or in a big armchair . . . without saying a word."[17]

The same French architects who positioned sofas in every room of all the important new residences of the turn of the eighteenth century were responsible for a very basic change in the design of those homes: they began to invent new kinds of rooms. These were in general intimate spaces, intended for the private use of those who lived in the home, spaces where outsiders were rarely if ever invited.

Among the innovative rooms found on the floorplans of eighteenth-century French residential architecture are, for example, *cafés*, tiny coffee rooms for those so devoted to the perfect cup evoked in the 1696 article in the *Mercure galant* that they wanted to savor one after every meal in intimate surroundings. There were in addition reading rooms and writing rooms, one of which was the boudoir, created to provide women with the same kind of private space men enjoyed in their studies or offices, as a room in which women could read and write and enjoy the pleasures of introspection without fear of interruption.

In all these spaces, cotton was the upholstery fabric of choice, sofas and very capacious armchairs the dominant furniture. In all these spaces, behavior considered remarkable when the dauphin first exhibited it—spending a good part of a day simply lost in one's thoughts—was seen as the norm. These were some of the earliest rooms expressly designed for those who were in no way professional scholars but who desired spaces that facilitated interior life. We know from floorplans that these new intimate spaces soon began to be included in homes all over Europe.

The private rooms of eighteenth-century residential architecture are perhaps the most intriguing legacy of the emergence of a modern consumer society. Exotic commodities and novel public experiences seem to have helped create among those who first enjoyed them in public the desire to broaden the sphere of the private in their lives. They wanted to enjoy more intimate space as well as the furnishings and decoration that could make it appealing—all of which indicates that they were granting increased importance to the interior life for which the new spaces made room in their homes.

CHAPTER FOUR

The Senses in Religion: Listening to God in the Eighteenth Century[1]

PHYLLIS MACK

I myself will see [God] with my own eyes—I, and not another.
— Job 19:27

My sheep hear my voice, and I know them, and they follow me.
— John 10:27

O taste and see that the LORD is good.
— Psalm 34:8

Let him kiss me with the kisses of his mouth.
— *Song of Songs* 1:2

We can become ". . . unto God a sweet savor of Christ."
— II Corinthians 2:15

INTRODUCTION

The Enlightenment was once defined as the cradle of modern secular society, when the religious culture of the pre-modern era was fatally undermined by the new mechanical philosophy and the corrosive criticism of the *philosophes*.

Even members of the clergy assumed that the time when God spoke directly to human beings belonged to a distant, pre-Enlightenment past. Thus the Anglican clergyman William Law interrogated a young woman who believed that God had commanded her to become a Quaker. He wondered how she knew that the voice she heard had actually come from God:

> You say, "God condescended to declare His will" . . . Do you only mean that such thoughts came forcibly into your mind, as when in other cases a person may say, the devil tempted or prompted him to do so or so? . . . If you heard such a voice, how did you know that it was God's, how comes it that you was not in some degree of astonishment and doubt about it?
> Law [1729] 1994: 27

These skeptical voices have moved some critics to argue, not only that *belief* in the supernatural declined during the Enlightenment, but that the *capacity* for such belief was lost. So the Jesuit philosopher Michel de Certeau claimed that the supernatural became inaccessible to the sensibilities of eighteenth-century thinkers, as it has to modern twentieth-century people. "The sacred text is a voice . . ." he wrote. "The modern age is formed by discovering little by little that this spoken Word is no longer heard . . . One can no longer hear it" (*The Practice of Everyday Life*, quoted in Schmidt 2000: 28–9).

The current upsurge of religious belief and practice in many parts of the world has led contemporary scholars to re-think the secularization paradigm and to approach the subject of religion and the supernatural in a radically different way; not as a relic of the pre-modern era but as a constitutive element of modernity.

> It is . . . a mischaracterization of the Enlightenment to regard it as something that existed only outside and in opposition to the churches. For example, almost all of the major faith traditions in the eighteenth century had internally generated reforming movements: Pietism within Lutheranism; Jansenism within Roman Catholicism; Methodism within Anglicanism; and international revivalism within Calvinism.
> Hempton 2005: 114

Many scholars now view eighteenth-century Christianity as a movement away from superstition, ritual, dogma, and the visual extravagance of the baroque, and toward a more inward spirituality centered in language and focused on the sense of hearing. This was true of Catholics as well as Protestants. Partly in response to Protestant preaching, but also influenced by mysticism and ascetic theology, many Catholic thinkers rejected baroque piety and adopted a calmer, more individualistic approach to spirituality. They abolished religious holidays, processions, and pilgrimages, disassembled altars and forbade worship of the relics of saints (Klueting 2010: 144–5; Lehner 2010: 21). Catholic worship began to be focused on the liturgy and sacraments, but especially on sermons. The architecture of churches changed, with large open naves to accommodate crowds of listeners, and more windows to let in light. Many reformers accused the Jesuits of encouraging superstition, but the Jesuits themselves mounted an evangelizing movement against what they considered to be ignorant and unorthodox beliefs and superstitions, like ringing bells to ward off storms, that survived under the aegis of the Catholic Church (Desan 1990: 38; Laven 2006: 710–11).[2] The Jesuits were also one of the main users of devotional prints, small pictures combining image (the Virgin, the saints) and text, which were produced by the hundreds of thousands for distribution to the devout masses; this production slackened after the decline of the Jesuits in the early eighteenth century and their suppression in the 1760s and 1770s (Po-Chsia Hsia 1998, 2005: 166–7).

An equally important movement within Catholicism was Jansenism. The Jansenists, followers of the Belgian reformist priest Cornelis Jansen (1585–1638), condemned the Jesuits' attempts to appeal to audiences by theatrical means: dramatic sermons, processions, images of saints, and plays performed in Jesuit colleges. Like many Protestant Calvinist groups, the Jansenists were motivated by a deep pessimism about human nature and the senses, which they believed were subject to corruption. Their religiosity emphasized personal austerity and inward prayer, and their preaching appealed to spirit and mind rather than the senses, as they attempted to inculcate an interior spirituality stripped of superfluous rituals and superstitions (Desan 1990: 39; Kostroun 2011: 99).

European Jews experienced their own Enlightenment (Haskalah) led by the German philosopher Moses Mendelssohn, who stressed the importance of inward religiosity and social ethics rather than strict outward observance. Mendelssohn emphasized practical rather than theoretical knowledge. He also pleaded for a straightforward, literalist reading of the Talmud and the Bible, rejecting both the obscure interpretations of the rabbis and the esoteric parables and symbolic diagrams of Jewish mysticism (kaballah). Mendelssohn believed that the Hebrew language had singular qualities that enhanced oral expression. "The spoken word's advantage is immediate understanding: the speaker's voice makes the words comprehensible so that it 'enters the listener's heart to arouse and to instruct him'" (Sorkin 2008: 186). Mendelssohn was especially interested in the structure of poetry as the most effective medium of "practical knowledge."

Biblical poetry, unlike classical literature, was intended "not for the ear of the auditor alone, but for his heart. [The words] will ... produce in him joy and sorrow, timidity or trust, fear or hope, love or hate, as is appropriate to the intention and to install in him the honorable attributes ... as stakes and nails that are implanted, as a peg that cannot be moved" (Sorkin 2008: 189–90).

Among Protestants, an informal movement called Pietism or "heart religion" began in Lutheran Germany in the 1730s and 1740s and spread to several countries, including England, Holland, America, and Eastern Europe. The movement attracted many sorts of Christians, including some, like the Anglican Dissenters, who were allied with official Churches and others, like the Moravians, who stood well outside the conventions of the main religious denominations. Drawing on English Puritanism, Lutheranism, and mysticism, Pietists de-emphasized doctrine and ritual in favor of edifying preaching, devotion, and Bible reading, all tending toward an experience of spiritual rebirth (Sorkin 2008: 120). There was a new stress on individual worship and a greater emphasis on sound as well as sight, the voices of the minister and congregation preaching and singing the evangelical message, the good news of Christ's coming. In these religious communities, the sermons, prayers, and hymns were often noisy, as in Methodist outdoor meetings.

Sometimes, but more rarely, it was the *absence* of noise that prevailed: a rapt gathering in a neighbor's sitting room or tavern, listening to a Bible reading, or a silent meeting of Quakers, waiting to be filled by the Inner Light (Schmidt 2000: 50–2).

"The *Noise* of Joy," wrote the Methodist-turned-Moravian John Cennick,

> properly begins when a Sinner repents, but at that time he knows little of it; on the contrary, he hears only the *Noise* of the Enemy, who crieth after him, the *Noise* of a guilty Heart, and of a clamorous and false World; but he shall hereafter hear *the Noise of them that keep Holy-day*; himself shall sing for Joy and clap his Hands, and leap for very gladness of Heart.
>
> Cennick 1754: 12

A NEW SPIRITUAL AESTHETIC

The prominence given to hearing in eighteenth-century religious culture has been studied in depth by several historians, notably Leigh Eric Schmidt (Schmidt 2000). A related issue preoccupied Protestant religious leaders and

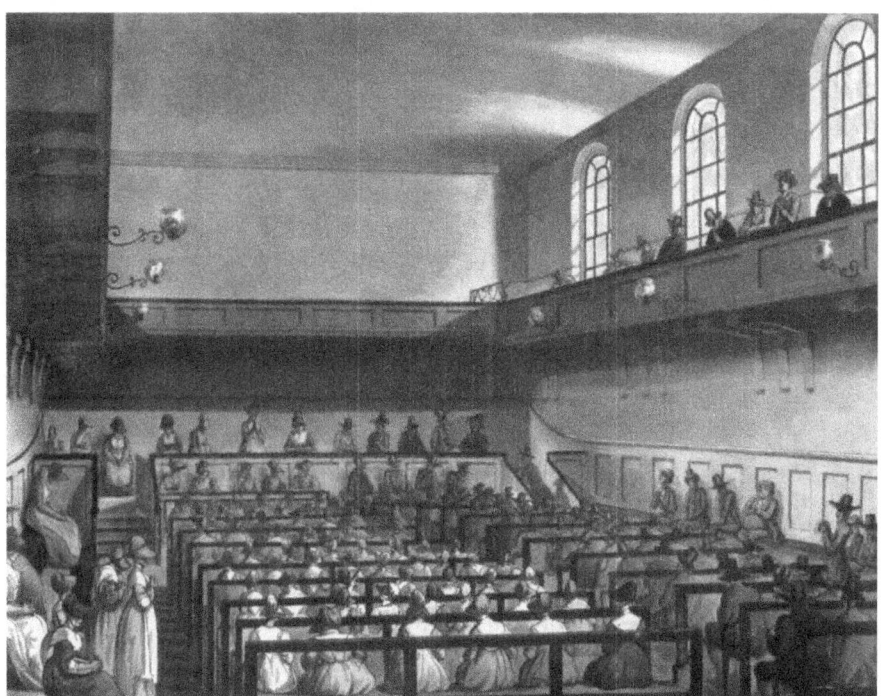

FIGURE 4.1: William Henry Pyne and William Combe, "Quakers' Meeting" (1809). From *The Microcosm of London or London in Miniature* (Volume II ed.), London: Methuen and Company, 1904, Plate 64.

thinkers during the Enlightenment: the artistic education of the senses as a means of enhancing spiritual perception and insight. We normally think of the Reformation as anti-art, focused on the pulpit rather than the communion altar or statues of saints, and we imagine pious Protestants mulling over sermons and religious texts rather than fine-tuning their aesthetic sensibilities through their engagement with paintings, poetry, or music. In fact, religious leaders were intensely interested in different kinds of artistic media, offering their adherents what amounted to an education in spiritual aesthetics: that is, a way of looking, listening, and singing that would refine sense perception, encourage spiritual insight, and promote contact with the supernatural.

This spiritual aesthetic was vastly different for different groups of Protestants, even for members of the same religious community. Compare, for example, two Methodist texts focusing on the senses of taste and touch, each referring to the same biblical passage in the *Song of Songs*.³ First, a hymn by Charles Wesley, "To be sung at the tea-table":

> How pleasant and sweet
> In his name when we meet
> Is his fruit to our spiritual taste!
> We are banqueting here
> On angelical cheer
> And the joys that eternally last.
>
> C. Wesley [1767] 1825: no. 146

Second, a passage from a letter by an unknown Methodist woman to Charles Wesley: "How sweet was Jesus Christ to me . . . I sat under his shadow with great delight and his fruit was sweet to my taste I could then say his left hand was under my head and his right hand doth embrace me and his banner over me was love" (early Methodist volume). The two texts suggest widely different modes of perception, the woman's celebration of the poem's erotic lyricism vs. the suppression of eroticism in the hymn (making it appropriate to sing at tea parties). The texts also raise questions about the role of gender in shaping the Methodists' religious sensibility. Of the hundreds of sermon texts produced by (male) Methodist preachers, references to the *Song of Songs* are extremely rare.[4] Yet the sermons and other writings produced by Methodist women are full of imagery from a poem which, more than any other biblical language, is permeated by images of nature, love, and sensuality. This suggests that avenues of sense perception and sensuous expression may have been explored differently by Methodist women and by men. In any case, the point to note here is that for both writers, the route to spiritual insight was neither in dogma nor in ritualized behavior, but in an empathic, imaginative identification with the divine as manifested in the Bible and in art.

In the remainder of this chapter, I shall proceed with a general discussion of the senses and Christianity, and the attempts of religious leaders to educate ordinary people in refining their sense perceptions in order to achieve greater openness to the divine. I will then focus on the prayers, poetry, and hymns of two Protestant groups, Methodists and Moravians, each of whom placed great emphasis on artistic expression (especially poetry and congregational singing), but who held very different views about the role of sensuality and sensuous experience in religion.

EDUCATING THE SENSES

The senses have always been a means of enabling and expressing humanity's relationship to God, as we see in the biblical passages quoted at the beginning of this chapter. "For everyone who partakes only of milk is not accustomed to the word of righteousness, for he is an infant. But solid food is for the mature, who because of practice *have their senses trained to discern good and evil*" (Hebrews 5:13–14; italics mine). However, theologians and biblical commentators were also suspicious of the senses as "floodgates of sin," leading to idolatry (the worship of statues and paintings) or to sacrilegious practices. "Guard we the windows of our soul," wrote the seventeenth-century Puritan Isaac Ambrose. "It is incredible, what a deal of pollution and ill the Devil conveys insensibly into the heart, through these floodgates of sin, and therefore we had need to watch over the Senses" (quoted in Kadane 2012: 48).

For mainstream religious thinkers like the Anglicans or Methodists, the common approach was to read sensuous biblical language symbolically; so the phrase, "Let him kiss me with the kisses of his mouth" in the biblical *Song of Songs* was interpreted as metaphor or allegory, the woman symbolizing the Israelites and the man symbolizing God or Jesus. Other religious thinkers had a more ambiguous and experimental understanding of biblical texts. The Moravians, a community that originated in Germany and spread to England, America and elsewhere, often depicted Jesus as female and maternal and the worshipper as an infant being reborn from Christ's bloody side wound (or "womb"). Moravian teachings also blurred the line between metaphor and actuality: "it is clear not only that [the Moravians'] desire for Christ was expressed in erotic metaphors but that these metaphors were sometimes taken quite literally ... One example is Zinzendorf's teaching that men are essentially female and that men were to become women upon death" (Peucker 2006: 60–1).[5]

Whatever their understanding of sensuous symbolism, most eighteenth-century thinkers embraced the Lockean principle that the senses are our sole basis for apprehending reality. This means that, since God is a spiritual being and thus not directly perceivable by the senses, He remains, now and forevermore, a mystery. "No man has a natural idea of God," wrote the Methodist leader John Wesley; "there is no image of God stamped on man's soul; by nature every man is an atheist" (Mack 2008: 33). Many religious thinkers explained the limitation or corruption of the senses as a punishment for Adam and Eve's sin. In Eden, wrote Wesley, "... heaven and earth and all the hosts of them were mild, benign, and friendly to human nature" (J. Wesley 1747, Preface). Eve's sin put an end to this epistemological paradise. "Hence, at present, no child of man can at all times apprehend clearly, or judge truly. And where either the judgment or apprehension is wrong, it is impossible to reason justly. Thus it is as natural for a man to mistake as to breathe" (J. Wesley [1777] 1960).

The concept of a mind whose only contents are the (often false) impressions received through sense perception also affected the Methodists' conception of original sin, or "spiritual diseases." In their view, we are born with polymorphous desires for gratification and engagement which are stimulated by the cacophony of sounds and sights in modern life. Our promiscuous sense perceptions, undisciplined by any innate tendency to seek God or virtue, seduce, confuse, and ultimately damn us. Yet our sense perceptions are supremely important to our salvation, because it is through the thoughts and emotions generated by the senses that we begin to understand our own unworthiness and our need of Christ's redeeming sacrifice, "seeing at present the soul can no more love than it can think, any otherwise than by the help of bodily organs."[6] Thus Wesley rejected the mystic's goal of effacing sense perception to achieve a higher reality, while the Methodist Mary Bosanquet Fletcher argued that, "the mind is the mouth of the soul, therefore the food my mind receives [through the senses] is that on which my soul must feed whether it be healthful or poisonous. And that all my success in the spiritual life depends on this" (Tooth 1796–7).

Methodists and others believed that we can begin to educate and purify our sense perceptions (and by extension our ideas), by simplifying our daily routines. Thus Wesley linked spiritual health to everyday actions like the consumption of caffeine, which unsettles the nerves and distorts perception, as well as the ability to lead a useful life. By such simple techniques of physical and mental discipline, Wesley aimed to train body and mind as instruments of spiritual enlightenment and virtuous activity, shaping his followers' responses and capabilities by inculcating restraint, promoting health, and regulating physical and sensory stimulation. Through a regimen of diet, exercise, and general moderation (including outdoor exercise and the use of fewer blankets at night), the mind's reactions and responses could be conditioned, not only to assist spiritual progress but to sustain it for the long term.

A more internalized method of educating the senses was by learning to read and pray with the heart and not the intellect. The Pietists de-emphasized doctrine and liturgy and focused their energies on practical Christianity or "heart religion," using devotional prayers and practices, including the writings of Catholic mystics, that would help the worshipper live a fuller, more ethical spiritual life. William Law's immensely popular work, *A Serious Call to a Devout and Holy Life*, counseled readers to seek truth with the heart rather than the head. "Reading is *eating*" he told a friend who had sent him some books, "and therefore I only read such books as have food suited to the state of life and hunger that is in me. I leave learning to the learned, and reasoning

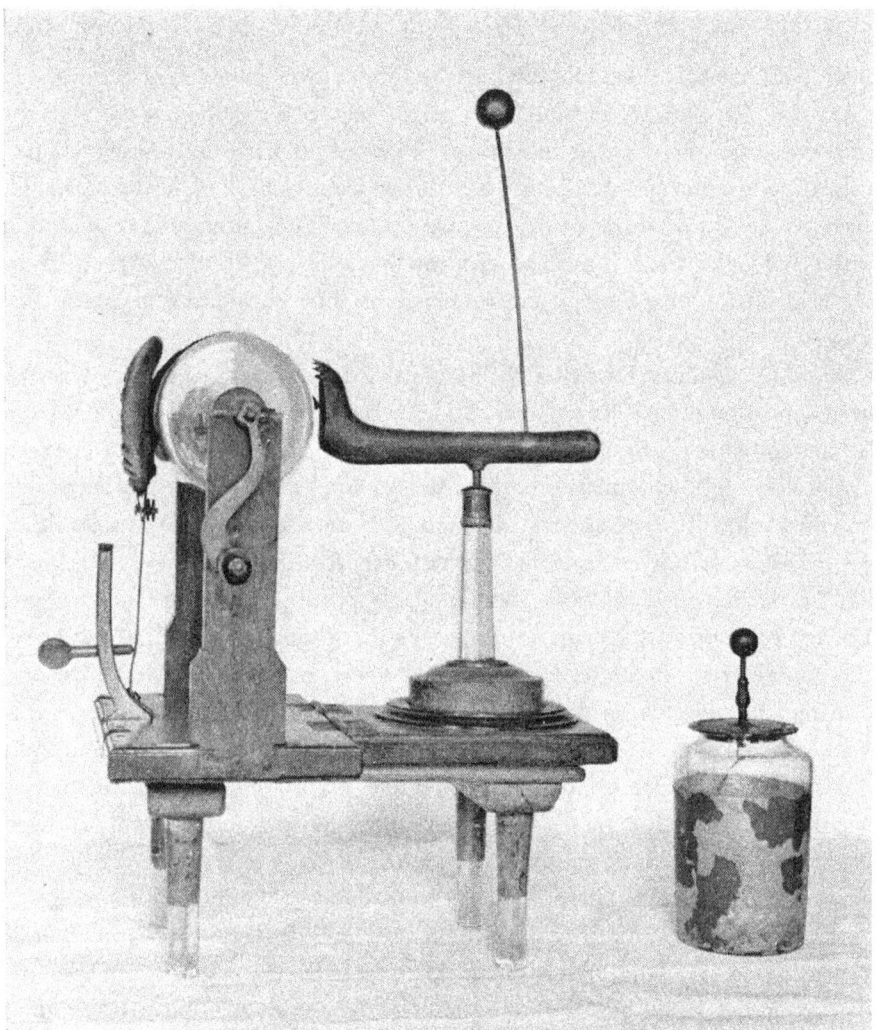

FIGURE 4.2: Electrical machine designed by John Wesley for the treatment of melancholia. Wellcome Library, London.

to those that seek help from it" (Rivers 2008: 645). According to the Moravian leader Count Zinzendorf, "we do not have to see God to sense him, just as we do not have to see our souls to know that we have souls. We know that there is a God because we feel God in our hearts. Religious experience is different from physical experience, but it is truly an experience nonetheless" (Atwood 2004: 44–5).

METHODISM AND MUSIC

Eighteenth-century spiritual seekers did not wait passively for a divine visitation. Through meditation and prayer, they tried to tune out the ambient cultural static: the noise of the city, the buzz of pointless conversation. They tried to sleep and eat only as much as was needed for physical alertness (though even Wesley found it impossible to give up tea). They attempted to read and listen with the heart and not the intellect. They considered the ethical implications of their own experiences and insights. But mainly, it seems, they sang.

For the Anglican Dissenter William Law, the chanting of psalms was the necessary beginning of personal devotion. His reasons are interesting. Far from being anomalous or unnatural, like traditional miracles or acts of extreme self-denial, he argues that music is both natural and uplifting, universally accessible and miraculously joyful and transformative. "For there is nothing that so clears a way for your prayers, nothing that so disperses dullness of heart, nothing that so purifies the soul from poor and little passions, nothing that so opens heaven, or carries your heart so near it, as these songs of praise" (Law 1729: 128–9). The rise of congregational hymn singing, of which the Methodists are a prime example, was a notable feature of many Protestant churches at this time. Though not recognized within the Established Church until the nineteenth century, hymns were one of the distinctive marks of Anglican Dissenters, Methodists, and Moravians; "like the familiar letter . . . [the hymn] allowed [the writer] to treat a substantial theological subject without the loss of personal, or even autobiographical, immediacy" (Hindmarsh 1996: 257). Among Methodists, the thousands of hymns published by John and Charles Wesley constituted an immense effort to convey theological principles to the ordinary worshipper, to create a sense of communal solidarity, and to generate certain affective states. Whether sung or read, they expressed the synthesis of interiority and community that was the essence of the evangelical experience.

Methodist hymnbooks included songs written by the Wesleys (chiefly Charles) as well as songs by the Moravians and other English writers; some fifty-seven published collections of hymns over a period of 53 years (Hempton 2005: 68–73). Many of Charles' hymns were written to dance hall music or popular songs; one was composed on the spot to a melody Charles had just heard sung by a bunch of drunken sailors (Tyson 1989: 21). John Wesley was fascinated by the psychological effects of different kinds of music. In his view, simple melodies had profoundly affected the nervous systems of ancient peoples, but this effect had been diluted by the addition of complicated harmony and counterpoint in modern composition. Wesley wanted hymns to be like the songs of simple Celtic peasants, where the melody "is not only heard but felt by all those . . . whose taste is not biased (I might say corrupted) by listening to counterpoint and complicated music" (J. Wesley 1835: 457). The new hymns were thus both powerful and dangerous: not only might they allow the listener to be swept away by the music rather than the message; they might also inflate the egoism of the singer.

> Still let us on our guard be found,
> And watch against the power of sound
>   With sacred jealousy;
> Lest haply sense should damp our zeal,
> And music's charms bewitch and steal
>   Our heart away from thee.
>   Hildebrandt and Bederlegge 1983: 326–8

The fact that Wesley was so suspicious of the dangers of singing shows that he thought there was a spiritual process also at work.

Beyond the music itself, Charles Wesley's hymns stressed the importance of the sense of sight in the drama of atonement. In "A Passion Hymn," writes the historian Joanna Cruikshank, he took the reader or singer deeper and deeper into the heart of Jesus' suffering, through the stages of being a witness, feeling responsibility for causing Jesus' agony, and praying to experience the suffering himself:

> See there! His temples crown'd with thorns!
> His bleeding hands extended wide, . . .
> The fountain gushing from His side!
> [Now the shift: We caused Christ's suffering.]
> Beneath *my* load he faints and dies:
> I fill'd His soul with pangs unknown;
> I caused those mortal groans and cries,
> I kill'd the Father's only Son.
> . . .
> [Then, empathy]
> Give me to feel Thy agonies . . .
> I fain with Thee would sympathise,
> And share the sufferings of my Lord.

As Cruickshank analyzes the hymn, the listener or singer must stop, pay attention, and watch while Jesus passes by. "The sensation of seeing is carefully evoked by the detailed naming of Christ's body—face, limbs, back, temples, hands, feet, side and brow—and the description of how each part suffers" (Cruickshank 2009: 52–3, 63, 64).

Methodist theology and practice are usually (and rightly) viewed in relation to the traditions of Pietism and Protestant Dissent. Ironically, the hymns are also reminiscent of a movement that began 200 years earlier, that of the Counter-Reformation Society of Jesus. Like the Methodists, the Jesuits promoted emotional training and discipline through educating the senses. In Ignatius Loyola's *Spiritual Exercises* (1548), the worshipper is instructed to meditate on certain objects and symbols in order to experience the smell of hell or the beauty of Christ.

> The first point consists in this, that I see with the eye of imagination those enormous fires, and the souls as it were in bodies of fire. The second point consists in this, that I hear with the ears of the imagination the lamentations, howlings, cries, the blasphemies against Christ . . . The third point consists in this, that I smell with the sense of smell of the imagination the smoke, brimstone, refuse and rotting things of hell . . .
>
> Loyola, quoted in Fulop-Miller 1956: 7, 10

The *Spiritual Exercises* was a manual of spiritual activity, not a book to be read. It was followed not only by novices in the Jesuit Order, but also by a wide audience, even including some Protestants.

The culmination of the Christian's spiritual transformation is a direct experience of God, what D. Bruce Hindmarsh calls "the evangelical sublime." Hindmarsh quotes Edmund Burke's statement that power produces the sublime as an accurate description of the evangelical experience: "Whilst we contemplate so vast an object . . . of almighty power, and invested upon every side with omnipresence, we shrink into the minuteness of our own nature, and are, in a manner, annihilated before him . . ."[7]

The ensuing spiritual rebirth created wholly new capacities for spiritual perception and moral judgment that religious leaders called "spiritual senses." Wesley wrote,

> It is necessary that you have the *hearing* ear and the *seeing* eye . . . that you have a new class of senses opened in your soul, not depending on organs of flesh and blood, to be "the *evidence* of things not seen." And

till you have these internal *senses*, till the eyes of your understanding are opened, you can have no apprehension of divine things, no idea of them at all.[8]

The spiritual senses should not be understood as mere metaphors, however. The minister John Fletcher argued that this would be showing contempt for the Word of God. The soul acquires spiritual senses in the same way that an infant gradually becomes aware of his own natural senses. The most imaginative rendition of this process came from John Fletcher's wife, Mary. Although she herself was not a biological mother, Mary Fletcher's perception of the infant's development shaped her understanding of the individual's spiritual relationships. In private notes on the communion of spirits, Fletcher meditated on the mother-child relationship as emblematic of the growing intimacy between the worshipper and God:

> When an infant is born into this world . . . it could have no communion with [its mother] but by *one sense* that of feeling but now it is enabled both to see, hear, and make itself heard by her . . . And may we not suppose if the use of sight and hearing as well as the powers of understanding are so improved by our birth into this lower world, that some powers analogous to the above are (at least) equally opened on the entrance of a spirit into a heavenly state: though perhaps small in the beginning, like the infant, compared with the measure that is to follow.
> Fletcher, *Autobiography* 23.6.3–4

THE MORAVIANS: RELIGION AND TRANSGRESSION

In the recently published correspondence of the Anglican and Methodist leader John Fletcher, there is a long letter written to his friend Charles Wesley in March 1761. The letter describes Fletcher's encounters with a demon or incubus who repeatedly tortured him in bed at night.

> . . . the noise of something which approached beat my ears and the sensation of something which settled itself along the length of my back eat upon me physically for several minutes so that I was more dead than alive: I often have experiences of this kind and if my good angel does not waken me . . . the Incubus . . . falls upon me again in my sleep and sometimes gorges me at his leisure for a part of the night.
> Forsaith 2008: 126–7

The letter is shocking to the student of eighteenth-century religion because it comes from the pen of an ordained and highly educated theologian and writer, one who presumably had left the world of magic and demonic energy far behind. The passage is easily dismissed as a hallucination, perhaps the result of Fletcher's excessive fasting or his fragile state of health. I believe it would be more fruitful to see it as an instance of what the anthropologist Michael Taussig calls "transgression": the element of disorder, agony, and horror relating to the human body that is a central feature of many religious cultures. Taussig notes the aversion to the idea of transgression in modern spiritual life.

> ... it would seem that the aversion to trying to think through the nature of transgression in religion ... could be attributed to the influence of taste and morality in modern times simply closing down massive areas of human experience ... by the combined action of Christianity and Enlightenment in harness with the utilitarian postulates of capitalist common sense.
>
> Taussig 1998: 352

The concept of transgression is a good place to begin an analysis of the Moravians, because the intensity of Christ's pain and the worshipper's ecstatic contemplation of His blood were the prime motifs of the Church's liturgy and practice. Moravian theology was centered on the meaning of the atonement, symbolized by the wounds of Christ. The senses of sight and touch were especially acute as worshippers visualized themselves held inside Christ's side wound or gazed at paintings of his bloody crucifixion. These images and practices are particularly fascinating because they were built, not only around traditional themes of sinfulness and punishment, but on the miracles of birth, infancy, and erotic love. For the Moravian worshipper, Jesus' agony is not only a punishment for humanity's sins; it is a celebration of their mutual love and joy. So Jesus speaks to the worshipper as a familiar friend:

> Do you want me? Do you receive me? Do I suit you? Am I acceptable to you? Do I please your heart? See, here I am! This is the way I look ... I have sweated the sweat of fear and anguish, the sweat of death, the sweat of the strife of penance; I have laid down my life for your sake ... Does this suit you? Is this important to you? Are you satisfied with me?
>
> Atwood 2004: 104

Moravian hymns and litanies celebrated Christ's humanity to a far greater degree than those of other Protestant groups. They did this as members of an advanced, highly artistic culture, in which hymns, liturgies, poetry, paintings, and costumes inspired both the Church's blood-and-wounds theology and the worshipper's capacity for aesthetic appreciation and erotic worship.

T. M. Luhrmann's description of today's fundamentalist Christians surely has affinities with the Moravians' attempts to cultivate the sensory perception of Jesus as more vivid than their ordinary sensory life. Luhrmann describes the modern fundamentalist's experience of hearing God's voice as hyper real: "this way of understanding God insists on a reality so vivid that it demands a willing suspension of disbelief while generating direct personal experiences that make that God real and integral to one's experiences of self" (Luhrmann 2012: 301). Similarly, the Moravian litany, along with many hundreds of hymns, was intended to bring the worshipper to a more intense identification with the bleeding Christ as both lover and mother. Moravians also collected small cards on which were depicted people in the postures of daily life, sitting inside Christ's side wound or vulva, within which he nurtured the unborn Christian soul and through which he gave birth.

Painting, music, and costumes were all designed to make the individual's relationship to Jesus more real than so-called real life. Conversion was depicted as a physically blissful event: "And as soon as they are with [Jesus] there is an embrace, a kiss . . . thus he draws like a magnet, rises them all up to himself, lays them . . . deep in his holy side, so that a soul in that hour and at that moment . . . can say: much happiness to eternal life, if only my whole life could remain like this!" (Atwood 2004: 92). Communion was viewed as the worshipper's union with Christ as husband, "a conjugal penetration of our bloody husband" (Podmore 1998: 135). John Wesley, who had initially been attracted by Moravian spirituality, was appalled, and quoted Zinzendorf as saying that Jesus was incarnated a man so that the "male member" might be sanctified, and born of a woman so that the female genitals might also be honored. "Were ever such words put together before from the foundation of the world?"[9]

Music and art were fundamental elements of Moravian worship. From 1727 to 1760 the Brotherhood (*Brudergemeine*) wrote, translated, or adapted thousands of hymns, many of which were distributed to people outside the community. Music was so vital to Moravians that the organist "also has an office of the Spirit and must be led by the Mother [Holy Spirit]." Zinzendorf reminded children that singing had been a natural expression of religion since the days of Moses, Miriam, Deborah, and David. With such singing "come beautiful thoughts and blessed expressions into the heart; nourishment that comes indeed from the Savior himself." Indeed, Zinzendorff wrote many songs

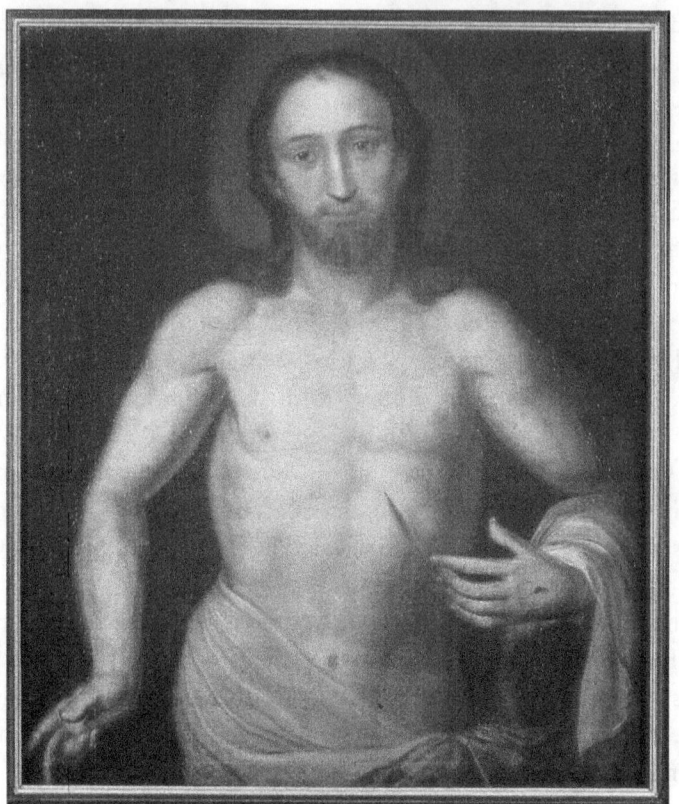

FIGURE 4.3: Johann Valentin Haidt (1700–80), *Jesus Showing His Sidewound*, n.d. Oil on canvas, 31 × 26 in. Moravian Archives, Bethlehem, Pennsylvania.

and lessons for infants in utero (Atwood 2004: 71). Moravians were also urged to paint pictures of Christ both on canvas and inside their hearts, so that art would transcend the antagonisms in Christianity.

Zinzendorff mounted thirty-eight religious paintings on the staircase of the Moravians' house in London. The pictures presented the visualization of wounds which the worshipper should "taste, see, smell, and touch" through the Eucharist and prayer. The artist was ordered to paint Christ's suffering on the cross so that everyone would be moved to feel astounding pity, "... and when the preacher's mouth will remain quiet, the painter's hand will still preach." The community of Herrnhaag (Germany) was famous for the vividness of its religious art. Paintings and transparencies were used frequently in worship, and the white walls of a Moravian *Saal* (worship room) served the

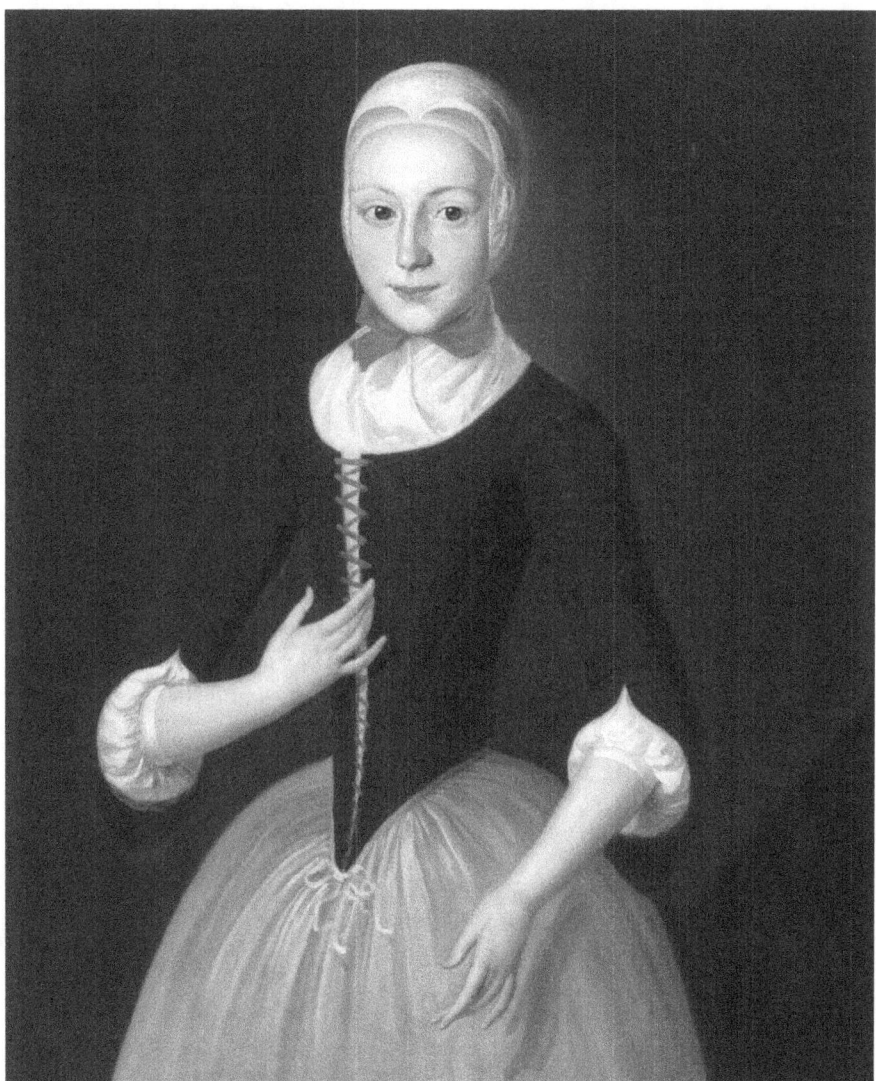

FIGURE 4.4: John Valentine Haidt, *Young Moravian Girl*. Smithsonian American Art Museum (Gift of the American Art Forum).

same function as the white walls of an art museum (Atwood 2004: 85–6). Adornment and pleasure were extended to the clothing worn by the congregation in public: there were ribbons—red for young girls, green for older ones, pink for single women, blue for married ones, and white for widows (Atwood 2004: 190; Schuchard 2006: 20, 118–25).

Moravian hymns of the 1740s were replete with images of marriage and of Jesus' side wound ("doves in the cleft of the rock") often taken from the *Song of Songs*. "O Husband with a hole! O what an incomparable ray! Kiss us, you cold little mouth! O corpse! Spread further in this church hall. We are lying here like the child . . . Kiss us, you cold little mouth!" The marriage hymns also emphasize passivity, the ecstatic submission of the worshipper to Christ:

> Lying in his arms,
> As his spoiled little darling.
> When he wants to kiss and embrace me,
> Then I am passively his sweetheart.
>
> Mack 2008: 44–5

Sally Cennick was an English Moravian who expressed her love for the great "Gardener of the universe" in a highly aesthetic mode, merging Jesus's "sore affliction" with her own erotic passion, highlighting the contrast between Jesus' red blood next to his white skin, his wounds like red flowers, the romance of "soft sensations" and "pleasing converse" as she mingled her tears with Jesus' bloody sweat:

> Red and white my Jesus' wounded Body,
>   Which in gardens' flowers excel,
> Lillies fair: and full blown Roses ruddy
>   Yield their odoriferous smell,
> Deep engraved upon thy corpse so sweetly,
>   Wounds like roses, fresh, and set completely,
>   . . .
> Hence it is that I with bride's affection,
>   To these places oft retire,
> With my Bridegroom in his sore affliction,
>   Here love's fervor I admire,
> Soft sensations in the pleasing converse
>   As these gardens I in spirit traverse
> With my Lord on Olivet,
>   Mingling tears with bloody sweat.

The letters of John Cennick (Sally Cennick's brother), a former Methodist who became a Moravian preacher, expressed the combination of awe and sensual comfort found inside Jesus' wounds. He wrote to the community where he preached:

> I feel I am a poor little bad Child, but I will not go away from the wounds of the Lamb, and tho I feel I am often too big and too great to get in yet, I will abide by them and kiss them, and pray the Lord to make me like a dear little Bee that can go in and out and suck the honey from all his wounds which are like so many pretty roses about his lovely Body.[10]

*

The hymns of Methodists and Moravians suggest the extraordinarily wide range of views and practices relating to the use of senses in eighteenth-century religious life. Indeed, it is hard to imagine a stronger contrast than that between the relatively pallid lyrics of a Methodist hymn to be sung while drinking tea with Moravian pain-filled ecstasies. The contrast is even more striking when we compare these Protestant and Pietist forms of expression with the torrid sensuality and monumentality of earlier Counter-Reformation art.

What do these very different renditions of Christ's sensuous humanity tell us about the needs and goals of the communities for which they were written? Many Anglican Dissenters shared the Methodists' appreciation of the need for total spiritual renovation. Where they differed was in the scope of their apostolic ambition. Instead of embarking on a mission to seek out, chastise, and awaken all the unconverted, they worked quietly from within their own churches and parishes. The hymns of Isaac Watts and Philip Doddridge were intended not to arouse the masses but to stir the hearts of individual, settled congregations. Isaac Watts's hymn, "The New Creation," asks God to give him spiritual senses:

> Renew mine eyes, and form mine ears,
>   And mold my heart afresh;
> Give me new passions, joys, and fears,
>   And turn the stone to flesh.
>
> Watts, Book 2, Hymn 130

Doddridge's hymns were designed to be sung following his own sermons. Many are contemplative and gently eloquent:

> When Death o'er Nature shall prevail,
> And all its Powers of Language fail,

> Joy thro' my swimming Eyes shall break,
> And mean the thanks I cannot speak.
>
> Doddridge 1776

Moravian music was also intended for stable religious communities, but unlike Anglicans, the Moravians followed a communal lifestyle in which sexuality was both celebrated as the highest expression of spirituality and strictly regulated in daily life. Members lived in groups of married and unmarried men and women, and males and females of all ages ate, worked, and worshipped separately; even their corpses were buried in separate parts of the cemetery. Marriages were arranged by the community, the partners selected by lot, and the unmarried were celibate. Because sex between husband and wife was also an enactment of the union of the church and God, Moravian marriage counseling was highly developed and sought after by followers of different Churches.

John Wesley opposed not only the eroticism of Moravian hymns and the "fondling" language of his brother Charles's Methodist hymns; he also opposed what he called "nambi-pambical" writing about a "meek" or "gentle" feminine Jesus. (Here he might have been negatively influenced by his rejection of Moravian beliefs, insofar as he saw their doctrine of stillness—the opposite of apostolic activism—as linked to their feminization of Christ and the Holy Spirit, whom they viewed as a mother.) Even the hymns written by Wesley's contemporary, Isaac Watts, were more delicately erotic than those of the Methodists:

> Come, let me love: Or is thy mind
> Harden'd to stone, or froze to ice?
> I see the blessed Fair One bend
> And stoop t'embrace me from the skies!
> O! 'tis a thought would melt a rock,
> And make a heart of iron move,
> That those sweet lips, that heav'nly look,
> Should seek and wish a mortal love!
>
> Jeffrey 1987: 92

John Wesley edited out many of Charles' more morbid verses that expressed the worshipper's despair and longing for death (C. Wesley 1989: 24–5). And while some hymns depicted the suffering Christ as vulnerable and in need of the believer's pity, the image of blood (used 800 times in the later hymns) was far more often a redemptive image of cleansing and renewal (C. Wesley 1989: 37). Moravians described their ecstatic and passive contemplation of their "bloody and juicy" husband Christ on the cross, and the Anglican Isaac Watts wrote more discreetly of the bleeding Christ as a lover:

> Did pity ever stoop so low,
> Dress'd in divinity and blood?
> Was ever rebel courted so
> In groans of an expiring God?
>
> Jeffrey 1987: 92

Methodists, in contrast, sang in full voice of the blood of the atonement, the blood that renews the sinner and imbues him with the strength to achieve the goal of sanctification.[11]

> He shed His blood to wash us clean
> From all unrighteousness, and sin,
> To save from all iniquity;
> Jesus hath died for us; for me.
>
> C. Wesley 1989: 39

The minister John Fletcher equated the marital embrace with absorption of the blood of Christ, not as a prelude to ecstatic union but as an anointing for battle: "Go meet the Bridegroom . . . hold up the vessel of your heart to the streaming wounds of Jesus, and it shall be filled with the oil of peace and gladness. Quit yourself like a soldier of Jesus."[12] The sanctified Christian does not simply yield to her divine husband; she is a heroic lover, armored and vigilant, ready to do battle with the unconverted elements both outside herself and within her own psyche.

CONCLUSION

There were many modes of religious belief and behavior, like the cult of relics and extreme physical self-mortification, that were rejected by the denizens of the Enlightenment. Yet many worshippers sought and found what they perceived as a direct, sensuous experience of the supernatural and the sacred. They also considered such experience as basic to the virtuous person's life as a Christian. Unlike the spectacular and melodramatic art and pageantry of the baroque church, which dazzled the passive viewer and induced a kind of self-alienation, hymn-singing or the contemplation of a painting hung in a gallery or private house both reflected and stimulated the singer's or viewer's individuality, her personal sensibility and emotions; a goal that was profoundly in tune with the Enlightenment emphasis on sensibility. As the religious writer William Law put it, "Singing . . . as it is improved into an art . . . is not natural. . . . But singing, as it signifies a motion of the voice suitable to the motions of the heart . . . is as natural and common to all men, as it is to speak high when they threaten in anger, or to speak low then they are dejected and ask for a pardon. All men are therefore singers" (Law 1729: 130).

The project of training the senses had many iterations during the eighteenth century. Common to all of them was a belief in the enhanced sensory perception that was available to the individual who emerged from ordinary existence to life as a Christian. Personal engagement with biblical texts and with different forms of art was intended to help ordinary people experience their material and spiritual worlds more fully and accurately, and in accordance with the theology and practices of their respective communities. Religion was not conceived by these men and women as a mere belief system—an assent to a doctrine or admiration of a minister's sermon—nor was it only an enhancement of the worshipper's own spiritual sensitivity. For evangelical Christians, it was a promise of self-transformation and a call to activism in the service of God. So Mary Fletcher wrote in her commentary on Psalm 90:14 ("O satisfy us early with thy mercy; that we may rejoice and be glad all our days"):

> . . . have we increased in faith the senses of the soul do we *see* more of God in every Providence . . . and do we *hear* more of God inward . . . do we *taste* more fine if we open the bible . . . do we *smell* the sweet odour, prefer him to our chief delight . . . in a word do we *feel* more tender conscience, endearing love, heavenly order, now let us apply our hearts to . . . devote our every talent to the Lord.[13]

Rather than restrict themselves to a symbolic understanding of religious art and writing, religious Protestants experienced the languages of poetry, art, and music as a stimulus to a more intimate engagement with biblical texts, and they used their own developing aesthetic sensibilities to generate new perceptions, new kinds of religious experience.

In her path-breaking study of evangelicalism in modern America, T. R. Luhrmann describes the role of discipline and conscious effort in developing what evangelicals believe is the capacity to talk with God and to literally hear His voice (Luhrmann 2012). The process involves learning to focus on the sounds and voices inside one's own head, being especially attentive to those voices whose counsel feels both authentic and ethical. This surely works as a description of efforts of eighteenth-century Protestants, whether Methodists or Moravians, to attune themselves to God's voice in their hearts. What makes the current experience of religious fundamentalists modern is that it takes place in a world where doubt of God's existence is part of the general atmosphere. The vividness and specificity of the voice(s), the concentration with which the listener strains to hear them as coming from outside as well as inside her head, is a way of pushing against this atmosphere of doubt. The Age of Enlightenment thus marked the beginning of a transition from the culture of pre-modern Europe, where God was assumed to exist even though He did not always appear, to our own modern Western world, where doubt of God's existence and the desire to hear His voice survive with equal intensity.

CHAPTER FIVE

The Senses in Philosophy and Science: Blindness and Insight

LISSA ROBERTS

It was Immanuel Kant's genius to resolve one of the great philosophical debates of his age by assigning the human senses and understanding interdependent positions in his scheme of reason. "Without the sensuous faculty no object would be given to us," he wrote, "and without the understanding, no object would be thought. Thoughts without content are void; [sensuous] intuitions without conceptions, blind" (Kant [1781] 1855: 46). Kant couldn't have chosen a more fitting expression, for his words force us to ponder what it might mean to make knowledge dependent on sensory perception and simultaneously claim that, without conceptual guidance, the senses are blind. A similar ambivalence appears later in his first *Critique* where Kant argued that "the senses do not err, not because they always judge correctly, but because *they do not* judge at all" (Kant 1781: 209, original emphasis). According to this image, the senses are virtuously productive precisely because of their inability to produce meaning. What role, then, did they play in Enlightenment "philosophy and science"?[1]

This chapter aims to make visible the senses' role in Enlightenment science and the philosophical discussions that attended its practices. It does so by focusing on three fields of endeavor: mathematics and the Enlightenment's "quantifying spirit," natural history, and the Enlightenment's "philosophy of manufactures."[2] The first draws our attention to the complex relations between the senses and contemporary modes of abstraction, particularly in terms of how doing mathematics engaged the senses and the consequences of employing quantification as a means to know and govern both nature and society. The second reflects the fact that natural history was the "big science" of its age. It attracted huge investment as it situated its practitioners at the confluence of efforts to examine nature in its most intimate detail and global breadth in order to tie the economy of nature to the economies of nations. The third examines the complex relationship between material and knowledge production on the eve of the industrial revolution, focusing particularly on ways in which knowledge and claims of knowledge ownership were used to mechanize or otherwise discipline manual labor. It was here especially that social and geographical distinctions came to be asserted regarding the embodied situation of reason, skill, and mechanical work.

Among the characters inhabiting this chapter are a number of blind practitioners, whose presence serves a variety of purposes. These include pointing to how loss of vision was related to scientific knowledge production: in some cases responsible for innovative and productive reliance on other senses, in other cases celebrated by biographers as affording intensified mental concentration or as a heroic element of sacrifice in the name of scientific progress. But their inclusion is also meant ironically to remind us of historians' traditional tendency to ignore or erase the active role played by the senses in the history of science; recovering their stories can help us gain new insights into the actual practices through which natural inquiry engaged with the world. And, in a further irony, we might see them as pushing us to look beyond vision to the active role played by the other human senses in the production of (embodied) knowledge. This is especially so for natural history, which (too) many commentators have explicated by privileging visual observation. But focusing exclusively on the visual not only obscures the deployment of other senses as investigative instruments. It runs the danger of narrowing our own historical field of vision in two ways. First, it analytically separates the realm of observation from the bodily engagement required to make observation and inquiry possible. Second, it cuts our appreciation of the investigation of nature off from the contexts of application in which it was often practiced and from the purposes to which it was seamlessly connected.

This chapter concludes with a reminder that such separations are as much a product of history as of historiography. For Enlightenment science and philosophy rested on discipline and distinction. It was a small step from considering the sense organs as instruments in need of calibration and control to comparing the bodies of others (whether slaves, sailors, artisans, laborers, or "exotic" foreigners) to automatic machines that mechanically performed the tasks required of them. Just as Kant declared the senses blind without the guidance of understanding, so did those who claimed to speak in the name of reason argue that artisanal and bodily labor needed to be disciplined by rational observation and management.

THE ENLIGHTENMENT'S "QUANTIFYING SPIRIT"

As secretary of the Académie des sciences, Bernard Le Bovier de Fontenelle (1657–1757) was positioned to judge the fruitfulness of various trends. Convinced of mathematics' growing power and impact, he ushered in the eighteenth century by remarking that a "work on ethics, politics, criticism and, perhaps, even rhetoric will be better, other things being equal, if done by a geometer." In 1990 a team of historians used this comment to introduce their influential volume on "the quantifying spirit of the eighteenth century" (Fontenelle 1719: 14; Frängsmyr et al. 1990: 1). What follows does not argue against the increasing presence of quantification during the eighteenth century. Rather, it initiates the recovery of one of this story's key elements, which contemporary mathematical philosophers and too many historians since have obscured: the sensuous engagement essential to pursuing mathematics and nature's quantification.

The question of whether a quantitative approach to nature allowed it to be "seen" more clearly is not only a retrospective one. It formed a central debating point between those like Jean le Rond d'Alembert (1717–83) who championed mathematical physics' revelatory powers and those like Denis Diderot (1713–84) who argued for investigating nature's qualitative heterogeneity, a stance more aligned with chemistry and natural history. Attending to prominent blind mathematicians and how their biographies have been presented helps set the claim of clarity through mathematical abstraction in sharper relief. Examining the rise of projects aimed at understanding nature statistically takes the discussion farther by indicating how qualitative and quantitative analysis came together by the end of the century to "see" nature in a way that made it ripe for exploitation.

Nicholas Saunderson

When Newton published his *Principia* in 1687, the mathematization of nature seemed assured. Three mathematical laws now held the universe together, stretching far beyond human perception's reach. But Newton proved unable to express all natural phenomena mathematically; most notably, the complexities of chemical attraction eluded his efforts. As if to underscore his failure to tame this sensibly heterogeneous realm mathematically, Newton's successors to Cambridge University's Lucasian Chair in mathematics contributed little to their field's advance during the eighteenth century. William Whiston (1667–1752) made his mark with the creationist *New Theory of the Earth* (1696). Nicholas Saunderson (1682–1739), blind since early childhood, left only the posthumous *Elements of Algebra*. This book is of interest for its discussion of "palpable arithmetic," which involved wooden boards of Saunderson's design, into which raised pins could be set and threaded together to form tactilely apparent geometrical shapes or afford processes of haptic calculation (Colson 1740: xx–xxvi). Saunderson remains best known, however, for his fictional appearance in Diderot's *Lettre sur les aveugles* (1749) in which he declares with his final breath that it is nature which is truly blind. How could a divinely designed world permit his monstrous existence? Perhaps the appearance of natural order is no more than a fleeting phenomenon (Diderot 1749: 307–11; Tunstall and Diderot 2011).

The non-materiality of mathematics, contrariwise, assured its analytical reliability for Saunderson. Despite its reputation as an abstract discipline, however, his practices indicate its grounding in sensible experience. Along with his palpable arithmetic, Saunderson larded his textbook with problems set in taverns, markets, and country fields to ease his students into the rarified world of mathematical abstraction (Gibbon 1766: 157–8; Hutton 1795; Saunderson 1740: 109–10 *et passim*). As his former student Lord Chesterton recollected, Saunderson "did not have the use of his eyes, but taught others to use theirs" (Baker 1897).

Leonhard Euler

If Saunderson is remembered as the blind preceptor of Cambridge, Leonhard Euler (1707–83), who went blind in stages, is considered one of the century's greatest mathematicians. Euler's first bout of blindness came in 1735. Francis Horner, Euler's English translator, hagiographically attributed this to his unremitting work ethic. Nicolas Fuss, Euler's assistant, continued in this vein, emphasizing further that he was undeterred by what others would have experienced as an insurmountable handicap (Euler [1765] 1822: x–xi; Fuss 1786: 7).[3] In 1766 illness finally left Euler completely blind. Far from defeated, his biographers claimed, sensible disencumberment freed him to produce some of his most valuable work (Calinger 1996: Section VI, 2007; Fuss 1786: 26; Horner 1822: xi, xx).

This image of the disembodied hero fits with the abstract nature of much of Euler's mathematics. But it would be wrong to consider all his work in these terms. Euler spent much of his time on projects that were thoroughly grounded in or intended for application in the material world. Nonetheless he was convinced that mathematics could uncover fundamental truths that eluded sensible experience. Perhaps the most dramatic case entails his involvement with attempts to measure the Earth. The eighteenth century was an age of global exploration in which mathematics played various key roles. Without seaworthy vessels, reliable navigational techniques and dependable instruments, setting sail would have been fruitless; without exacting measures and triangulation methods, mapping the globe and calculating its contours would have been impossible. Euler gained an international reputation for his mathematical "theory of ships" and contributed to numerous projects related to these endeavors (Nowacki 2008; Schaffer 2007).

This conjuncture of physical and mathematical activities was recognized in contemporary accounts of expeditions to measure the Earth published by scholarly societies such as the *Académie des sciences*, but in a way that equated the physical challenges of making measurements in the wild with the exertions of *in situ* mathematical calculations. The twin themes that repeat throughout these tales involve overcoming physical obstacles that impeded progress and overcoming errors that impeded mathematical exactitude; both called for heroic effort (Terrall 2006). Though Euler didn't physically join any expeditions, he saw to it that their data reached his desk where he continued the work of determining their meaning.[4] This was expedited in 1735, when he became director of the St. Petersburg Academy's geography section, its most heavily funded division. In this position he translated data from the Great Northern Expedition, which was meant to open Russia's east to profitable exploitation, partially by providing the measurements needed to map Russia's empire (Lincoln 2007: 107–21). The resulting *Atlas Russicus* appeared in 1745, reportedly leaving Euler partially blinded by his exhausting efforts. As his mathematical prowess helped translate Russia's wild landscape into a series of orderly two-dimensional representations, so was his own vision diminished. At almost the same time, he could boast of Russia's cartographic prowess and bemoan the sensible cost he had paid to help realize it.

Calculating Nature's Storehouse

A major motivation behind government-sponsored explorations of nature was a desire to assess the value and exploitability of available resources, and to

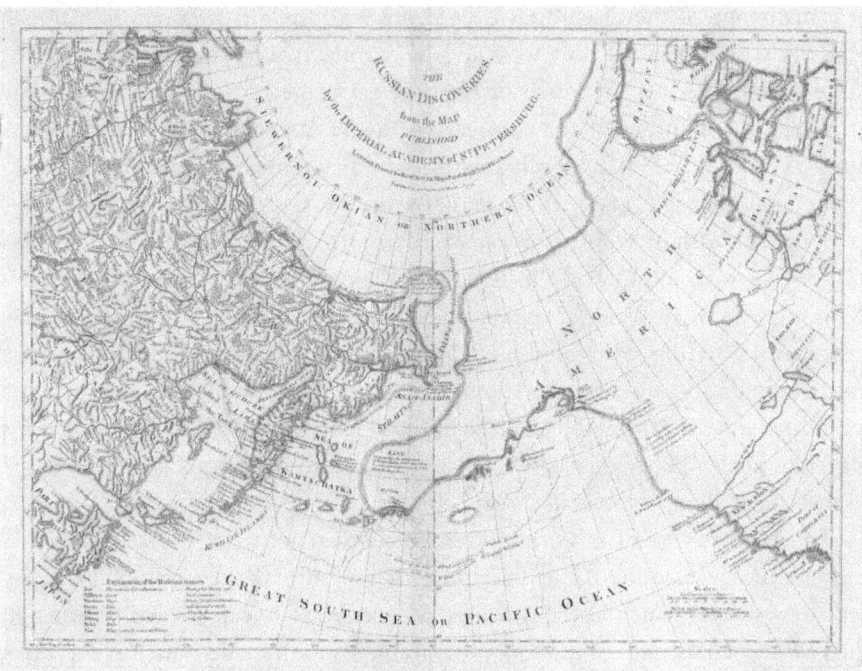

FIGURE 5.1: Thomas Jefferys, *The Russian Discoveries, from the Map Published by the Imperial Academy of St. Petersburg* (London, 1776).

catalog that information for future use (Jones 2008). It also set the stage for translating nature's heterogeneous richness into recordable and manipulable quantities. We might consider this in Heideggerian terms of modern technology as enframing the world as "standing reserve" and directing our vision of both nature and ourselves exclusively toward the use to which they might be put. Historically technology came thus to speak through science's demand "that nature report itself in some way or other that is identifiable through calculation and that it remain orderable as a system of information" (Heidegger 1977: 23).

Governmental urges and this way of seeing came together with particular prominence in relation to the theory and practice of the cameral sciences, forming what contemporaries called the "statistical gaze" (Bödeker 2001: 169). According to Henry Lowood, "the result was quantification and rationalization as applied to both the description of nature and the regulation of economic practice" (Lowood 1990: 316). We recall, however, that statistics could be qualitative as well as quantitative: some sought to capture sensibly heterogeneous evidence while others homogenized such testimony through quantification. What matters is that both resulted from the same will to have "nature report itself" in a way that could be ordered for management and use. While foresters were taught to place statistical emphasis on the quantity and volume of standing wood, for example, a survey of forests taken in the Palatinate around 1770 recorded that the "woods in places [were] so ruined that ... hardly a single bird can fly from tree to tree" (Lowood 1990: 318). Both resource abundance and scarcity pointed the way toward efforts at control.

Statistics was, in fact, a science taught in universities and practiced in various ways throughout Europe during the eighteenth century (Johannisson 1990; Török 2011). Working in tandem with fields ranging from public administration (*Polizeiwissenschaft*) and agriculture to forestry, mining and technology, it aimed to depict a territory and all its resources—both natural and social—by marrying attention to particularities with political arithmetic.[5] As a tool of governance and economic stimulation, it had a mixed record (Johannisson 1990; Wakefield 2009). But as a way of envisioning the world, it had profound effects. Through statistical tables, an area under consideration—whether a state, region, forest, or population—could be "seen" and examined as a quantitatively homogenous whole. Simultaneously, its qualitative particularities were also cataloged and compared. This allowed for scrutiny from a distance, affording local access, management, and exploitation. When placed in the context of a quantitatively expressed whole, perceived differences were brought into sharper relief, allowing for comparison and discrimination. What Linnaeus advocated for the classification of nature could thereby be extended to the social world. A proliferation of ethnographic studies helped to classify peoples in complex systems of sociocultural, economic, and political hierarchies (Koerner 1999; Sörlin 2000). The body politic thus gained a powerfully structured sense of itself.

EXPLORING NATURAL HISTORY

"Natural history is nothing more than the nomination of the visible" (Foucault 1973: 126). Foucault's well-known definition faces a number of challenges, ranging from the presence of blind naturalists to the globally extensive economy of sensuous engagement that encompassed eighteenth-century natural history. Indeed the century opened with the blind naturalist Georg Everhard Rumphius' (1627–1702) *Ambonese Curiosity Cabinet* (1705), whose frontispiece portrait does nothing to hide his condition; Rumphius sits in his study, working with his hands.

While his study could be anywhere, the "curiosities" that fill Rumphius' book all hailed originally from the seas around Ambon. Their discovery, harvesting, preservation, packing, transport, cataloging, and representation all required work in which various people and sense-infused processes were involved. Rumphius' collection was far from the only one made possible by sensibly engaged fieldwork carried out far from the European metropole. Likewise, he was not the only naturalist whose blindness provides us with insight into Enlightenment natural history. Recovering the sensuous engagement effaced by Foucault's definition thus requires a more thorough examination of the actors and activities involved in producing natural historical knowledge. This section begins with a small number of European naturalists and their "gaze." It then charts the geographically and bodily distributed activities that, in practice, composed the enterprises of eighteenth-century natural history.

Observing Blind Naturalists

A number of historians have recently focused on the acts of attention and observation, especially in relation to natural history, too often obscuring the complexities of bodily engagement in favor of emphasizing vision, the written word and "the mind."[6] Lorraine Daston, for example, refers to "heroic observation"—that is, "a kind of mental as well as visual dissection" as the recognized mark of "genuine naturalists" during the eighteenth century. And while naturalists used instruments to magnify the microscopic and reveal the hidden, the most crucial tools for attending to detail and certifying attention, she tells us, were "techniques of description"—the journal, the table, and the illustration. These means of capturing, intensifying, and preserving the visible continued a process that began with visual scrutiny: the more single-mindedly observation was pursued, the more other sensations receded from conscious experience. Hence did some of the Enlightenment's most famous naturalists such as René Antoine Ferchault de Réaumur (1683–1757) and Charles Bonnet (1720–93) owe their reputations to both their prolixly detailed publications and their claimed willingness to forgo eating, sleeping, and other creature comforts as they observed insect behavior for hours. Not only were they described as oblivious to discomfort and pain during such bouts of attention, they paid for their scientific heroism with permanent loss of sight (Daston 2008: 107–13).

If Réaumur and Bonnet were (described as) willing to sacrifice their vision for what thus seems to have been the century's visual science *par excellence*, their fellow naturalist François Huber (1750–1831) was blind long before the

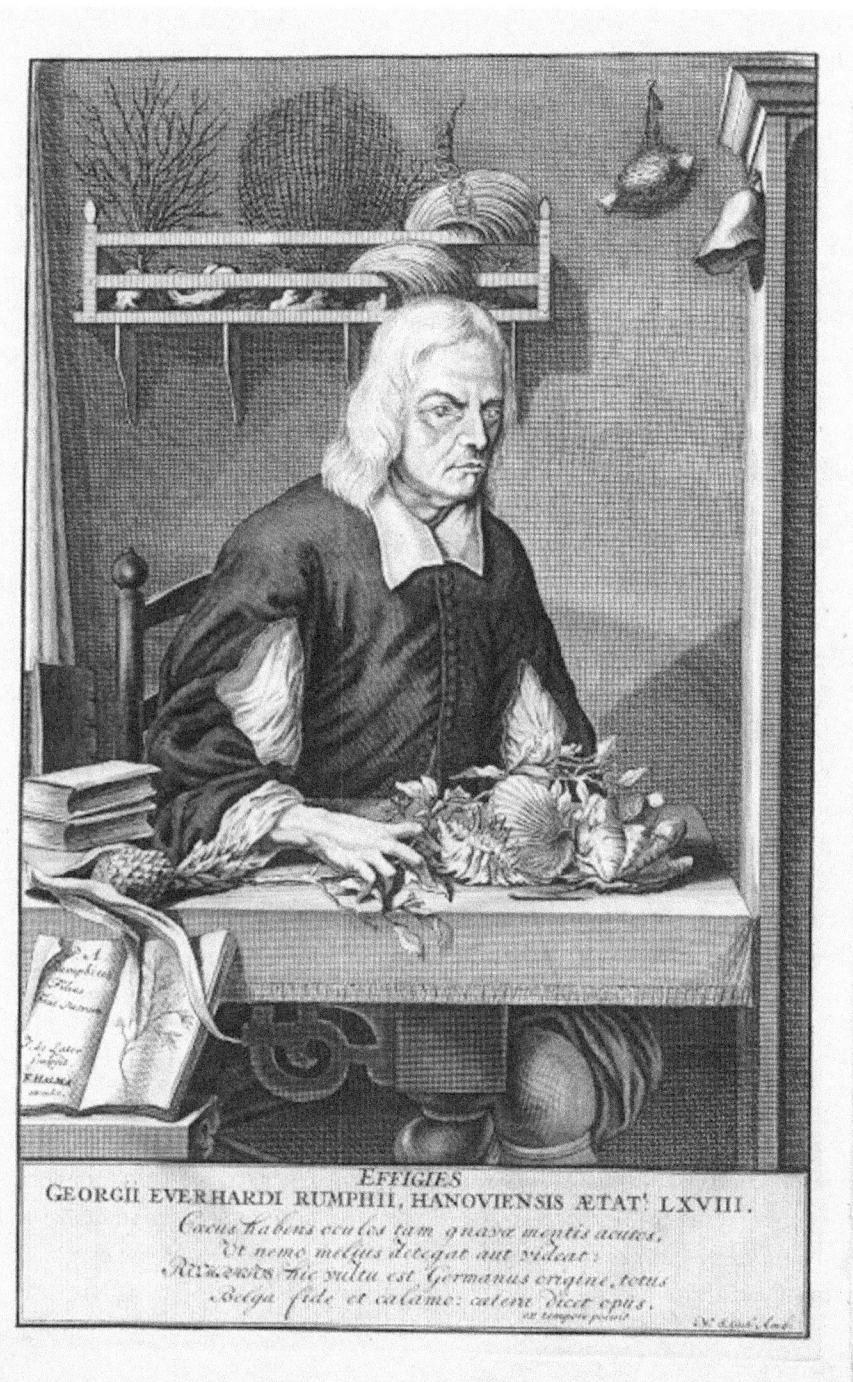

FIGURE 5.2: Frontispiece from G. E. Rumphius, *Amboinsche Rariteitkamer* (Amsterdam, 1705).

publication of his *Nouvelles observations sur les abeilles*. But, as Huber freely admitted, the luster of his efforts included the reflected glow of his servant's selfless collaboration. In his book's introduction, Huber describes how he trained François Burnens (1766–1828), a pleasurable task because of Burnens' curiosity, intelligence, dexterity, and dedication. It was Burnens who fashioned their instruments, helped design and carry out new experiments, and willingly suffered multiple bee stings to obtain the observations on which Huber's book depended (Huber 1792). We find here a set of practices that depended on the coordination between a recognized naturalist and his servant, as well as between the hand, eye, and mind. This invites us to question narratives that project the invisibility of technicians, assistants, and exotic "others," as well as the dualism of Cartesian epistemology that posits a distinction between mind and body or thought and sense (Roberts *et al.* 2007; Schaffer *et al.* 2009; Shapin 1989).

In an essay which historicizes "observation," while remaining predicated on the body-mind split, Patrick Singy points to Burnens having been read out of the annals of natural history by elite naturalists such as Bonnet and Jean Senebier (1742–1809), who refused to grant him any status beyond serving as "Huber's eyes" (Singy 2006). It is just this "reading out" that has allowed eighteenth-century natural history to be definitionally circumscribed by the table and its visually-based categories. But as recent reassessments of Carl Linnaeus (1707–78) have helped us appreciate, both Linnaeus' own conception and practice of natural history were a far cry from this portrayal. Here we find observation bracketed by the mobile engagement of all the human senses, reflecting the fact that most naturalists spent only a fraction of their time in the library. Eighteenth-century natural history was, rather, embedded in an active world of travel and multi-sensual involvement.

Natural History in Action

Linnaeus aimed at investigating nature's oeconomy so as to harness it for Sweden's oeconomic well being (Koerner 1999). His natural history, then, was not simply a matter of cataloging nature's three kingdoms with standardizing nomenclature, but entailed a policy of exploration in search of exploitable natural resources and domestic environments in which to transplant useful resources and augment national self-reliance. It was, essentially, a naturalist program of import substitution.

Linnaeus began working toward this goal with a grueling journey to Lapland in 1732. Reading his travel journal reveals how such fieldwork

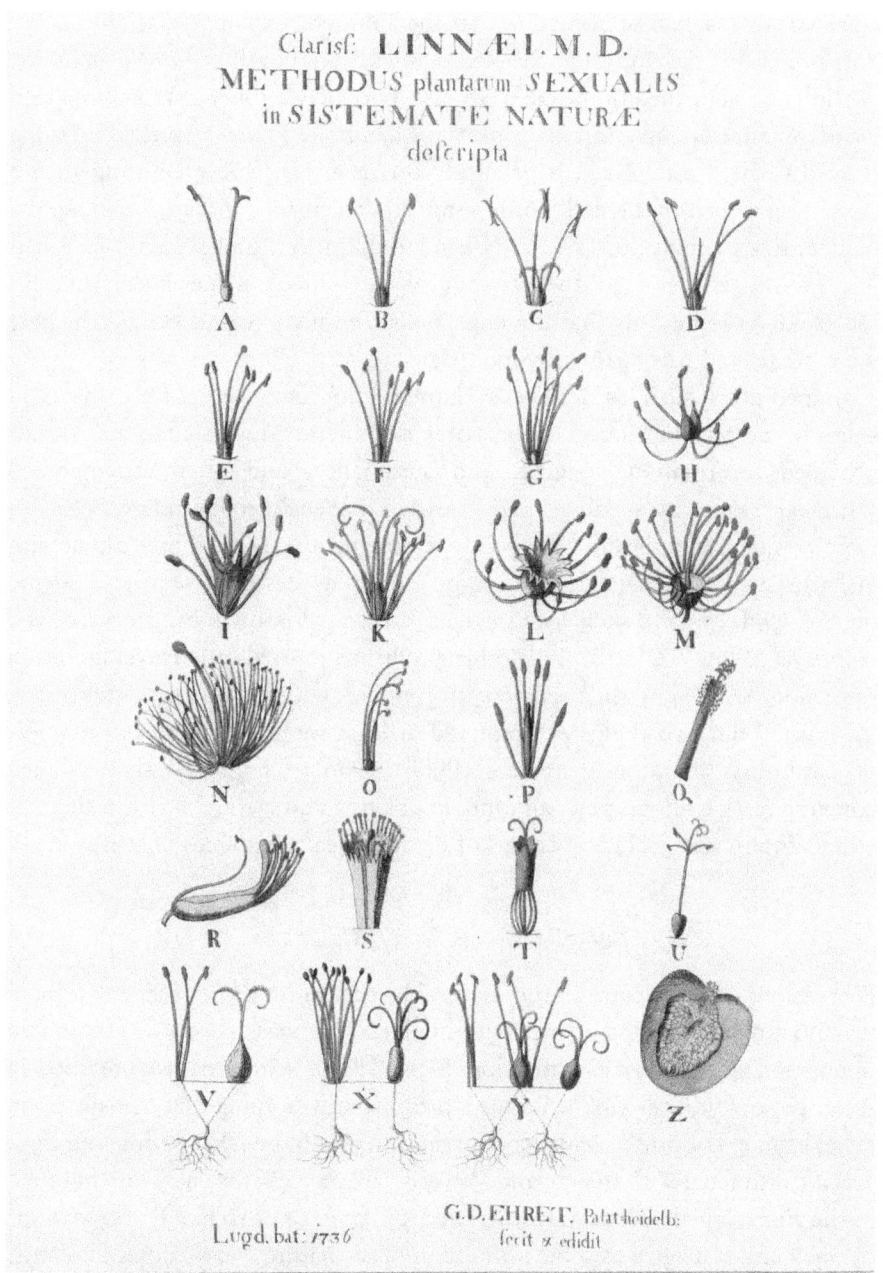

FIGURE 5.3: *Caroli Linnaei Classes S. Literae*, plate by Georg Dionysius Ehret depicting the characters used in Linnaeus' classification system for *Genera Plantarum* (Leiden, 1737). With thanks to de Beer Collection, Special Collections, University of Otago, New Zealand.

engaged all his senses, sometimes to the point of exhaustion (Blunt 2001: *passim*). Bodily discomfort and sickening sensations enveloped the most taxing portions of his expedition, but were also part of his more narrowly defined work. While examining an owl's nest, for example, Linnaeus picked up what proved to be a rotten egg. It promptly broke in his hand, "emitting such a disgusting stench that I shall not attempt to describe it for fear of making my readers sick" (Blunt 2001: 43). Scientific publications and reputations might have valorized vision as the warrant of disciplinary achievement, but his recollections remind us that the engagement with the world on which these were predicated was adamantly multi-sensate.

Expeditions such as Linnaeus' Lapland journey were rarely made in solitude, despite the heroic claims of many literary representations. Locals provided information, lodging, and sustenance, and often accompanied European explorers as guides and brawn. Linnaeus' fleeting reference to his Lapp companion indicates how bodily engagement was distributed along with tasks in such circumstances; the Lapp's burdens deserved only parenthetic notice, while details such as Linnaeus carrying his own baggage received emphasis (Blunt 2001: 50). Like other published journals and travel literature that flourished alongside eighteenth-century natural history enterprises, his journal did two things. It preserved at least some of the sensual richness of naturalists' bodily experiences (Philip 1994). Simultaneously it joined contemporary ethnographic literature in positing and hierarchically evaluating ethnic differences, including claims of distinct local economies of sense.[7]

Natural History's Sensory Geography

Discussions of eighteenth-century natural history must acknowledge that there was no single definition of what it entailed. This wasn't only a question of opposition to Linnaean classification (Sloan 1976). While Spanish botanists in America sought to discipline nature's profusion by arguing that "smell, color, taste, lushness or other accidents of plants, are of no use when setting out their specific differences" (Lafuente and Valverde 2005: 139), the entry on "botany" in the *Encyclopedia Britannica* offered a different approach: "The sensations of smell and taste give us some intimation of the nature and qualities of plants. An agreeable taste or smell is seldom accompanied with noxious qualities; on the other hand, when these senses are disagreeably affected, the qualities are generally more or less noxious, being either purgative, emetic, or poisonous" (*Encyclopedia Britannica* 1771–3: 632). So too was there debate regarding whether "savage taste" was pure or degenerate, how that differentiated exotic "others" from Europeans and whether such tastes ought to be emulated, adapted, or shunned (Norton 2006; Spary 2009).⁸

A further debate that divided European naturalists involved the geography of their discipline's method. At mid-century, Joseph de Jussieu (1704–79) justified his career by expansively claiming that "it is only by travelling, by passing through forests and fields, that one can conduct research that is useful to botany" (Safier 2008: 203). Georges Cuvier (1769–1832) sought contrarily to limit natural history's space of knowledge production. "The traveller can only travel one road; it is really only in one's study that one can roam freely throughout the universe" (Outram 1996: 62–3). Significantly, he directed his remarks to Alexander von Humboldt (1769–1859), whose name has come to stand for a stream of nineteenth-century research that valorized *in situ* bodily engagement with nature. But associating the embodied character of natural historical fieldwork with Von Humboldt's romantic travels and the work of those who followed him shouldn't eclipse its eighteenth-century presence.⁹ Not only did Linnaeus dispatch his disciples around the world to explore nature, the scale of expeditions such as those discussed in the previous section indicates that natural history was the century's "big science" (Raj 2000).

Recovering its sensuous character thus requires that we survey the various locations inhabited by its practices. This includes ships as both vehicles of global transportation and sites of natural historical work. Exotic plants and animals had to be cared for while on board; some ships were outfitted with greenhouses for this purpose. What began as on-land fieldwork thus continued en route as naturalists and their assistants struggled to keep their specimens intact and alive, gaining hands-on experience that was as useful as other forms of natural historical observation (Chambers 2000: 129; Sorrensen 1996). Frequently enough the perils of sea-borne natural historical practice were dwarfed by the physical challenges of survival.¹⁰ But calibrating the care of exotic plants and animals to ambient circumstances was challenging, even at the best of times. This was no simple matter of intellectual understanding.

Once on land, European naturalists and their assistants could begin hunting out specimens and knowledge—processes contoured by local climates, cultures, and the involvement of local residents in the production, circulation, and use of natural knowledge. Various historians have written on the important roles played by indigenous peoples, Creoles and African slaves in the western hemisphere, in areas ranging from pharmacology to agricultural improvement (Cañizares-Esguerra 2005; Carney 2001).¹¹ Direct testimony of how the senses were engaged in these activities is not always easy to find, however, because of illiteracy among many indigenous groups and slaves and the too-frequent undervaluing of their experiences by European witnesses and commentators.[12]

Some documents do exist, however, to offer a glimpse of indigenous peoples' and African slaves' investigative encounters with nature (Cañizares-Esguerra 2005: 67; Equino [1814] 1999: 82–3; Gordon and Krech 2012; Musselman 2009). Despite rhetorical conventions that often color such narratives, placing them in a broader, comparative context would enable us to trace how such sensuously informed reports were commissioned, ignored, used, co-opted, and translated by Europeans. Such an exercise would have to confront the importance of varying local environments and cultures. What holds true for eighteenth-century natural history and intercultural exchange in colonial Spanish America, for example, where complexly hierarchical multi-cultural societies inhabited environments ranging from unexplored jungles to Europeanized urban centers, does not hold true for China and Japan. Both these countries, whose central governments closely monitored interaction with foreigners, boasted well-established cultures and economies, including active traditions in natural history that attracted extensive European interest. We can begin to appreciate this by bringing together the experiences of Linnaeus' student Carl Pehr Thunberg (1743–1828), who combined botanical research with his duties as surgeon at the Dutch East Indies (VOC) factory in Japan, with the world of Japanese natural history.

Collaboration with Japanese counterparts was eased by basic agreement regarding what natural history entailed. *Honzogaku* also linked natural inquiry and fieldwork to issues of (nationally oriented) utility, with special attention to the development of local resources to replace imports; as such, it ranged from *materia medica*, through botany, zoology, and mineralogy, to agriculture and mining. At the same time, it overlapped with the aesthetics of gardening and pictorial arts.[13] This meant that, whether Thunberg did his own fieldwork, went on forays accompanied by Japanese, or relied on specimens, information, books, and illustrations presented to him by his Japanese hosts, similar sense-based experiences and evidence were involved. Plants and their fruits were experienced, described, and compared in terms of color, smell, and taste, as well as in relation to their use (Thunberg 1796: 62, 66, 81–2, 158, 186).

The cultural distance some European observers nonetheless constructed between Asian and European investigations and representations of nature by the turn of the century cast a formative shadow on subsequent history. This can be seen by turning to China's port city Canton, which provided numerous opportunities for inter-cultural exchanges related to natural history (Fan 2004). While foreigners' access to China's vast territory was severely limited in the eighteenth century, gardens owned by wealthy Canton merchants and notables, commercial nurseries, herbalists' shops, and urban markets all provided contexts for intelligencing and fieldwork.

Of special interest were the Cantonese workshops in which much otherwise non-transportable knowledge was pictorialized so as to render it immutably mobile. Among the visitors to such ateliers was John Barrow (1764–1848), who accompanied Lord McCartney on his mission to Beijing (1792–4) and published an account of his travels in China (Barrow 1804). Barrow found it vital both to describe the manual skill demonstrated by Chinese illustrators and to assert their absolute lack of originality and understanding, whether in terms of representational art or the natural phenomena they were charged to portray. In fulfilling commissions from European customers, Barrow claimed, Chinese artisans could copy models with exacting fidelity, but never rose above the brute use of bodily skill—a point to which we will return (Barrow 1804: 327). These hands-on craftsmen, he averred, could never be natural historians. It is in this insistent separation of the European mind and the Oriental hand that we find the origins of praise for "mindful attention" which some historians have celebrated as the central hinge of scientific observation.

THE ENLIGHTENMENT'S PHILOSOPHY OF MANUFACTURES

The English mathematician, naturalist, and experimental philosopher John Gough (1757–1825) wrote a memoir in 1802 in which he explored the thermo-elastic properties of natural rubber (caoutchouc). Though not well known today, Gough helped set the stage for an important transition in industrial and manufacturing history through his recognition that "heat increases the pliancy of the substance" (Gough 1805: 289).[14] Various Europeans had been testing rubber for use in products ranging from tubing to waterproof clothing since La Condamine's report on South American practices in 1736 (Reisz 2007), but it suffered from vulnerability to ambient temperature. This would finally be overcome once the process of vulcanization was perfected (1839–44), the understanding of which was greatly assisted by the work of Gough and the physicist James Prescott Joule (1818–89), who acknowledged his debt to Gough in his publications.

Three things are of special interest in this story, beginning with how Gough performed his experiments:

> Hold one end of the [rubber] slip . . . between the thumb and fore-finger of each hand; bring the middle of the piece into slight contact with the edges of the lips . . . and you will immediately perceive a sensation of warmth in that part of the mouth which touches it, arising from an augmentation of temperature in the Caoutchouc: for this resin evidently grows warmer the further it is extended; and the edges of the lips possess a high degree of sensibility, which enables them to discover these changes with greater facility than other parts of the body.
>
> Gough 1805: 289–90

The methodological principle behind Gough's approach involved his understanding that investigating nature depended on a prior knowledge of one's body and the ability to deploy its various parts as effective scientific instruments. Though obscured by a growing reliance on laboratory instrumentation and measures, quantification and an "objective" style of reporting that increasingly came to characterize scientific publications in the nineteenth century, a researcher's sensuous engagement remained as much a practical requisite for the field of experimental physics as for other experimental sciences such as chemistry (Roberts 1995). In this case, Gough advised recourse to the lips' "high degree of sensibility."[15]

Gough's experimental work gains extra meaning when we turn to this story's other two points of interest. First, this well-respected natural philosopher had gone blind by the age of three. Alongside his work in experimental physics, nonetheless, Gough was a highly proficient mathematician, an accomplished naturalist who identified plants by examining them with his tongue, and a successful teacher (Nicholson 1861). Among his best known students were the color-blind John Dalton, famous for his atomic theory and work on color-blindness, and William Whewell (1794–1866), who in 1833 coined the term "scientist", which so many have blindly applied retrospectively to natural investigators before that time.

The final point takes us back to Gough's memoir in which he presented his sensibly based findings as facts. Importantly, this was only Gough's first step; he next interpreted these "facts" as resulting from rubber's mutual attraction with caloric. Insisting thus that his experimental results be understood mechanically, he translated them into a vision of nature that neither he nor anyone else could see (Gough 1805: 293–4).[16] Between fact and theoretical understanding yawned a sensibly unbridgeable gap. In this regard, Gough's interpretive practice reflected a key epistemological challenge that faced Enlightenment philosophers with an interest in sensationalism. For despite sensationalism's fundamental claim that *nihil est in intellectu quod non prius in sensu*, two critical problems haunted much of the age's epistemological inquiry. First was the relationship between sense perception and (complex or abstract) ideas. Second was the relationship between sensations and the external world that apparently occasions them (O'Neal 1996; Roberts 1985; Seigel 2005).

Of note is that this proved to be more than just a philosophical puzzle. For developments in the fields of mechanical construction and manufacture entailed analogous discussions regarding the relationship between mechanical work and rationalizing management. As we shall see, this often led to assertions of a hierarchical distinction between (artisanal) labor—seen as repetitively mechanical, bodily activity—and theoretical understanding, which granted ascendency to European elites who claimed a (cultural) monopoly on this mental capability (Roberts *et al.* 2007). While the reduction of workers to "appendages of the machine" is generally associated with nineteenth-century industrialization, the roots of this revolution can be found in what is here called the Enlightenment's philosophy of manufactures.

Enlightenment Sensationalism

Diderot signaled sensationalism's difficulty to account for the relationship between sense perception and ideas in his *Encyclopédie* article on Locke; Locke "seems often to have taken for ideas of things those which are not nor could be in accordance with his [sensationalist] principle" (Diderot [1765] 2013, ix: 626). Contemporaries generally grappled with how to relate sense perceptions and reason in one (or a combination) of three ways. The first revolved around a question initially posed by William Molyneux in 1688: would someone born blind and able to distinguish tactually between a ball and a cube, be able to distinguish between them visually upon gaining the sense of sight (Degenaar 1996; Locke 1690; Riskin 2002)? At stake here was whether different sense perceptions could give rise to the same idea and, if so, how to account for it. Invariably, affirmative answers required recourse to the intermediary action of some kind of mental faculty, which either opposed or could not be fully reconciled with sensationalism.

The second way involved invoking sense-based analogies or metaphors to explain the transition from sensation to (complex) thought. It was described, for example, in terms of mental attention to "vibrating strings" or to the striking of an internal bell, or depicted in terms of the mind as "a moving picture [*tableau mouvant*] that we constantly try imitatively to paint."[17] As evocative as such language was, this approach joined the first in not resolving the gap between sense perception and mental attention and reflection. Finally, the third option involved designating signs as the intermediaries between sense perception and reflection. Much of this was developed in the context of theorizing about the origins of language, a discussion of which would take us too far afield. What matters here is that turning to signs and language as the habitual glue which holds sensual experiences together and allows for mental analysis could not resolve the relation between sense perception and thought in favor of an unmitigated form of sensationalism (Kuehner 1944; Rosenfeld 2001).

This leaves us with the second sense-related specter which hung over epistemological discussions of the age: the relationship between sense perceptions and the external world. Etienne Bonnot de Condillac (1715–80) introduced his *Essai sur l'origine des connaissances humaines* with these words: "Whether we raise ourselves, to speak metaphorically, to the heavens, or descend into the depths, we never leave ourselves. And it is never anything but our own thoughts that we perceive" (Condillac 1746: 1–2). Apparently unable to escape this solipsistic trap through direct philosophical reasoning, he turned to a popular dramatic vehicle in his *Traité des sensations*. While the Pygmalian myth was frequently adapted on stage, in music, and literature during the eighteenth century, Condillac explored the connection between sentient humans and the external world through the conceit of a statue brought to life one sense at a time (Carr 1960; Condillac 1754; Lajer-Burcharth 2001). In his telling, only one sense enabled the statue to distinguish between itself and the world beyond: touch (Condillac 1754: 219–28).

Importantly, Condillac situated the statue's touch in its hands. But the hands did not maintain their heroic status for long. Associated with work at a time when labor's management was becoming an increasingly pressing requirement for meeting the challenges of manufacture and the market, touch—embodied and represented by the hand—was quickly surrounded by a disciplining economy of reason (Arendt 1958: 79–93; Roberts *et al.* 2007). For Condillac (as later for Kant), it remained the job of mental attention to assemble, compare, and judge manually-borne experience in order to produce understanding. And in the name of enlightenment, the editors of the *Encyclopédie* gave artisanal work a voice by subjecting it to the reasoned presentation of a dictionary written by *une societé des gens de lettres* and illustrated by plates that rendered it static and mechanical (Roberts 2012; Sewell 1986; Stalnaker 2010). As d'Alembert wrote, "In the workshop it is the moment that speaks, and not the artisan." That moment had to be captured and analytically deconstructed, he argued, so that it could be re-presented in a rationalized way (Alembert [1751] 1929: 146).[18]

Automating Bodies, Mechanizing Work

The implications of this mode of representation and its reflection in the Enlightenment's philosophy of manufactures can be understood by turning to a highly fashionable trend during the eighteenth century, which embodied the tensions and ironies attending manufacture's fundamental dependence on the senses. The age was rife with automata; they appeared in shop windows, on stage, and in domestic cabinets. So too did they serve as tools for explaining the structure and function of the human body and as models for rationalizing production.[19] Lacking the sense perceptions which, as illustrated by Condillac's statue, fed an individual's identity and independence of thought, automata and machines could be counted on to perform as their masters required. If it wasn't possible to replace manual labor by such mechanical contrivances, the ideal came to be that of making it as mechanical as possible by disciplining the deployment of workers' senses and isolating it from workers' disruptive ability to reflect and judge. The disciplined use of workers' senses might even be valorized as skill. Workers' reason, contrariwise, was seen as best transferred to the rhythms of machinery and a cadre of managers. As the Scottish philosopher Adam Ferguson wrote, many mechanical arts "succeed best under a total suppression of sentiment and reason . . . [m]anufactures . . . prosper most, where the mind is least consulted, and where the workshop . . . be considered as an engine, the parts of which are men" (Schaffer 1999: 129; see also Koepp 1986; Picon 1992).

If anyone personified the pursuit of automation in eighteenth-century Europe, it was Jacques de Vaucanson (1709–82). Famous for his mechanical flute player, duck, and drummer, Vaucanson aspired to leave his mark on medicine and industry as well. Combining his knowledge of anatomy and mechanics, he embarked on an extended program to produce *anatomies mouvantes*—life-like models that replicated functions such as respiration and blood circulation (Doyon and Liaigre 1995: 110, 145). Inspired as a youth by the industrial machinery of Lyon, Vaucanson sought to mechanize the city's silk industry after being appointed Inspector General of silk works in 1741. Lyon's workers responded by running him out of town in 1744. Motivated in turn by what he saw as their ignorant recalcitrance and the inconsistent quality of what they produced, Vaucanson carried on, convinced he was working in the public interest.

The primary problem with the French silk industry, he argued, was that it had been left "in the hands" of workers who were "incapable of correcting themselves and generally poorly disposed to being instructed." Not only did they fail to accept rationalization of their activities, they persisted in practices that destroyed their own sensible capabilities—continuing to draw silk threads out of boiling water with their fingers, for example, until they lost all feeling. The best solution, Vaucanson concluded, was to perfect their machinery to the point that sensible human body and mechanical apparatus formed an integrated whole (Bertucci 2013; Vaucanson 1749: 154, 150). He further advocated that standardizing quality at a high level for a competitive price required housing silk production in large factories. Only there was it possible to employ machines and utilize the guiding intelligence of managers. This would ensure the proper distribution of work such that "each worker constantly repeats one simple operation" and a superior grade of silk could be produced in a shorter period of time (Condorcet 1785: 163).

Projects such as Vaucanson's were both increasingly numerous and subject to a number of challenges as the century went on. Reform-minded projects were often initiated or supported by government agencies and scientific societies that aimed beyond restructuring individual enterprises to institute new market and sociocultural relations (Schaffer 2007). But manufacturers were sometimes reluctant to adopt the unproven management, methods, and machinery these initiatives entailed; many were themselves products of a system that recognized artisanal work as an amalgam of bodily sense and practical reason and as a source of innovation (Epstein 1998; Vicente 2006). This was often matched by the mundane impossibility of replacing workers, whether because of their inimitable sensible engagement, traditional rights, control of trade secrets, or the limitations of available material and management technologies to effect mechanization successfully. The solution found in the nineteenth century ultimately involved the victory of a manufacturing regime that substituted quantity for quality as its goal and measure of success. In such a context, issues of sensible discernment on the workfloor were overshadowed by protocols of standardization.

Automation's Global Reach

Our discussion of the "philosophy of manufactures" began with the interaction between a blind experimenter and a substance whose trajectory linked European natural inquiry with global networks of exploration and trade. So too did the philosophy of manufactures generally build on a global geography, one in which sensible engagement was crucial. The ships that sailed between Europe and far-flung destinations to identify new lands and resources, or trade for dye-stuffs, cotton, and silk were manned by motley crews whose embodied knowledge and skills kept them afloat, but who also provided a constant source of concern to officers and the navies and companies they represented. Elaborate systems of corporal management and punishment were used to keep such threats in check. Much of these systems rested on sociocultural distinctions, structured in terms of taste and refinement in relation to indigenous or adopted climates of habitation. The senses of slaves and colonials were thought to operate differently than those of metropolitans. But even if workers and sailors hailed from the same city or province as the upper classes, their bodies were taken to respond differently than their more genteel counterparts, which was bound to affect their general comportment and capabilities (Delbourgo 2006a; Land 2001; Linebaugh and Rediker 2000; Parish 2006; Spary 2009, 2012).

Finally, culture was seen as having a formative or constraining impact as well. Hence, as European views of China grew more negative, so too did descriptions of the relation between the sensible bodies and minds of the Chinese (Hsia 1998: 18). John Barrow, quoted previously, had much to say on this score. He commented, for example, that Chinese arithmetic was easier than its European counterpart, ironically suited for use by the blind, despite the fact that it engaged Chinese eyes much more than their minds. Similarly, the Chinese were able to "extract from the three kingdoms of nature the most brilliant colours, which they have also acquired the art of preparing and mixing . . . yet they have no theory on colours." Given this attitude it was no wonder that Europeans thought Chinese artisans had to be carefully instructed by Europeans when contracted to produce illustrations for the western market, though what they produced was technically superb. "The coloured prints of Europe that are carried out to Canton are copied there with wonderful fidelity. But in doing this, they exercise no judgment of their own . . . [Chinese artisans are] mere servile imitators" (Barrow 1804: 298, 327).

Viewing China as so densely populated with machine-like human labor, Barrow questioned the value of introducing labor-saving mechanization there (1804: 311). European "philosophers of manufactures" increasingly voiced the opposite sentiment regarding their own domestic workforces. Though the very word "manufacture" denotes manual labor, Andrew Ure (1778–1857) finally defined its ideal as totally dispensing with the work of the hand; "productive industry should be conducted by self-acting machines" (Ure 1835: 1). The mechanical looms powered by this ethos were matched as the

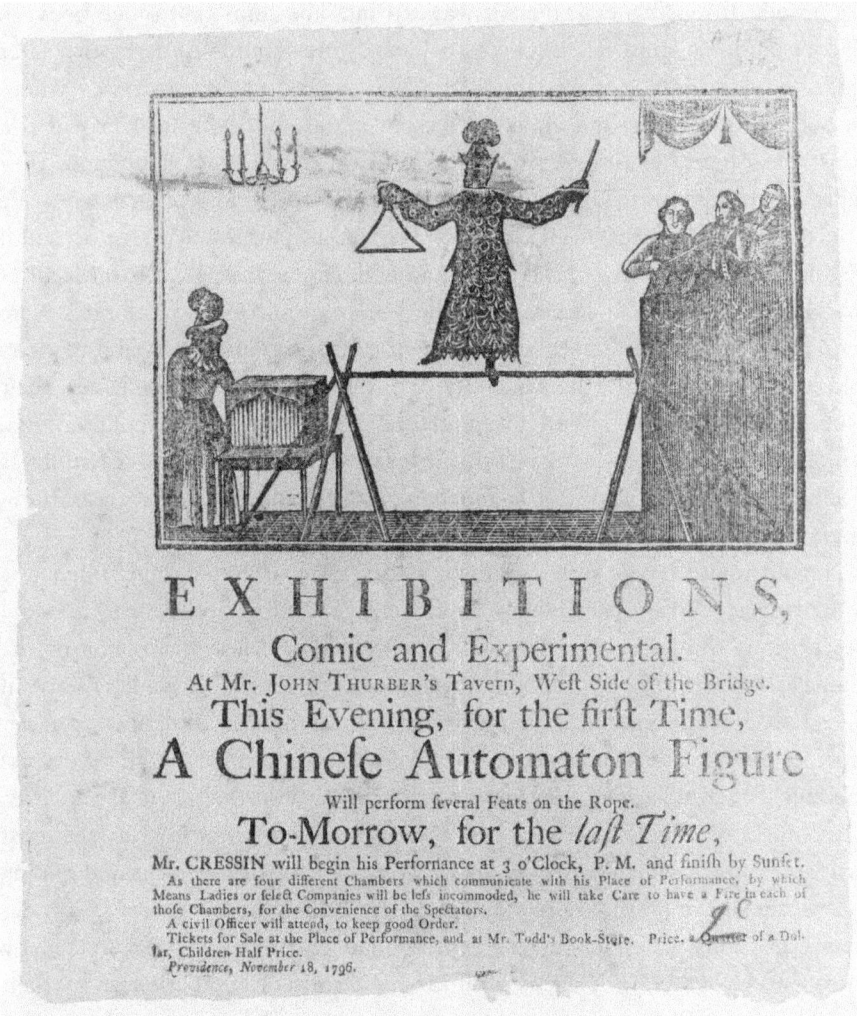

FIGURE 5.4: Advertisement for Mr. Cressin and his Chinese automaton, Providence, RI, 1796. Rhode Island Historical Society.

nineteenth century progressed by European imperialism's industrially driven policies, which brought more and more of the world into its gambit. With this in mind, the most appropriate symbol for the philosophy of manufactures' Enlightenment roots is perhaps not Vaucanson's mechanical duck (Riskin 2003b), but the mechanized "otherness" of Mr. Cressin's "Chinese automaton" which performed with thoughtless precision before tavern audiences in New England as the century came to a close.

CONCLUSION

In his study of the five senses, Michel Serres (b. 1930) breaks away from their previous philosophical representation. Where Kant saw blindness, Serres sees the senses as transforming the external world into information—softer than conceptual knowledge, but crucial for actively inhabiting the world. Against Merleau-Ponty's analytical substitution of language for sensation, he endeavors to re-establish the primacy of the senses, presenting them as moving beyond the strict limits of their physical embodiment to mesh seamlessly with the world they engage (Serres 1985).[20] But even if we grant his philosophical assertion that the senses are "capacities for doing, for becoming" (Serres 1985: 156), we cannot ignore that our "becoming" unfolds through history. This chapter has suggested countless ways during the Enlightenment in which information and knowledge based on sense perception were used, not to reinforce an initial openness of our sensuous relation to the world, if such is the case, but as a means of discipline. Qualitative description joined quantitative analysis to transform nature into a storehouse of exploitable resources. Not content to project this view onto nature's three kingdoms, enlightened Europeans created socially and geographically distributed hierarchies in which to situate their fellow humans in terms of how they were taken to live through their senses. Slaves and manual workers alike were considered too sensuous to be left to their own devices. Their bodies had to be managed "for the good of all" and their knowledge was rarely recognized as anything more than information, which needed to be disciplined by the reason on which the "enlightened" claimed a monopoly. Rather than opening up to a world of boundless creativity, the senses and their embodiment were to be constrained through rationalization and mechanization, all in the name of productivity. While science and technology were thus celebrated as ushering in an age of unending progress, a very human price would have to be paid (Condorcet 1794).

CHAPTER SIX

Medicine and the Senses: The Perception of Essences

PATRICK SINGY

According to many historians of medicine, the Enlightenment physician "was a thinker not a toucher" (Porter 1993: 185), an armchair practitioner who considered "a manual method of diagnosis beneath his dignity" (Reiser 1978: 22). The victim of a "monumental taboo against touching the human body" (O'Neal 1998: 476; see also Brockliss 1994: 79–80; Nicolson 1992: 109–10), he "virtually omitted any kind of clinical investigation, in the sense of observing and examining the patient" (Shorter 1993, 2: 784). Many textbooks on the history of medicine add that physicians began to use their senses only after the French Revolution, on the cusp of modernity. Enlightenment medicine would thus stand in opposition to modern medicine like "word-oriented, theory-bound scholastics" to "touch-oriented, observation-bound scientists" (Reiser 1978: 19).

If this account were correct, the present chapter would be blank, or at least very short. But the perennial idea that Enlightenment physicians avoided using their senses in their medical practice needs to be thoroughly revised. A rapid survey of medical books published in the eighteenth century suffices to reveal the importance of the senses in Enlightenment medicine. Open Samuel August

Tissot's *Avis au peuple sur sa santé*, arguably the most successful and influential medical book published in the Enlightenment, and you will find numerous references to medical symptoms and signs that could only be grasped by means of the senses, such as the pulse, the color and consistency of urine, or the smell of the breath (Tissot [1761] 1993). In another book Tissot laid out for medical students how they should proceed in a medical examination: after a few preliminary questions addressed to the patient, the medical student must, among other things, examine the breathing, the pulse, the strength and temperature of the patient, the state of her mouth (dryness, color of the tongue, taste in the mouth), as well as the appearance of her face and eyes. In many diseases, "it is also very necessary to palpate with precision the lower abdomen to investigate the state of the viscera" (Tissot 1785: 121–3; on the medical training of the senses in the Enlightenment, see also Lawrence 1993). Tissot's reliance on the senses was nothing original and had its roots in the strong empiricism of Hippocratic medicine (cf. Jouanna 1999: 291–322).

The senses had a role to play in the three branches of Enlightenment medicine. For the prevention of diseases, they could be used to identify unsanitary conditions. Non-potable water, for instance, was recognized "by its weight, color, taste, smell, heat, or some other sensible quality" (Buchan 1774: 49). For the treatment of diseases, the senses could help build a pharmacopeia. For instance, at the end of the seventeenth century, Dr. John Floyer published a two-volume work whose subtitle promised the discovery of "the virtues of vegetables, minerals, and animals, by their tastes and smells" (Floyer 1687–90; see Jenner 2010). Finally, and most importantly, as we will see throughout this chapter, the senses were crucial for diagnosing diseases.

A few historians have begun to revise the traditional description of Enlightenment medicine as a purely scholastic enterprise, and have convincingly demonstrated that "the contact with the patient's body [was not] marginal in medical practice in eighteenth-century Europe" (Keel 2001: 182). While necessary, this empirical revision of the dominant historiography remains insufficient. Instead of asking, *how much* did Enlightenment physicians use their senses, we need to ask a different question: *how* did they use their senses? For while it would be inaccurate to reduce Enlightenment medicine to a lofty, purely theoretical enterprise, it would also be problematic to jump to the conclusion that there is no significant difference in the practice of medicine between the Enlightenment and the modern era. In the first section of this chapter I describe what I call the "experience of perception" of Enlightenment medicine and science, an experience that helps us understand the peculiar way in which Enlightenment physicians used their senses. In the next sections I show how this experience of perception concretely played out in the quotidian practice of physicians. I focus on three medical practices, chosen for their historical and historiographical importance: consultation by letter, percussion of the chest, and pathological anatomy.

ENLIGHTENED PERCEPTION[1]

In order to understand how physicians in the eighteenth century saw, touched, smelled, heard, or tasted, we must begin by considering how they conceptualized the objects they tried to grasp with their senses, i.e., bodies and their diseases.

One might say that in Enlightenment medicine, bodies were transparent. What Michel Foucault called the "theory of representation" of the classical age (Foucault 1966), and what eighteenth-century aesthetics called "the principle of imitation" (see for instance Batteux 1746), was a structure of perceptibility in which some things, directly perceptible through the senses, represented other things, which could only be grasped by the understanding. To look at a painting (Arasse 1996), to listen to a piece of music (Goehr 1992: 139–47; Johnson 1995), and to examine the body of a patient, meant to see or hear *through* them in order to grasp the signified thing itself.

For eighteenth-century physicians, the signified thing was the disease. Diseases were not abnormal modifications of physiological phenomena, as they have been since the nineteenth century. A disease was an "essence," in the sense of an abstract entity, a sort of Platonic form existing outside the physical world, a pathological species "inserting itself in the body, where it is possible" (Foucault 1994: 138). To be sick was to be in "a polemical situation" (Canguilhem [1943] 1998: 13) since it involved a fight between the *res naturales* (the "natural things" that compose the body) and the *res contra naturam* (the "things against nature," i.e., the diseases). By definition, diseases were ontologically different from the nature they attacked.

This means that they had their own coherence, independent from physiological variations. Pinel explained that disease "must be considered neither like an endlessly moving picture [*tableau*], nor like an incoherent assemblage of reappearing affections that one needs to fight always with remedies, but like an indivisible whole from its beginning to its end, a regular ensemble of characteristic symptoms and a succession of periods" (Pinel 1797, 1: vij). The notion of "critical days" held, for instance, that a disease belonging to species X would have a crisis on the seventh day after its outbreak, then another one on the fourteenth, and would disappear on the twenty-first: "this numerically fixed duration [was] part of the essential structure of disease"

(Foucault 1994: 10–11; on critical days see for instance Aymen 1752; Bordeu [1754] 2013, iv: 471–89; Camino 1799). Any evidence to the contrary could easily be explained away, either by blaming the physician who missed the exact day of the outbreak of the disease, or by invoking the "complications" that disturbed and altered the regular course of the disease. In any case, most eighteenth-century physicians subscribed to the idea that "it is certain that there is something constant and uniform, in the character of the generality of diseases" (Zimmermann [1764] 1778, 1: 51).

In order to be able to recognize which species of disease his patient was suffering from, the physician had to take into consideration what was perceptible in or on the body of his patient. But what exactly was he supposed to look for? Foucault called eighteenth-century medicine a "botany of symptoms" (1994: xiv), implying that at that time only symptoms mattered. But it would be more accurate to talk of a *botany of obvious perceptions*. In the eighteenth century symptoms were necessarily perceptible, since they were defined as "obvious and sensible changes" (Sauvages 1771, 1: 28), and this is why they were so important to physicians. But any pathological fact that was easily perceptible also had to be included in the definition of disease: "The definition [of a disease] is defective, if it contains obscure and hypothetical things, like the internal seat of the disease that the senses cannot perceive in a living man. But one must include the seat of the disease in the definition when it is sensible, or when we know it from the sufferer's account" (Sauvages 1771, 1: 28). The criterion that marked what elements had to be included in the identification of a disease and what elements had to be excluded was therefore not based on the nature of these elements (are they symptoms or not?), but on their perceptibility (are they easily perceptible or not?).

In this epistemological context, perceptual details were problematic. Far from being the indicators of the quality of an observation (as they became in the nineteenth century), in the Enlightenment they had to be excluded rather than sought for. The great theoretician of observation Jean Senebier (1742–1809) explained that "although small differences deserve attention, one should not use them too often, because they are not perceptible [*sensibles*] enough, and can mislead" (1802, 2: 56). Tissot (1728–97) advised that in the clinic "it is on the essential characteristics of the disease, on those that enable one to distinguish it from any other and to make one grasp its true cause, that one must most insist" (1785: 124–5; see also Frank 1790: 25; Pinel [1793] 1980: 54). Tissot's colleague and friend Johann Georg Zimmermann (1728–95) warned that someone "who is too minute in his observations, without doubt, often sees things which are not perceived by others; but, at the same time, he is often in danger of mistaking his own ideas for reality" ([1764] 1778, 1: 111; see also Double 1811, 1: 43–4). To take details into consideration was even a sign of one's lower condition. Using an argument based in part on a gender divide in perception, Zimmermann explained that:

> Men of narrow genius, often see, in certain objects, many things, which a superior genius passes over without observing them; but these things are usually such as a man of refined genius should avoid seeing. This minuteness seems to be the lot of little minds. Women have, on a thousand occasions, a finer eye than the men; but it is for things that are made to be seen only by women. A mind, formed for more elevated views, ought to pass over these objects; because it is not destined to dwell on such minutiae.
>
> Zimmermann [1764] 1778, 1: 113

This disdain for details was not limited to medicine, or even to science. In eighteenth-century aesthetics details played a similarly problematic role. As Sir Joshua Reynolds explained in his *Discourses on Art*, "some circumstances of minuteness and particularity frequently tend to give an air of truth to a piece. . . . Such circumstances therefore cannot wholly be rejected." Yet in typical eighteenth-century fashion he added that "the general idea constitutes real excellence. All smaller things, however perfect in their way, are to be sacrificed without mercy to the greater" (Reynolds [1797] 1988: 58). Too many details in a musical piece could also easily blur the representation. Joseph II's famous complaint, "Too many notes, my dear Mozart," expressed something shared by many, and even in the early nineteenth century Frenchmen continued to react similarly to Beethoven's music (Johnson 1991, 1995: Chs. 15, 16).

Because the physician's senses focused on easily perceptible pathological facts, their sharpness was not relevant. The great nosologist François Boissier de Sauvages (1706–67), who relentlessly insisted on the necessity of observation in medicine, explained that the apparent characteristics of diseases, on which his entire nosology rested, were "even within women's reach" (1732: xv). The physical preconditions for good senses were essentially negative: it was necessary that "the senses have never suffered from any weakening or diminution" (Musschenbroek 1769, 1: xviij). For instance, physicians who wanted to take the pulse had to be careful "not to do anything that could make the tip of the fingers calloused" (Fouquet 1767: 13; Landré-Beauvais 1809: 21). It was also recommended to use one's senses at specific times of the day, when they were supposed to be functioning better (Senebier 1802, 1: 185). Yet, as surprising as it might seem to us, the best senses were not the most sensitive ones, but the most ordinary ones. Senebier explained that an observer should "perceive like the crowd," for this was a guarantee that his senses were not the source of illusions and mistakes (1775, 1: 98; this phrase was not included in the 1802 edition). The anatomist Joseph Lieutaud (1703–80) put Senebier's advice into practice: "Although I have ... very good eyesight that makes me see the smallest parts, I always put these parts under the eyes of all those who were near me, and I reached a conclusion only when their unanimous judgment [*sentiment*] conformed to mine" ([1742] 1766: xiij; see also Carrard 1777: 5). Deficient senses were not senses that were insufficiently trained and that made the observer miss minute details, but senses that were subject to illusions or literally extra-ordinary.

In eighteenth-century medicine the senses were in the background of the experience of perception. Not only did they not need to be hypersensitive, but some epistemologists, like Senebier, even argued that they *should not* be hypersensitive. There is therefore no irony in the fact that the empiricist philosopher Etienne Bonnot de Condillac (1715–80), who claimed that knowledge comes from sensations, had himself very bad eyesight (Voltaire 1953–65, 30: 143). Nor is it paradoxical that Sauvages, who suffered from "some weakness in the eyes," wanted to base his work on experience, which he said "consists in observing with attention, by means of the senses such as sight, hearing, touch, etc., the spontaneous facts that occur in the universe" (Sauvages 1771, 1: 5; on Sauvages's bad eyes, see Ratte 1771, 1: xvj).

What distinguished the true physician from the amateur was not the sharpness of his senses, but his ability to combine perceptions and grasp the essence of diseases. It is at this noetic level, not at the level of the senses, that the distinction was made. The accomplished physician could discover "all the relations that would not strike the eyes of a less educated man" (M.*** 1756: 31). The symptoms and signs of diseases formed, "by their diverse combinations, separated pictures [*tableaux détachés*], more or less distinct and strongly marked, depending on one's more or less exercised vision, and on whether one has had an extensive or superficial education" (Pinel 1797, 1: vj). Impostors might pretend they are sick by faking several symptoms, but even if each particular symptom were perfectly faked, "the physician who knows, as it must be, the combination of symptoms, will easily expose these deceits, because there is never the necessary liaison in the symptoms we see in those impostors" (Sauvages 1771, 1: 108).

In one of the most important eighteenth-century books on the pulse, first published in 1756, Théophile de Bordeu (1722–76) gave an account of the practice of the taking of the pulse that confirms both the less than crucial importance of the sensitivity of the senses and the fundamental role of the mind in the experience of perception of the Enlightenment. He explained that:

> the most perceptive and the most confident physicians as regards this kind of knowledge, are those who have the mind the most filled with all the images of the different kinds of pulses; those in whom these images are so well put, so well arranged, that there could hardly be any confusion, and that memory distinctly displays to them the idea of the species of pulse resembling the one they are touching.
> Bordeu [1756] 1818, 1: 263

An acute sensitivity at the tip of the fingers was *not* necessary for taking the pulse:

> The natural disposition of the organs, their finesse, their aptitude, contribute infinitely to make one feel well the nuances that differentiate the pulses: *but it is not impossible to perceive these nuances without this tactile finesse*. Thus the specific knowledge that physicians can acquire on the pulse, must be attributed less to a peculiar sensitivity of their touch, than to their experience.
> Bordeu [1756] 1818, 1: 262, my emphasis

The physician had to "have in mind the standard piece or pulse, to which he can relate the one he wants to judge." The difficulty was not so much to *feel* the pulse, as to *compare* what was felt with the memory of the standard pulse. The physician had to receive passively an impression from his sense of touch, at the same time that he had to use actively his memory to recall the sensation corresponding to the standard pulse. Once these two sensations were in the physician's mind, it was the turn of the faculty of attention to work: "It is easy to understand that attention is divided between these two objects, and that the operation by which the soul draws a parallel between the present pulses and an *absent* pulse, presupposes a considerable effort" (1: 263).

Medical practice in the eighteenth century was obviously something quite intellectual. But it was a practice nevertheless, based on sensory perception. Enlightened physicians were not afraid to touch bodies. They only claimed that the senses had to be at the service of the mind. As we will see in the rest of this chapter, this was the practice of progressive physicians like Tissot, Morgagni, or Auenbrugger—of physicians who touched their patients, who relentlessly

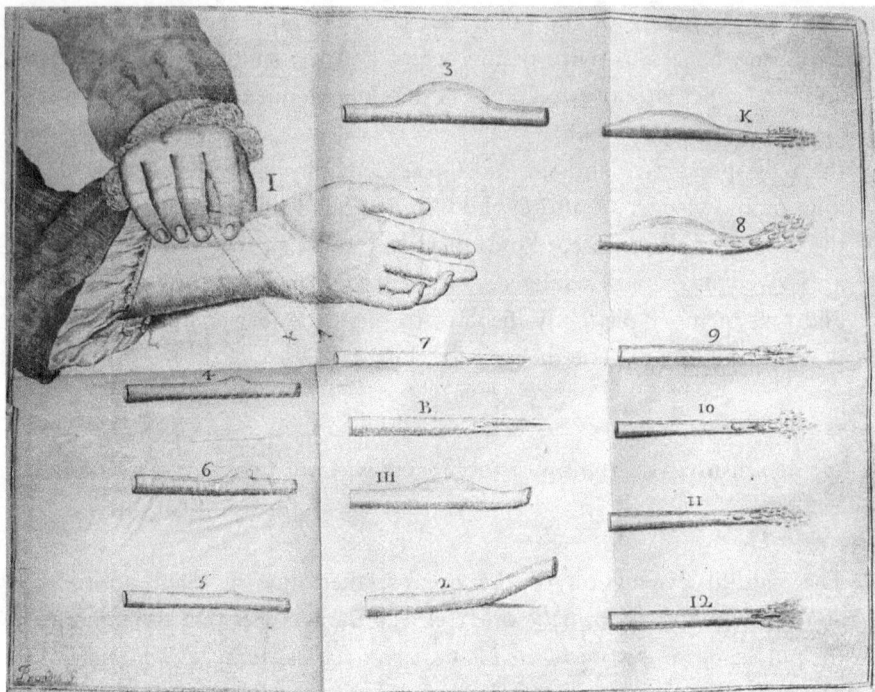

FIGURE 6.1: Fold-out plate from Fouquet's *Essai sur le pouls* (1767). Copperplate engraving by Brondes. Courtesy of Ebling Library for the Health Sciences/Rare Books & Special Collections, University of Wisconsin-Madison.

warned against the spirit of system, who frequented hospitals, and who opened up corpses.

CONSULTATION BY LETTER

Since at least the time of Galen (129–c. 217), physicians have practiced consultation by letter. In the literary genre called the *consilia*, the ordinary physician would write to another physician, usually someone of great reputation, to ask for his advice on a difficult case. The consulted physician would reply without ever seeing the patient, basing his judgment only on what he read in the letter (see Agrimi and Crisciani 1994). This practice seems to have blossomed in the eighteenth century, probably for material reasons such as the development of the postal service. It also became more common for the patients themselves to write the letters rather than to go through their ordinary physicians, perhaps because of the spread of medical knowledge among the lay public (see Brockliss and Jones 1997: 536).[2]

In the eighteenth century, some of the most respected physicians published their consultation letters, such as Friedrich Hoffmann (1660–1742) and Herman Boerhaave (1668–1738) (Hoffmann 1754–5; Boerhaave 1743). Other no less famous physicians, including Giovanni Battista Morgagni (1682–1771) and Théodore Tronchin (1709–81), had prepared their consultations for publication but died before they had time to publish them. In the Enlightenment, probably all physicians of a certain stature gave advice to sufferers they had never seen, and did so without any bad professional conscience.

Some historians of medicine have claimed that the widespread use of consultation by letter in the Enlightenment proves that at that time "physical examination . . . was quite secondary" (Porter 1993: 183; see also Nicolson 1993: 809). Yet the reading of such letters shows that very often the ordinary physicians, or the sufferers themselves, would not only communicate how the sufferers said they felt, but also the results of their physical examination. Hoffmann asked that the letters he received include, among other things, "the structure of [the sufferer's] body, the disposition of the vessels and the nerves, . . . the constitution of the parts [of the body], . . . the pulse, . . . whether the internal parts are not threatened by dangerous inflammations," etc. ([1734] 1754–5, 1: xj–xij). All this information required some kind of physical examination.

What is more, consultation at a distance was also practiced by those who could never avoid the materiality of the body: the surgeons. In his *Opuscules de chirurgie*, Sauveur-François Morand (1697–1773) explained that surgeons needed to be able to write correctly because they have to write consultation letters (1768, 1: 125–6). In order to help the countryside surgeons who did not have as much practice as surgeons in large cities, Henri-François Le Dran (1685–1770) wrote a book of fictional consultations in the form of a correspondence between a surgeon from the provinces and a surgeon from Paris. Even though the letters were not real, they were meant to represent a realistic situation (Le Dran 1765). Pierre Fabre (1716–93) transcribed real consultation letters in his *Traité des maladies vénériennes* because "they are paintings [*tableaux*] which make a much greater impression on the memory of young surgeons than the most extensive reasoning" ([1758] 1773: 50).

The publication of consultation letters was not thought to be a pompous display of theoretical knowledge. There could not be any work more *practical* than such books. A compilation of eight volumes of consultations from several physicians of the Montpellier school was "the treasure of the clinical practice of one of the most famous schools in Europe."[3] Referring to the consultations of Paul-Joseph Barthez (1734–1806), Jacques Lordat (1773–1870) thought that "if one could gather together all of them, they would constitute an almost complete

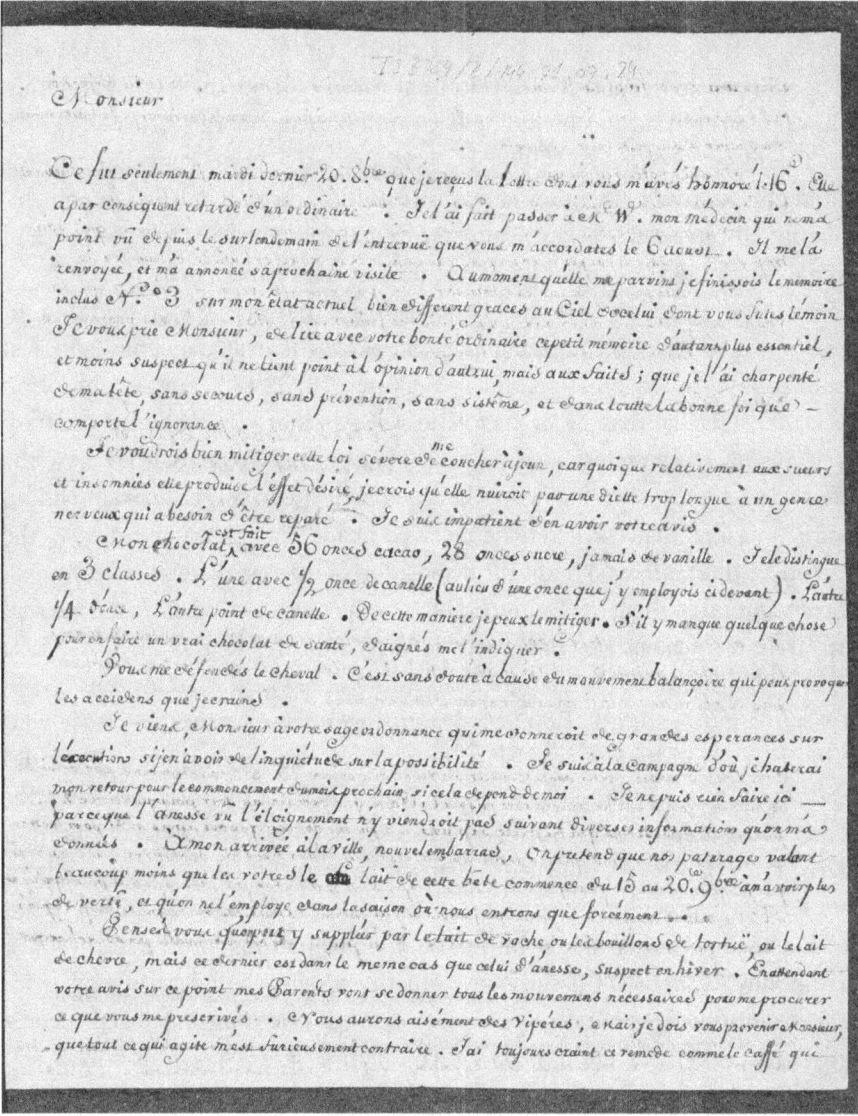

FIGURE 6.2: Two pages of a consultation letter from Lavergne l'aîné to Tissot, Lyon (France), October 25 [1772]. Bibliothèque cantonale et universitaire, Lausanne, Fonds Samuel-Auguste Tissot, 3784/II/144.01.07.24.

treatise of practical medicine, that would almost have the advantages of teaching at the bedside" (Lordat 1818: 98). What characterizes consultation by letter is not the absence of physical examination, but the possibility of its communicability.

The division of labor upon which the practice of consultation by letter rested was clear: the job of the writers of a consultation letter was limited to "a simple description," as the editor to the English edition of Boerhaave's *Consultationes* said (in Boerhaave 1745: 33, note a). Monsieur V., ordinary physician to Madame M., wrote a letter to Louis-Jean Le Thieullier (d. 1751) in which he said he "simply laid out" the symptoms, "without any reasoning, as it must be done when one writes to people of your rank" (Le Thieullier 1739–47, 2: 373). Nacquart went so far as to say that it was more difficult to write a good letter to a physician than for the latter to give his advice. Yet the difficulty should in principle be easy to overcome:

> In order to write well [the report on the sufferer], one would only need to transcribe what one had under the eyes, and to become the historian of the disorders which constitute the disease. But instead of a simple, faithful, bare report, one inserts commentaries and thoughts in every line; in general, one even says what one thought instead of what one saw. It matters much less to the physician to know what one has decided, than to have a material on which to establish his judgment.
>
> Nacquart 1813, 6: 38

Lurking in this comment is the accusation of spirit of system. In that respect, the less educated one was, the better. Zimmermann shared with his readers his experience with people of high intellect: "I have often been consulted by men of fine genius: all that I required of them, when they wrote to me, was, to give me pure and simple nature in their letters. I was sure it would be impossible to understand them, if they mixed any of their genius with their complaints" ([1764] 1778, 1: 161; see also Knott 2010: 664, on Benjamin Rush making a similar remark).

The sufferers very well understood that accuracy was on their side. They were the ones who could write "in all the good faith belonging to ignorance."[4] The ordinary physician, on the other hand, might already have an idea about the disease, and in his report would then "so well arrange the symptoms . . . that he forces the consulted physician to make the same mistake he made."[5] The parents of a young sick woman asked a friend of theirs to write to Tissot, because they knew that physicians "cannot help making their opinion known, and presenting things as they see them."[6] "I have expressed myself as I felt," said a sufferer, "whereas a professional physician [*homme de l'art*] would perhaps have written a report according to his ideas."[7] The disease belonged to the patient, and the ordinary physician was an intermediary that would only distort sensations he himself did not sense: "My disease is internal, only I can feel it; I also thought that only I could describe it."[8] Writing a letter of consultation required skills that were more negative than positive: it implied a restraint (of interpretation, of knowledge) more than any special ability.

Physical examination was often necessary, but, since the focus had to be on pathological facts that were easily perceptible (rather than on details that would have required special training to be perceived), there was no epistemological need for the consulted physician to see the patient with his own physical eyes or to touch him with his own hands. Others, including the sufferers themselves, could easily report to the remote physician what they felt with their fingers and saw with their eyes. Tronchin asked a patient to give him more information about the "gland on the bone of the leg" that this patient had described in a previous letter.[9] For another patient, he asked the ordinary physician "to press on the small lobe of the liver, when the patient lays on his back," in order to discover "the calculus concretion by the resistance one remarks and by the pain one causes."[10] A physician wrote to Tissot that "the sufferer has been palpated with attention, and we have not found any congestion in the region of the liver, nor pain or sensibility."[11]

As for the consulted physician, his job was the same as the one of a physician who would have been at his patient's bedside: to recognize the essence of a disease, visible by the eye of the mind after having been extracted from a collection of perceptions. The only difference is that the perceptions upon which his diagnosis was founded were second-hand. The editor of the posthumous letters by Barthez explained that the study of books of consultation letters had a goal that was "approximately the same as the one of clinical exercises," that is, "to learn to recognize, amidst the accidental symptoms, and despite the complications, the diseases of which one has read the history" (Lordat 1810, 1: 7). The editor of another edition of the same letters to and from Barthez advertised that "here . . . one contemplates with secret pleasure the physician whose trained sight and extensive gaze [*regard étendu*] glide over all the symptoms and sort out immediately the place and the cause of the lesion" (Saint-Ursin 1807, 1: xiv). This trained sight and this extensive gaze had never actually had the sufferers in front of them, but that did not matter: they were the sight and the gaze of the eye of the mind.

Medical consultation by letter was unproblematic in the eighteenth century because the physical distance between sufferers and consulted physicians was a continuation of the epistemological separation between the "botany of obvious perceptions" (directly accessible through the senses of anyone) and the diseases (only visible to the eye of the mind of expert physicians). The peculiar configuration of the experience of perception in the Enlightenment easily accommodated a practice like consultation by letter.

PERCUSSION OF THE CHEST

Percussion of the chest is a diagnostic technique that consists in tapping the chest with the fingers in order to elicit a sound that can reveal the presence of a disease inside. In the same way that the sound is different when one taps an empty barrel or a barrel with something in it, the chest sometimes emits a different sound when there is a disease in it or not. Unlike consultation by letter, percussion of the chest involves a direct contact between the fingers of the physician who diagnoses and the body of his patient. For this reason, this practice is sometimes described as being emblematic of nineteenth-century medicine. It was, however, invented in the middle of the eighteenth century. In 1761 Leopold Auenbrugger (1722–1809) published a short book in which he described this new diagnostic method (Auenbrugger 1761). Percussion became very popular after 1808, when Jean Nicolas Corvisart (1755–1821) translated Auenbrugger's book into French and added very extensive commentaries (Auenbrugger 1808; Corvisart 1808).

Before 1808, the interest in percussion of the chest seems to have been somewhat tepid. A progressive and representative eighteenth-century physician like Tissot, for instance, was only mildly enthusiastic about Auenbrugger's technique. In his *Avis au peuple sur sa santé* he mentioned percussion in passing, but added: "I doubt that this observation is generally true, and it would be dangerous to decide that there is no abscess in the chest, because the latter does not emit a muffled sound" (Tissot [1761] 1993: 90–1). Another sign

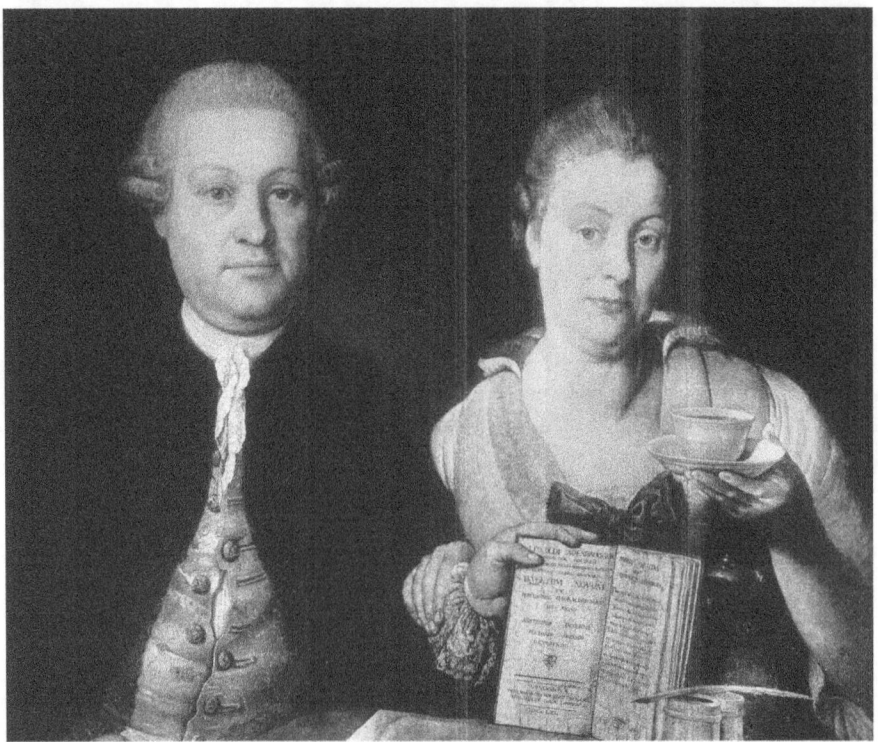

FIGURE 6.3: Leopold Auenbrugger and his wife. Photograph by V. A. Heck. Wellcome Library, London.

of the mild enthusiasm for percussion in the eighteenth century is that although Auenbrugger's book had been translated into French already in 1770, its translator, who was a physician, strangely confessed that he himself had not tried out Auenbrugger's technique (de la Chassagne 1770: 7).

A careful reading of Auenbrugger's book and a comparison with Corvisart's commentaries can help explain the historical fate of this book. More importantly, it can shed light on how physicians were supposed to use their senses in the Enlightenment. When one reads in parallel Auenbrugger's book and Corvisart's commentaries, a striking difference appears immediately: Auenbrugger never advises physicians to exercise their senses in order to practice percussion; Corvisart repeats it over and over again (Corvisart 1808: vii–x, 16, 31–2, 38 n. 1, 48, 90–1, 120, 130, 249–53, 260, 319, 328–9, 376, 425–6). John O'Neal has argued that "[w]hereas this injunction to use the senses is implicit in Auenbrugger's original text, it becomes explicit in Corvisart's translation" (O'Neal 1998: 484). But this interpretation makes Aueubrugger say what he never said, and fails to take into consideration the gap that exists, at the level of the experience of perception, between Auenbrugger and Corvisart.

Auenbrugger's silence as regards the training of the senses is not an oversight, but a direct consequence of the general eighteenth-century experience of perception. Auenbrugger did think that percussion of the chest required training, but what was to become sharper as a result of this training was not the senses, but the mind. He advised that physicians practice percussion on different individuals: "One must . . . percuss the thorax of many [healthy] individuals in order to know well the nature of the emitted sound, because of the different states of the body in diverse individuals" (Auenbrugger 1808: 28).[12] The function of the repetition of percussion is quite clear here. By listening to a multiplicity of different sounds that were, however, all coming from healthy chests, the physician learned to neutralize differences that were due to something other than a disease. An "obscurior sonus," for instance, could be heard in healthy individuals in the region of the heart and where there is a thick layer of muscles or fat, but also in patients suffering from nostalgia (1808: 14, 15, 171, 174); an "obtusior sonus" could be heard in healthy but fat people, as well as in patients suffering from dropsy of the pericardium (1808: 15, 400). In other words, the physician had to learn to sort out from the sound he heard what was accidental from what was essential, what was due to idiosyncratic but healthy characteristics from what was a true sign of disease. For Auenbrugger, training oneself in the practice of percussion of the chest had as its goal to form clear ideas of the sounds corresponding to essential diseases, in order to help distinguish later, in everyday practice, between the essential and the accidental. As a reviewer explained, this kind of exercise "is of a great usefulness for establishing a solid judgment" ("Review of *Nouvelle découverte de la percussion du thorax"* 1761: 109).

The exercise that Auenbrugger said was required was therefore of no help in perceiving small diseases. He for instance stated as a fact that "[p]ercussion cannot make one discover a slightly calloused lung, a small tumor," etc. (1808: 248). Corvisart interestingly commented on this concession, explaining that it depended on how well-trained one was in the practice of percussion: "The habit . . . of percussion must bring here remarkable modifications" (Corvisart 1808: 249). Corvisart was here introducing a new decisive factor: the sensitivity of the physician himself. Unlike Enlightenment physicians, their successors had to train their senses and learn to perceive better than the crowd.

Some historians have attempted to explain the lack of success of Auenbrugger's book in the eighteenth century by its concision. For instance, Stanley Joel Reiser claims that:

> Auenbrugger's treatise was too brief (only 95 pages in the original) to portray the specific differences in the percussive sounds that he claimed would allow physicians to discriminate among diseases. The delicate variation in sound that had to be distinguished to apply this technique was an obstacle to the learner, who required extensive explanations and examples to appreciate the shades of differences among the various possible sounds.
>
> Reiser 1978: 21

Reiser's point cannot really explain why it took so long—almost fifty years—before someone thought it was necessary to write long and detailed commentaries to Auenbrugger's *Inventum Novum*. The simplicity of Auenbrugger's opuscule must be taken at face value: Auenbrugger was simply not interested in the "delicate variation in sound" or the "shades of differences," and neither were his contemporaries. The goal for him was not to hear fine nuances of sounds, but to focus only on obvious sound differences, and to find, by an operation of the mind, the relations between these sounds and other obvious perceptions (like visible symptoms, palpable tumors, etc.), in order ultimately to reach a diagnosis.

Foucault thought that percussion was completely ignored in the eighteenth century, arguing that "[s]ounding by percussion is not justified if the disease is composed only of a web of symptoms" (Foucault 1994: 166). But since in the eighteenth century disease was not composed of a web of symptoms, but of a web of obvious perceptions, percussion could very well be used, on the condition that the sounds be obvious enough. When Auenbrugger heard a pathological sound, he heard one of the elements in the web of perceptions that pointed to a disease, and his diagnostic tool was therefore justified. Yet its importance was not paramount: in many cases the visible symptoms, the pulse, and other signs, were sufficient, while the sounds emitted by the chest were not clear and distinct enough. This is probably why eighteenth-century physicians showed a certain interest for percussion of the chest, but were never excessively enthusiastic. Auenbrugger himself ranked percussion under the taking of the pulse and the exploration of respiration as a means of finding the essence of a disease (Auenbrugger 1808: xxiv). As the first French translator of *Inventum Novum* said, percussion was "one more means that one can use, without any risk" (de la Chassagne 1770: 7).

PATHOLOGICAL ANATOMY

Pathological anatomy, like percussion of the chest and for the same reason, is often thought by historians to be antithetical to the eighteenth century. It is certainly true that pathological anatomy blossomed in the nineteenth century; but it nevertheless existed also in the Enlightenment, although it was structured in a specific way by the experience of perception of this period. In what follows I will focus on one disease, pulmonary phthisis, a common and dangerous disease in the eighteenth and nineteenth centuries (see Rey 1993).

Boissier de Sauvages is often thought of as a physician who was only interested in external symptoms, never in internal lesions. In his discussion of phthisis Sauvages listed the symptoms of this disease: "the emaciation of the body, with a slow fever, a cough, a breathing problem, and usually a spitting of pus" (1771, 3: 255). But he did not ignore organic lesions: "The opening of corpses reveals the lungs sprinkled with hard tubercles and diverse abscesses" (1771, 3: 256). He gave a list of twenty species of phthisis, of which only the last one is "deprived of ulcers in the lung." It was not, however, deprived of an organic cause, since "its cause is a white layer with which the lungs are usually covered after inflammation" (1771, 3: 267). Sauvages's senses penetrated inside the body.

Unlike Sauvages, Morgagni is supposed to be at the origin of modern medicine since he focused on organic lesions (see for instance Emch-Dériaz 1987: 146; Grmek 1991: 59–60, 69–70; Keel 2001: 184). Morgagni discussed phthisis in Letter XXII of his *De Sedibus et Causis Morborum* (1761), a letter that "treats of the hemoptœ [spitting of blood], of purulent and ill conditioned expectorations, the empyema [accumulation of pus in a cavity] and consumption [*phthisis*]" (1769, 1: 643). The common denominator of these diseases is a symptomatic similitude, not an organic lesion: the spitting or accumulation of

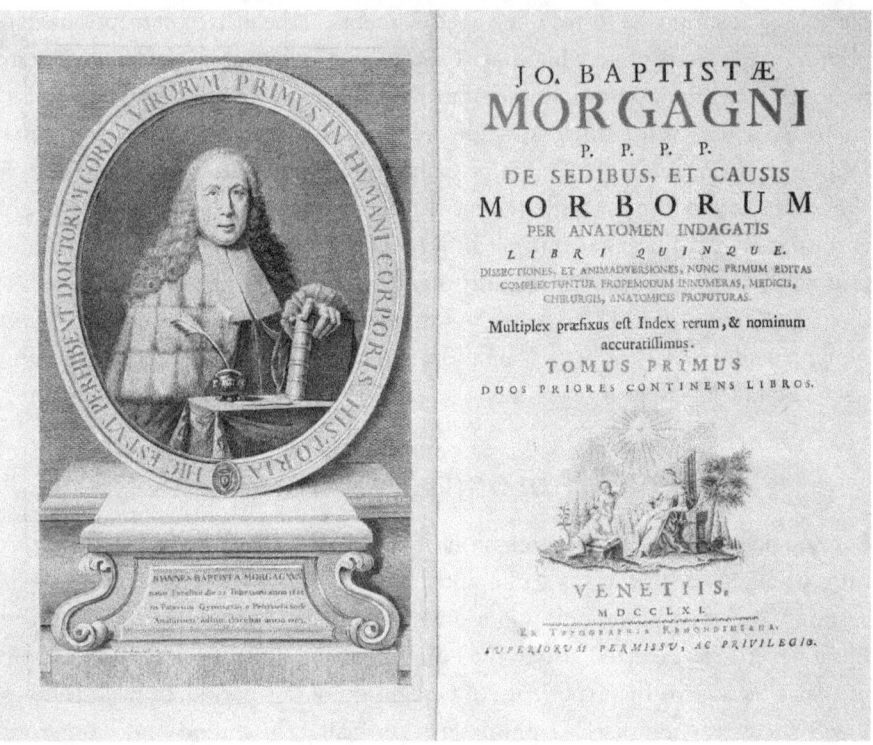

FIGURE 6.4: Title page and frontispiece with portrait of author. Giovanni Battista Morgagni, *De sedibus, et causis morborum* ... (Venice, 1761). Wellcome Library, London.

blood or pus. As regards phthisis, it is worth transcribing the entirety of one of Morgagni's cases. Typically, Morgagni began with a description of symptoms, most of which are the same as the ones offered by Sauvages:

> A strumpet, of about twenty years of age, had labored many months under a slow fever, a cough, an ill-conditioned expectoration, and a wasting of the whole body. She complained of a pain in the left part of the thorax, so that she could scarcely bear to lie down upon it. She was troubled with a difficulty of breathing. To which was added a copious spitting of blood: but this being checked, and two days after a south wind blowing hard, in which state of air those who labor under a similar disorder, for the most part, perish, death put an end to her disease.

After this description of symptoms, Morgagni turned to the description of the corpse. Here he provided more information than Sauvages:

The right lobe of the lungs adhered very little to the ribs. Both of them abounded with hard tubercles, which inclined to a white color, and resembled glandular bodies. Besides, the upper lobules of the lungs, on both sides, had other disorders in that upper part. For the right lobe, towards the sternum, contained a large hollow ulcer, and in this a purulent matter; but the left, towards the side, contained a hard substance, equal to the size of a large pear, which, in some measure, resembled the substance of the pancreas, when indurated; and in the middle of this substance was a small ulcer, full of pus. In the pericardium was a small quantity of serum: in the left ventricle of the heart was a small polypous concretion; in the right was one of a moderate size, the greater production of which was inserted into the neighboring auricle.

Morgagni 1769, 1: 654–5

Morgagni, like Sauvages, opened up corpses in order to find the "seats and causes of diseases," in other words the lesions that had caused the symptoms he had observed when the sufferer was alive. Obviously, these two physicians were committed to different projects: Sauvages wanted to build a nosology and his interest for lesions was only secondary, while Morgagni, without ever questioning the nosological knowledge of his time (Risse 1997, 2: 186), tried above all to find the possible organic causes of symptoms. But all the sick people suffering from phthisis, whether they were Morgagni's patients or Sauvages's, had similar symptoms: cough, spitting of blood or pus, fever, weakness. And almost all the corpses opened either by Morgagni or by Sauvages had tubercles in their lungs.

With his senses the physician could determine the location, size, color, and type of a lesion, but these perceptions were only some of the many elements that would enter into consideration for forming a diagnosis. A physician would also consider all the symptoms, the variety of sounds elicited by percussion of the chest, the different types of pulses, etc. The lesion that he could see with his eyes and touch with his fingers was a cause of disease, and for this reason it was diagnostically relevant, but it was not itself a disease.

Three important consequences follow. First, the same disease could be caused by different lesions, if these lesions caused enough similar symptoms. This is why neither Sauvages nor Morgagni thought that phthisis had to be caused necessarily by tubercles, even though this is what one could most often observe. Morgagni explained that "a pulmonary consumption [*phthisis pulmonaris*] may be brought on from other causes ... besides suppurated tubercles" (1769, 1: 660).[13] Second, and conversely, the same lesion could be found in different diseases, if enough symptoms were different. Finally, there could not be a disease if there were lesions but no symptoms.

The fact that some eighteenth-century physicians were more interested in opening corpses than others does not change the fact that their practice was governed by the same experience of perception. Sauvages's nosology was not in principle opposed to Morgagni's pathological anatomy, and there is in fact no doubt that Sauvages opened up many corpses. Philippe Pinel, who pursued Sauvages's nosological enterprise, also took into consideration organic lesions. In *La médecine clinique* his clinical cases typically begin with the history of the symptoms seen on the living patient, and end, if the patient died, with the description of what was found in his/her corpse (Pinel 1802). Morgagni's *De Sedibus* offered nothing else.

In the eighteenth century pathological anatomy was therefore welcome but not always necessary. It was welcome because it added more perceptible elements to the other elements from which the physician had to abstract diseases. But it was rarely necessary because the seat of diseases was usually not an essential part of their nature (see Foucault 1994: 8–9; Nicolson 1992: 109; Sauvages 1771, 1: 22–4). The ambivalent success of pathological anatomy in the eighteenth century mirrors the one of percussion of the chest.

Moreover, when enlightened physicians did quibble over pathological anatomy, it was not because they turned their eyes and hands away from bodies, preferring to build neat theories than to plunge their hands into nauseating corpses, but because the knowledge emerging from corpses was of dubious epistemological value. Lesions were problematic not because of their materiality but because of their indistinctness. Sauvages had said that physicians have to "deduce the characters of diseases from their constant phenomena and from their obvious symptoms" (1771, 1: 26). But what was observed in corpses was neither constant nor obvious. Johann Peter Frank (1745–1821) warned that when opening corpses "only the hand of the master will be able to avoid" taking the effects of diseases for their cause (1790: 35). There was also this important difficulty, which Morgagni had to address: "One can find in corpses . . . lesions that occurred only during or after death" (Morgagni 1820–4, 1: 60).[14]

Nineteenth-century physicians came to mock their predecessors for having been interested only in lesions that were "serious, visible, even extraordinary" (d'Amador 1837: 327). But this characteristic of Enlightenment pathological anatomy was not mere carelessness. It was the response to an epistemological requirement, which demanded that pathological facts be easily perceptible in order to be taken into account. Only big enough lesions could be safely counted among the pathological elements from which to deduce the species of a disease.

CONCLUSION

According to most textbooks on the history of modern medicine, consultation by letter was possible in the eighteenth century because physicians "relied heavily upon the patient's narrative as evidence." We are also told that it is "[t]he advent of pathological anatomy, auscultation, and the other techniques of physical diagnosis [that] changed this situation" (Reiser 1978: 196). This interpretation, which we have inherited from nineteenth-century positivism, rests on the common-sense opposition between heads and hands, theory and practice, or thinking and doing.

But this opposition is an inadequate lens for reading the history of medicine in the Enlightenment. Perception and the senses need to be historicized instead of being used as the markers of modern medicine. In the Enlightenment, consultation by letter, percussion of the chest, pathological anatomy, and many other practices were organized by the same experience of perception. This experience was transformed in the early nineteenth century, with a ripple effect on the practice of medicine (consultation by letter disappeared, pathological anatomy and percussion of the chest became quite different practices, etc.). Medicine did not go from a theoretical science in the eighteenth century to an empirical one in the nineteenth. Rather, the distinction between theory and practice is itself historically dated and cannot be applied to the Enlightenment without running the risk of anachronism. For Tissot, Auenbrugger, Morgagni, and their contemporaries, head and hand worked hand in hand.

CHAPTER SEVEN

The Senses in Literature: Pleasures of Imagining in Poetry and Prose

ROWAN ROSE BOYSON

Considering the role of the senses in literature invites a host of philosophical and historical questions. One might start by asserting that the indispensable tool of poems and novels is not scents or tastes or textures, but *words*. Literature, unlike sculpture and symphonies, is essentially immaterial, and it happens "in" the head. Yet such an assertion rests on covert historical assumptions, dating from the later Enlightenment: first, that one might naturally unify plays and poems and essays and novels, marked as "imaginative," through the category of literature, and second, that these literary products are predominantly experienced through silent and still reading. These assumptions have been questioned in recent years. In particular, book history has insisted that even silent reading requires a whole bodily repertoire of sensual practices: touching an embossed leather binding, squinting in candlelight, absorbing paper's sweet aroma (Price 2012). At the same time, literary critics have become increasingly aware of the way that eighteenth-century writers themselves reflected at length on how poems and fictions (and their siblings: painting, sculpture, theater) might stimulate or stymie the senses. Shaping the emerging literary domain and participating in a broader culture preoccupied with sensation and perception, Enlightenment writers went so far as to ask whether literary language might provide the condition for having any sensual experience at all.

This chapter traces some of the ways in which eighteenth-century writing discussed the senses, and it attempts to identify shifting tendencies towards and away from each of the senses. In the early eighteenth century, in line with dominant psychological theories, poems and plays were often understood to work by raising (visual) images in the mind. At the same time, whilst vision might be invoked as a kind of literal explanation for poetry's effects, "taste" had a huge significance as a metaphor for art and its appreciation. The dawn of aesthetics in this period, as a theory first of sensation in general, and then of art in particular, involved constant literary reflection on sensuality and about particular senses. Gradually a new parallel started to dominate aesthetic thought, the relation of poetry and music, wherein *sound* took on a new significance, particularly regarding the effects—cognitive and sensual—of meter, accent, performance, and rhyme. Sound came to be regarded as softening or disrupting visual forms of knowledge and communication, but this presupposes another breach: between science and clear vision on one side, and literature and the obscure on the other. Whilst this chapter focuses mainly on the discrete (biological) senses—indeed, the classical and medieval five-senses trope survived well into the late eighteenth century (Vinge 1975)—these five constantly flowed into and out of one another, and into their semantic relatives, *sensibility, sensuousness, sensationalism*. As Jane Austen intimated in her 1811 novel *Sense and Sensibility*, these words in this period were highly charged or "complex," as William Empson later described them (Empson [1951] 1995). The question of the specificity of sense-description versus broader ideas of "sensibility" was one that recurred throughout. Detailed sense-description could be a cause for literary disgust or celebration, whilst sometimes literature announced a desire to merge or blend sense impressions. Poetry is a particular focus of this chapter, being a form of writing that, perhaps more than any other, brings up issues of linguistic specificity and generality, and problematizes the distinction between description and lyric.

AUGUST AND DISGUSTED SENSES (*c.* 1670–1740)

The sensory deprivation caused by the 1666 London plague helped generate one of the first modern accounts of literature's ability to stir the senses. "Seeing then our Theatres shut up," wrote Dryden in the Preface to his *Essay of Dramatick Poesie* (1668), "I was engag'd in these kind of thoughts with the same delight with which men think upon their absent Mistresses" (Dryden 1971: 3). His *Essay* dramatizes four friends' arguments about the merits of drama, ancient versus modern, and French versus English, as they sit in a barge to escape an aural onslaught. "[T]he noise of the Cannon from both Navies reach'd our ears about the City: so that all men, being alarm'd with it ... went following the sound as his fancy led him" (Dryden 1971: 8). As they sail down the Thames, Eugenius, Crites, Lisideius, and Neander do not agree on much, but they do finally agree on what is "indeed rather a Description than a Definition" of a play: it "ought to be, *A just and lively Image of Humane Nature, representing its Passions and Humours, and the Changes of Fortune to which it is subject; for the Delight and Instruction of Mankind*" (Dryden 1971: 14–15). Dryden ushers in an Enlightenment of printed culture by extolling the poet's ability to provide a sensual truth and pleasure, a descriptive "liveliness" that may out-do reality itself: "The words of a good Writer which describe it lively, will make a deeper impression of belief in us than all the Actor can insinuate to us, when he seems to fall dead before us; as a Poet in the description of a beautiful Garden, or a Meadow, will please our imagination more than the place it self can please our sight" (Dryden 1971: 40). Neatly tied here with a semicolon are two aesthetic problems: the difference between what we see on the stage and what happens in our mind when we read, and the power of actual sights versus described sights. These two questions patterned many early eighteenth-century debates about poetry and drama, when a preoccupation with classical genre divisions and their rules came together with a preoccupation with the status of mental images in the new psychology that followed Locke. This blend of rules and psychology opens up an interesting paradox regarding the possibilities of sense-representation and sensuality in literature. On the one hand, the neoclassical turn away from the intricate conceits of Renaissance style, back to ancient conventions and a formal simplicity and calm, in some ways militated against sensuality, as did the strong theoretical preference for the "universal" and "typical" over the "particular." On the other hand, there was an enormous interest in how poetry and the other arts worked upon the senses, in relation to ancient sources and to the empiricist movement of late seventeenth-century psychology and natural philosophy. Arguably, in the hands of the great neoclassical critics René Le Bossu, Jean-Baptiste du Bos, and Nicolas Boileau in France, and John Dryden, John Dennis, and Joseph Addison in England, this duality brought "aesthetics" and even the category of "literature" slowly into existence.

In the quotation above, Dryden focuses upon the poet's ability to create "images." In considering the special importance of sight in this period, one must consider three words that launched a fleet of aesthetic treatises—*ut pictura poesis*, from Horace's *Ars poetica*. Usually translated as "as is painting so is poetry," this claim was also linked with another ancient commonplace attributed to Simonides, "poetry is a speaking picture, painting is mute poetry." Dryden's own contribution to this discussion was his introduction to his translation of the *Ars poetica*, "A parallel betwixt Poetry and Painting" (1695). One of the most influential *ut pictura poesis* treatises was Jean-Baptiste Du Bos' *Reflexions critiques sur la poésie et sur la peinture* (1719), which also raised the influential idea of a "sixth sense" on which critical judgments were based (Sambrook 2005: 111). These discussions were extended well into the eighteenth century, as for example in Charles Lamotte's *Essay upon Painting and Poetry* (1730), and James Harris' "Dialogue on Art" (1744) (Hagstrum 1958; Marshall 2005). In these treatises, an epistemological question (how do we perceive things in reality, and in imagination?) shaded into a literary question (how do we perceive things in imagination through poetry and fictions?). The conventional key terms of these accounts of description were always "strength," "liveliness," and "vividness."

David Hume argued in 1748 that "real" sense experience would always win out—"The most lively thought is still inferior to the dullest sensation" (Hume [1748] 1999: 96)—but earlier writers stressed that literary works could have an impact greater even than sensual existence. The essayist Joseph Addison commented, closely echoing Dryden, that "a Description often gives us more lively Ideas than the Sight of Things themselves" (Addison [1711–14] 1965, iii: 560). His major contribution to literary theory, the eleven-part *Pleasures of the Imagination* essay published in the *Spectator* in June and July 1712, began with an unabashed celebration of vision: "OUR Sight is the most perfect and most delightful of all our Senses. It fills the Mind with the largest Variety of Ideas, converses with its Objects at the greatest Distance, and continues the longest in Action without being tired or satiated with its proper Enjoyments" (1965, iii: 535–6). This focus on pleasure—and the effect of "Paintings, Statues, Descriptions, or any the like Occasion" on the reader's imagination and ideas—began to shut the door on the older rhetorical and persuasive models that had for so long dominated poetics (Addison 1965, iii: 537). Despite this emphasis on the centrality of (visual) "Images" in mental life, other senses were quickly brought into the analysis, implicitly acknowledging that the senses do not work in isolation. Within the first paragraph Addison redefines sight as "a more delicate and diffusive kind of Touch, that spreads it self over an infinite Multitude of Bodies" (1965, iii: 536), and later admits that sound or "a Fragrancy of Smells or Perfumes" could "heighten the Pleasures of the Imagination," working by helping us tune our attention into the scene (1965, iii: 544).

"Taste," not smell or sound, was however the key supporting sense for Addison and most other critics of the period. The operations of poetry were deemed to be "literally" involved with seeing, but taste rose to become the key "metaphorical" sense for art and writing. The link between physical "tasting" and an individual judgment of liking or disliking is longstanding in several languages: *de gustibus non est disputandam, chacun à son goût, sobre gustos no hay disputa* (Gigante 2005: 2). In *Spectator* 409, where Addison first promised his new theory of the pleasures of the imagination, the taste metaphor is acknowledged to be "general in all Tongues", but Addison claims his attempt to consider how writing affects "the Reader" as, in critical terms, "entirely new" (at least since Longinus) (Addison 1965, iii: 527, 530-1). And he was right: the idea that refined appreciation of poetry and the arts was based in a subjective, but potentially educable sense of "taste," which responded to the sublime, wonderful, and beautiful, was a source of proliferating and complex debate right up to and beyond Kant's great *Critique of Judgment* (1790). Perhaps the intellectual productivity of this idea was born of its paradoxical nature—how could this mark of cultural and even moral superiority be rooted in the damp feeling organ of the tongue? Many works of aesthetics trod a fine line to avoid taste's vulgar, bodily associations, like appetite and the distasteful, or *disgust* (Gigante 2005).

Whilst there is a traditional view of Augustan poetics as "hostile" to the senses, given its marked preference for generality over particularity (Damrosch 2005), the lower bodily senses nevertheless featured heavily in early eighteenth-century poetry. John Gay's and Jonathan Swift's poetry evokes the sights, sounds, and smells of cities, wine, and prostitutes. *Strephon and Chloe* (1734) is one of a number of "scatological" poems Swift wrote in his sixties, circulated in manuscript rather than addressed to a public, permitting indelicacy. Modeled on classical pastoral, the poem tells of the young swain Strephon's love for Chloe, a beautiful nymph, whose perfect *cleanliness* is stressed: "In Summer had she walk'd the Town / Her Arm-pits would not stain her Gown" (ll. 21-2). Strephon is full of nerves on their wedding night. Chloe pushes him away—because she has drunk too much tea, and quietly deploys a bed-pan. Strephon sniffs out this peccadillo, transforming his impression of his bride: "He found her, while the Scent increas'd / As *mortal* as himself at least" (ll. 185-6). The newly-weds soon cast off all embarrassment about bodily functions: they, "by the beastly way of Thinking, / Find great society in Stinking" (ll. 209-10). Prying in "The Lady's Dressing Room" (1732), Strephon shatters his own senses, first finding the magnifying glass that will help squeeze out the "smallest Worm in Celia's Nose" (l. 64), before experiencing the horrendous impact of her "reeking Chest":

> Thus finishing his grand Survey,—
> Disgusted *Strephon* stole away
> Repeating in his amorous Fits,
> Oh! *Celia, Celia, Celia* shits! (ll. 115–18)

The poet concludes that if Strephon would only *look* at his paramour, and "stop his Nose" (l. 136):

> He soon would learn to think like me,
> And bless his ravish't Sight to see
> Such Order from Confusion sprung,
> Such gaudy Tulips rais'd from Dung. (ll. 141–4)

Sight is the sense of "order" and perfection; smell is the sense of "confusion" and beastliness; in the grim slam of the final couplet, one of the oldest misogynistic arguments is sounded: woman is excrement (see Nussbaum 1984). Yet there is an interpretive challenge about the senses in satire: below the dirty jokes and apparent revulsion, is a deeper level of acceptance or pleasure announced? Swift's dark joke that Strephon and Chloe find "great society in Stinking" could be taken to imply the discovery of a level of true community underneath layers of social pretension. Adorno and Horkheimer, writing on the Enlightenment, argued that nasty jokes on stink involve a surreptitious enjoyment: the fantasy of the prohibited "mimesis," immersion in the earth and the other: "The prohibited impulse may be tolerated if there is no doubt that the final aim is its elimination—this is the case with jokes or fun, the miserable parody of fulfilment. As a despised and despising characteristic, the mimetic function is enjoyed craftily" (Adorno and Horkheimer [1944] 1997: 184).

Attending to Augustan poetics' avowed or explicit commitments, we might reframe the question not in terms of hostility to, or celebration of, the senses, but a search for the correct sensual proportion, informed by ideas about vision and "scope" emerging in natural philosophy and theology. The horrors of sensory magnification, the senses on the wrong scale, are well portrayed in Swift's *Gulliver's Travels* (1726), when Gulliver is repulsed by the intense smell and the coarse skin of the massive Brobdingnagians.

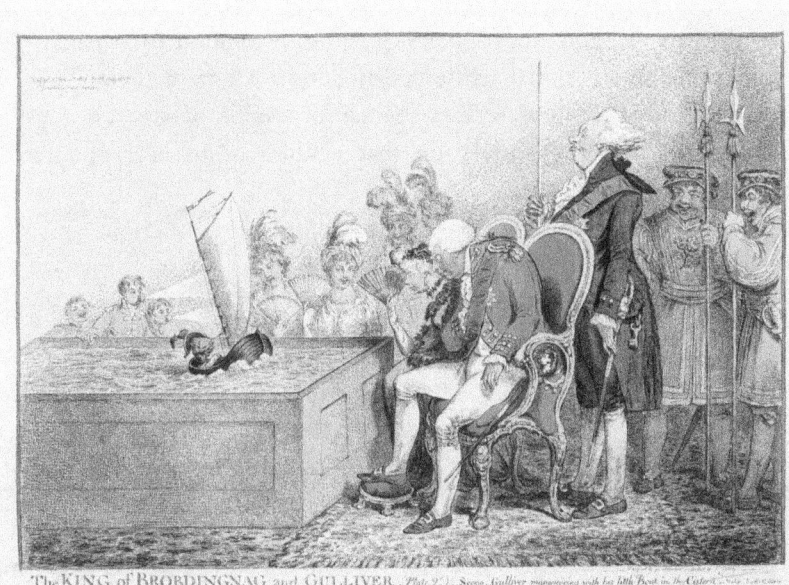

FIGURE 7.1: James Gillray, "The King of Brobdingnag and Gulliver" (1804). Credit: Victoria and Albert Museum. Swift's play with sensory scale remained a fertile ground for satirists over the coming century, as seen in Gillray's Swiftian caricature of George IV and Napoleon.

In Pope's *Essay on Man* (1733–4), the senses are the route to the appreciation of the divinely ordered cosmos, but again they must be correctly scaled:

Why has not Man a microscopic eye?
For this plain reason, Man is not a Fly.
Say what the use, were finer optics giv'n,
T'inspect a mite, not comprehend the heav'n?
Or touch, if tremblingly alive all o'er,
To smart and agonize at ev'ry pore?
Or quick effluvia darting thro' the brain,
Die of a rose in aromatic pain? (Epistle I, ll. 193–200)

This famous mockery of a sensitivity so acute it might suffer "aromatic pain" soon seemed somewhat outdated, if still funny, given the dramatic cultural transvaluation of sensibility in coming decades. Yet Pope himself hardly failed to recognize that poetry is the transcription of sensuality into words, noting, "What thin partitions Sense from Thought divide" (l. 226). In another passage, Pope describes the sensory skills of creatures, using a meta-poetic and multi-sensorial pun that enables us to hear and feel the senses in the "line":

> The spider's touch, how exquisitely fine!
> Feels at each thread, and lives along the line (ll. 217–18)

QUESTIONING VISION AND THE TURN TO DARKNESS (c. 1730–70)

A kind of "microscopic" perspective was much more positively considered from the 1730s onwards. James Thomson's *Seasons* (1727–30) used an Augustan refined poetic lens on a Newtonian, scientific cosmos. In this and other mid-eighteenth century poems of place and space (loco-descriptive and georgic), sight is the triumphant literary sense, in line with Addison's earlier arguments about sight as the chief source of "pleasures of the imagination." This accords with the broader status of vision in the Enlightenment, through which (as many twentieth-century scholars argued) a natural-philosophical confidence about man's powers to explore the universe became tied to ideological "ways of seeing," asserting ownership and control over land and populations (Barrell 1988; Foucault 1966). But the working of sensual "description" is complicated when taking poetic form: consider this audaciously close-up, almost impolite account of God's role in plant growth:

> By Thee the various vegetative Tribes,
> Wrapt in a filmy Net, and glad with Leaves,
> Draw the live Ether, and imbibe the Dew:
> By Thee dispos'd into congenial Soils,
> Stands each attractive Plant, and sucks, and swells
> The juicy Tide: a twining Mass of Tubes.
>
> Thomson 1972, Spring, ll. 561–6

This ugly-lovely sensory descent into soil and roots has, however, a fantastical, impossible quality. We are not actually "sensing" it but imagining it (Spacks 2009: 47). Thomson repeatedly plays with poetic limits, tempting us to call up "Infinite numbers, delicacies, smells, / With hues on hues expression cannot paint" (ll. 553–4), inviting us to "See" broad beautiful vistas, then suddenly reminding us that we are not present but reading, and of the inferiority of this experience (and his writing) to God's creation.

Mark Akenside's *The Pleasures of the Imagination* (1744) displays a similar push-pull relationship to sense description. The rich yet delicate sensuality in this poem is less insistently visual than in Thomson. It draws on a language of blooming, breathing, quickness, and thrilling, reflecting both the preponderance of flowers in the verse as well as Akenside's medical training in the new sciences of nerves and vitality. Consider this account of the senses:

> So the glad impulse of congenial powers,
> Or of sweet sound, or fair-proportion'd form,
> The grace of motion, or the bloom of light,
> Thrills thro' imagination's tender frame,
> From nerve to nerve: all naked and alive
> They catch the spreading rays . . . (I, ll. 116–21)

These lines portray sense-experience as intrinsically pleasurable, tactile, and almost erotic. Akenside's "Design" for the poem first sets out a psychological-anthropological account of poetry as a kind of bridge between the senses and morality. Lying between the "organs of bodily sense" and the "faculties of moral perception," the Powers of Imagination are "inlets of some of the most exquisite pleasures we are acquainted with" (Akenside 1857: 1). They had led "warm and sensible" men to try to find ways of "recalling" these delights—through painting, sculpture, music, and poetry (1857: 1). This complex relation between sense, imagination and morality leads to a later point in the poem when sound and taste are diminished in favor of a metaphorical or inward "sense": knowledge.

> . . . the beams of Truth
> More welcome touch his understanding's eye,
> Than all the blandishments of sound, his ear,
> Than all of taste his tongue. (II, ll. 100–3)

Knowledge, or "Science," which comes from and relates to God, is required to fully appreciate the perception of "the melting rainbow's vernal-tinctur'd hues" (II, l. 106, l. 104). In a virtuous circle, sense-pleasure indicates health and bodily wholeness: "The bloom of nectar'd fruitage ripe to sense, / And every charm of animated things, / Are only pledges of a state sincere" (I, ll. 367–9).

Sonically juicy with consonants, plosives and puns, this description generates synaesthetic pleasure of its own, and in so doing points up the moral (later adapted by Wordsworth and Keats) that "truth and good are one, / And beauty dwells in them, and they in her" (I, ll. 374–5).

Whilst Akenside purports to show that sensory pleasure in nature (rather than idle, "luxurious pleasure," I, l. 418) is healthful and God-given, an ambivalence or admonition about the secular pleasures of the senses was a theme of other writing of the mid century, and contributed to a subtle shift away from "sight" towards new ideals of obscurity and sublimity. Edward Young's *Night Thoughts* (1742–62) explicitly rejects the clarity of neoclassical light (Young [1742–5] 2008: 1). This sequence of long, personal, Christian meditations begins in a night-time waking state, and invokes not music or light for assistance but "*Silence,* and *Darkness!* Solemn Sisters!" (l. 28). For Young, only in solitary dark night can the individual imagination explore its place in the universe and man's eternal destiny: otherwise "In Sense dark-prison'd all that ought to soar" (2008, 60, II: 344). *Night III* presents the view that the senses offer not wonderful "particularity" or "difference" (as modern theories of the senses may claim) but only deadly sameness:

> A languid, leaden iteration reigns,
> And ever must o'er those, whose joys are joys
> Of sights, smell, taste: the cuckoo-seasons sing
> The same dull note to such as nothing prize,
> But what those seasons, from the teeming earth
> To doating sense indulge. But nobler minds,
> Which relish fruits unripen'd by the sun,
> Make their days various; various as the dyes
> On the dove's neck, which wanton in his rays.
>   Young 2008: 82–3, III, ll. 373–81

This is a performatively brilliant passage, in which prosody and diction enriches and complicates the basic didactic claim about the inferiority of sensual pleasure compared to mental or imaginative forms. The analogy between sensuality and overripe fruit in line 379 (possibly borrowed from Akenside), is anticipated by a pun on "must" in line 374, which leaves a damp, moldy aroma at the edges of our attention. Subtle colors (pale shades, dove-grey) and sounds (the half-rhyme of dyes / rays) also show the inevitability of the invocation of sensation, whilst asserting the power of "imagination" in poetic form to provide a "noble" and yet intense pleasure of its own.

The sublime, that central eighteenth-century aesthetic category and landscape style, had strong associations with both light and dark. In the French critic Boileau's groundbreaking translation (1657) of Longinus' ancient treatise *Peri hypsous*, the central example of sublimity was Moses' *fiat lux* (let there be light). By the middle of the century, and most notably in Burke's *Philosophical Enquiry into the origins of Our Ideas of the Sublime and the Beautiful* (1757), the sublime was linked to obscurity and darkness. Whilst it was linked to "sensationist" epistemology, it was ultimately a doctrine that could be said to go so far into the senses that it exploded them into something larger (Lamb 2005). "Vast Objects occasion vast Sensations, and vast Sensations give the Mind a higher Idea of her own Powers," wrote John Baillie in his 1747 *Essay on the Sublime* (Ashfield and De Bolla 1996: 89). The discourse of the sublime was influenced by both secular and religious debates, from nerve physiology to biblical and Judaic scholarship stressing the significance of music for a culture that prohibited images (for instance, Robert Lowth's influential 1753 *Lectures on Sacred Hebrew Poetry*).

The desire that literature should "return" to a more primitive or pure state of musicality was frequently voiced, offering an example of how ideas about the senses create and reshape literary genres. The mid-century emphasis on the indissolubility of poetry and music may be understood in terms of the "gradual ascendancy of the lyric" over this period (Keach 2005: 121). However, the ancient connection between poetry and song had never exactly been forgotten. For instance, it was made explicit throughout the whole period in a number of celebrated odes written for the feast of St. Cecilia, patron saint of church music. William Collins' 1747 "The Passions: An Ode for Music" joins that tradition, but pleads directly to Music, "Why, Goddess, why to us deny'd? / Lay'st Thou thy antient Lyre aside?" In the poetic climax where personified Joy plays Music's lyre, the half-erotic experience of sound is supplemented with a non-visual sensation, scent:

> While, as his flying fingers kiss'd the strings,
> Love fram'd with Mirth a gay fantastic round:
> Loose were her tresses seen, her zone unbound;
>   And he, amidst his frolic play,
>   As if he would the charming air repay,
> Shook thousand odours from his dewy wings.

One critic has recently argued that Collins performs Music's "return" to modernity, by using complex metrics and stanzaic patterning to generate ideas other than visual ones; the poem works in ways that are not only pictorializing or mimetic (Jarvis 2010).

A focus on *not*-showing, not-pictorializing, meant a revivification of the earlier *ut pictura poesis* debates about the relation of poetry and painting, in which painting had previously won out. Now poets were exhorted—notoriously by Diderot in the *Salon de 1767*—"Soyez ténébreux!" (Be obscure!: Diderot 1975: 147). The tide's turn against visuality was marked by Gotthold Ephraim Lessing's *Laokoon oder über die Grenzen der Malerei und Poesie* (*Laocoön: an essay upon the limits of painting and poetry*, 1766). Lessing's essay begins by analyzing the Laocoön sculpture's representation of the agony of the Trojan priest as he and his sons are attacked by sea serpents sent in revenge by Dionysus. From conversational beginnings, the essay builds up to the major theoretical claim that poetry and painting have different modes of operation: painting works in space, and poetry in time. Poetry works centrally through characterization and emotional effect; thus long passages of description are both tedious and practically ineffective. As René Wellek summarized approvingly: "Lessing is certainly putting his finger on the issue when he points to the difficulty of our forming a whole from an accumulation of traits ... Literature does not evoke sensuous images, or if it does, does so only incidentally, occasionally and intermittently" (Wellek [1965] 1983: 163). Against the idea that we could recreate the *Iliad* and *Odyssey* from "pictures" based on Homer's descriptions, Lessing attended to the tropes of "mist and darkness," and praised the non-visual imaginative procedure of the blind Milton's *Paradise Lost* (Lessing [1766] 1985: 94, 97). He criticized the "rage for description" in poetry, borrowing from Pope's editor Warburton to call such long poems a "dinner of nothing but soup" (Lessing [1766] 1985: 59, 106).

Though such ideas probably contributed to the revival of drama among young German writers as well as to the lyric surge, they did not put an end to questions and practices of description in writing. Thomson's *Seasons* were translated into French in 1759, influencing Jacques Delille's *Georgiques* (1760) and his later *L'homme des champs* (1800). George-Louis Leclerc de Buffon and the French *encyclopédistes* made descriptive language a major theme, because of its centrality to epistemological and methodological problems. They discussed style and the history of poetics as much as animals and rocks. Natural historians grappled with the uses of sensuality to "describe" the creatures and objects of the world. The question of how language can paint "in the mind's eye" continued to haunt all manner of literary and scientific writing (Stalnaker 2010; Wall 2006).

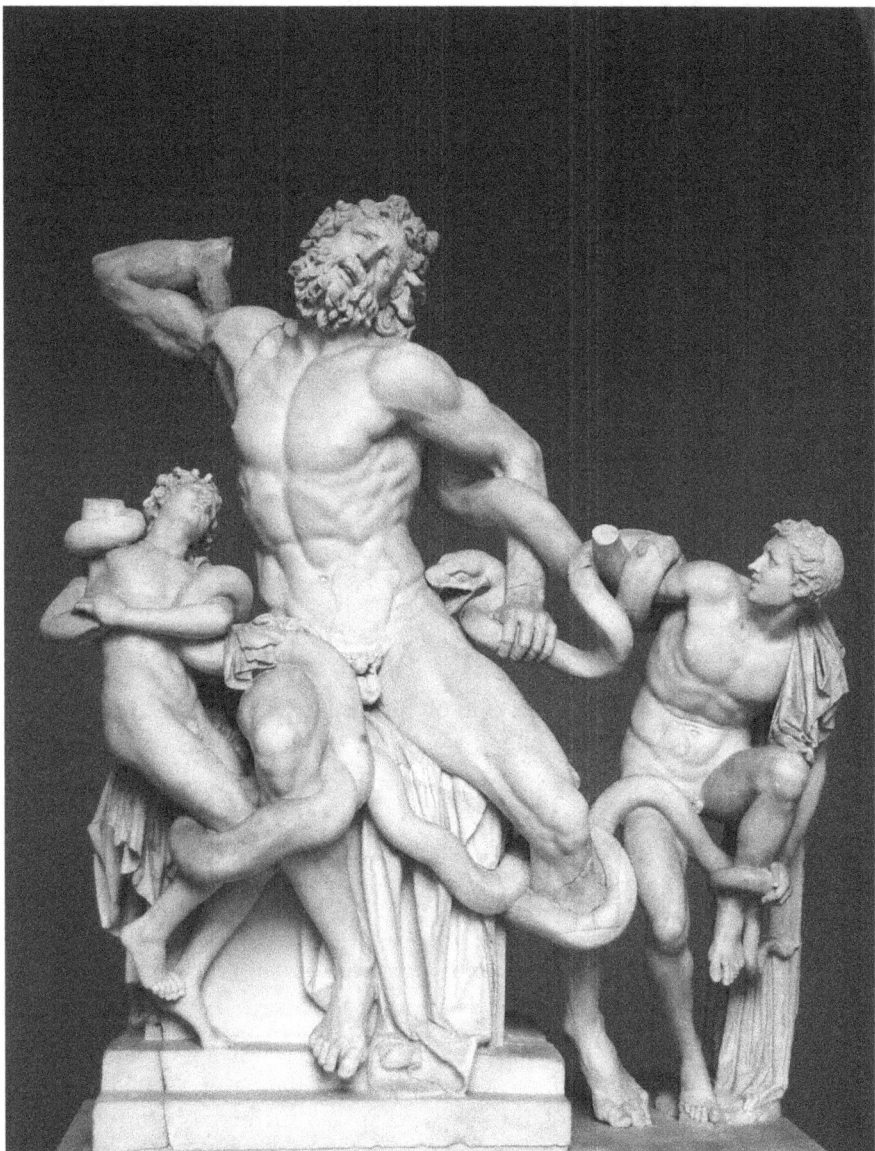

FIGURE 7.2: *Laocoön and His Sons*. Vatican Museum, Rome. Photograph: Dom Crossley (November 14, 2009). This monumental Roman sculpture, unearthed in 1506 and acquired by Pope Julius II, exerted enormous influence over Renaissance sculpture and later aesthetic theory.

SENSITIVITY AND SADISM (c. 1760–90)

Lessing's focus on pain and emotion in the Laocoön sculpture may be set alongside a major innovation of the mid eighteenth century: the cult of "sensibility," which was at once of, and not of, the senses. Some proponents of sensibility, especially those in Britain, sought to evade the sexual, mechanistic, even atheistic connotations of sensuality. Yet sensibility was associated with a heightened susceptibility to sense impressions, and had a bodily repertoire: blushing, fainting, crying, delicate appetite, slenderness, eroticism. Sensibility presents an interesting continuation of the shift from visuality towards obscurity and ineffability, and from clear and distinct senses towards their melding. Earlier we saw how Pope mocked the idea of a person so "tremblingly alive all o'er" that they would "smart and agonize at ev'ry pore," but already in Akenside we witnessed a more positive description of sound and motion "thrilling" from "nerve to nerve." Scholars have detailed the factors behind the rise of sensibility, particularly the new physiology of the nerves that can be dated to Isaac Newton's widely-read *Opticks* (1704) (Barker-Benfield 1992; Vila 1998). Newton speculated that light rays caused vibrations that traveled through the nerves into the brain and created the sensation of seeing, and thus, in a way, reframed "seeing" as a kind of "touching." Touch was the dominant sense and metaphor of sensibility, for it involved both notions of sympathetic human connection, and the sexual frisson that secretly ran through this ostensibly moral cult.

Sensibility was closely connected to a parallel literary innovation. The immense popularity of epistolary novels, beginning in the 1680s, reaching their height in the 1740s and enduring until the mid-1780s, reflected and generated new medical-moral theories around sensitivity as an indicator of moral refinement and virtue. Compared to the romance, the novel's generic predecessor, these purportedly real collections of "letters" between lovers and friends were built on notions of authenticity and intimacy. Sensibility was a quality of feeling and emotional response that was attributed both to fictional characters (pretty young women, troubled rakes), and to readers (increasingly female, as female literacy and authorship soared, but also male). Novels were meant to instruct their readers in propriety and sympathy, but they also risked inflaming them through scenes of high emotion and sexual trespass. Samuel Richardson's *Pamela, or virtue rewarded* (1740) presented the letters of a young maidservant who details her attempts to fend off the sexual advances of her master. Richardson's "Preface" promised moral instruction "*in so probable, so natural, so* lively *a manner, as shall engage the Passions of every sensible*

Reader ... without raising a single Idea *throughout the Whole, that shall shock the exactest Purity, even in those tender instances where the exactest Purity would be most apprehensive"* (Richardson [1740] 2011: 3). The "touching" (arousing) qualities of this fiction were highlighted by one Parson Tickletext in Henry Fielding's spoof, *Shamela* (1741). The sensory nature of words themselves was brilliantly explored in Laurence Sterne's own form of tickletext, the novel *Tristram Shandy* (1759–67), which used print to evoke sound and motion: famously, the whistling of Lillabullero and a cane sweeping through air (Tadié 2001).

Novel reading as a phenomenon helped elaborate the concept of sympathy in Scottish philosophy of the 1740s and 1750s, for example in David Hume's *Treatise of Human Nature* (1739–40) and Adam Smith's *Theory of Moral Sentiments* (1759). The "hard" senses of empiricism, associated with self-interest and skepticism, were transfigured into more ethereal "inner senses," "sixth" or "seventh" senses, or "internal senses" in Alexander Gerard's *Essay on Taste* (1759), following on from Francis Hutcheson's similar aesthetic-moral philosophy. Edmund Burke's essay on "On Taste," appended to the *Philosophical Enquiry into the Origin of our Ideas of the Sublime and Beautiful* (1757) made close, careful distinctions between the "senses" of men, which they shared and agreed upon, and their imaginations or "sensibilities," which might differ and be trained. In France, ideas of sensibility bloomed in a number of philosophical and literary texts, though the line separating sensibility from "sensationalism" and "materialism" was even finer than in England. The radical materialist and hedonist Julien Offray de La Mettrie virulently defended the senses as the only route to knowledge in *Traité de l'âme* (1745), and *L'homme machine* (1747), whilst Diderot explored the different qualities of the senses in the *Lettre sur les aveugles* (1749) and the *Lettre sur les sourds et muets* (1751) (Goodden 2001).

Rousseau's diverse writings emphasized experience rooted in "real" or "natural" senses rather than imagination, which, he (sometimes) argued, generated self-importance and insecurity. In the *Lettre à M. d'Alembert sur les spectacles* (1758), Rousseau decried theater's ability to inflame the imagination and generate sympathy with the unjust. In his educational treatise *Emile* (1760) he advised that the child should be protected from all novels until at least twelve, with the exception of *Robinson Crusoe* (which would teach Emile self-sufficiency). Yet his own novel, the runaway bestseller *Julie, ou la nouvelle Hélöise* (1761), was notorious for its addictive, imaginative impact. Julie herself is an ideal figure of sensibility, first as ardent and adored pupil of Saint-Preux, then as loving wife of Wolmar and mother of children. In that role she offers moderate delights to Saint-Preux—delicious suppers of local fish, soft cheeses, fresh greens and cakes, walks in her garden—meant to re-educate and reform his senses, enabling him to achieve personal and political renovation away from his destructive passion for Julie. Yet, the novel's ending, returning to the passion and fantasy of the two lovers, is ambiguous, suggesting the philosophical difficulties of identifying a "natural" experience of the senses free of imagination and language.

The sexual and philosophical side of sensibility and the senses continued to shape genres and aesthetic theories as well as contributing to the intellectual ferment of the French Revolution. The gentle titillations of "touch" in Richardson and Rousseau were sent in explicit, and often violent, directions with new libertine novels of sex and cruelty, such as Choderlos de Laclos' *Les Liaisons dangereuses* (1782). The gothic, pornographic novels of the Marquis de Sade, including *Justine* (1791) and *Juliette* (1797), turned the mid-century sentimental narrative of the young girl's "virtue" inside out, through thematizing the pursuit of pleasure, including via pain. In Britain, libertinism was present in milder vein in the learned doctor Erasmus Darwin's erotic-scientific poetry, often mocked, yet innovative and influential. Darwin's enthusiasm for new discoveries in botany, geology, and chemistry led him to produce didactic, encyclopedic poetry in neoclassical style. Floral scents described in "The Economy of Vegetation" (1791) are pleasurable but also insect-attracting: the biological purpose of the senses was Darwin's focus. "Nature may seem to have been niggardly to mankind in bestowing upon them so few senses, since a sense to have perceived electricity, and another to have perceived magnetism might have been of great service to them, many ages before these fluids were discovered by accidental experiment" (Canto I, Note to l.365). The idea of human progress as involving the expansion of the sensorium was one that recurred in Romantic and post-Romantic philosophy up to Marx.

"Sensibility" and "sensationalism" caused counter-reactions amongst both conservative and radical writers, particularly when it came to the question of woman, for whilst sensibility gave greater prominence to women's experience and women writers it also created an increasingly rigid ideal of womanhood, focused on the purported delicacy of their bodies. Mary Wollstonecraft powerfully denounced the reductive and irreligious association of women with the mere senses in her *Vindication of the Rights of Woman* (1792). Offering a kind of socio-biological analysis, Wollstonecraft claimed in Chapter 4 that women's "senses are inflamed, and their understandings neglected, consequently they become the prey of their senses, delicately termed sensibility, and are blown

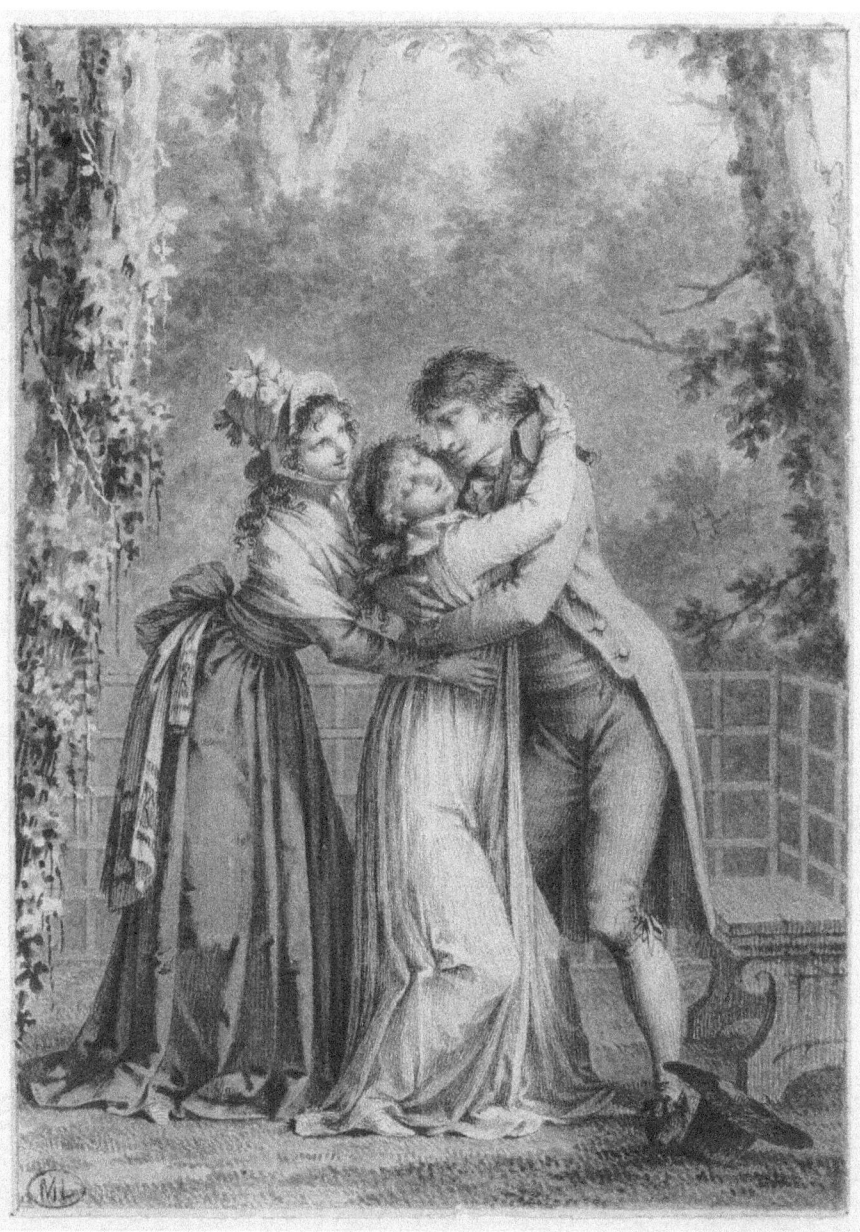

FIGURE 7.3: Pierre-Paul Prud'hon's "Le premier baiser de l'amour," ink and wash drawing (11.3 × 8.2 cm) produced between 1792–6 and engraved to illustrate an 1804 edition of Rousseau's *La nouvelle Héloïse*. Credit: Musée du Louvre, département des Arts graphiques, photographed by RMN. The novel's scene of Julie's fainting after first being kissed by Saint-Preux was particularly famous, and this later portrayal by the Romantic artist Prud'hon emphasizes through close physical touch the erotic bonds of sensibility uniting Julie, Saint-Preux, and Claire.

about by every momentary gust of feeling" (Wollstonecraft [1792] 1995: 136). Rousseau was both her hero and antagonist in this account, for she agreed that the healthy well-being of the body was a condition of equal social relations. Her novel *The Wrongs of Woman*, for instance, celebrates sensual experience, so long as it is based in "nature" (the scent of flowers and fresh air) rather than fashion and artifice, and is balanced by rationality. There are some similarities with the way Jane Austen satirically ranged "sensibility" against (good) "sense" in her novel of 1811, *Sense and Sensibility*, though in Austen's writing "sense" usually carries its old, metaphorical meaning, of practical, shared, or tacit understanding (Empson [1951] 1995: 306–10; Heller-Roazen 2007).

The status of woman was also a trigger issue for William Blake's critique of reductionist sensualism. His *Visions of the Daughters of Albion* (1793) echoes Edward Young's ideas about the way sensualism might restrict or limit a broader imaginative or spiritual existence, but goes further in linking scientific concepts and power relations. His character Oothoon, raped by Bromion, laments the doctrine of the five senses:

> They told me that the night & day were all that I could see;
> They told me that I had five senses to inclose me up.
> And they inclos'd my infinite brain into a narrow circle. (Plate 2, ll. 30–2)

She demands to know how the infinitely various modes of experience can be reduced to a five-senses categorization:

> With what sense does the bee form cells? have not the mouse & frog
> Eyes and ears and sense of touch? yet are their habitations
> And their pursuits, as different as their forms and as their joys.
>   (Plate 3, ll. 1–6)

SENSUAL AMBIENCE (*c.* 1790–1810)

Retrospective definitions of Romanticism (for it was not a term employed by the English writers under discussion) have either admired its attempt to render the particularity of sensual experience, or alternatively attacked its sensuality as effeminate or immoral (Babbitt 1919). Yet what, if anything, was distinctive about literary references to the senses around and after 1790? As this chapter has shown, the verse of Pope, Young, and Collins may be seen to possess the "lyrical," sensuous qualities often thought of as "Romantic," whilst critiques of "sensualism" appear in many later writers, including Blake and Coleridge.

Three ideas may be considered: a political slant to sensation; a more explicit relation to scientific practices and languages, especially of experiment and chemistry; and what has often been called a "subjective" turn in philosophy, which had many poetic parallels. The familiar yet indispensable "Preface" to Wordsworth and Coleridge's *Lyrical Ballads* gives a first route into these aspects of Romantic-period senses. Though their literary manifesto mostly uses the word "sense" in that Austenite notion of good sense, or for poetic meaning, plural "senses" sometimes appear: "The objects of the Poet's thoughts are every where; though the eyes and senses of man are, it is true, his favourite guides, yet he will follow wheresoer he can find an atmosphere of sensation in which to move his wings" (Wordsworth [1850] 1974: 167). This seemingly accidental distinction between vision and the other senses is developed explicitly in Wordsworth's *Prelude*:

> I speak in recollection of a time
> When the bodily eye, in every stage of life
> The most despotic of our senses, gained
> Such strength in *me* as often held my mind
> In absolute dominion. Gladly here,
> Entering upon abstruser argument,
> Could I endeavour to unfold the means
> Which Nature studiously employs to thwart
> This tyranny, summons all the senses each
> To counteract the other, and themselves,
> And makes them all, and the objects with which all
> Are conversant, subservient in their turn
> To the great ends of Liberty and Power.
> But leave we this: enough that my delights
> (Such as they were) were sought insatiably.
>   Wordsworth [c. 1805] 1979, XII, ll. 127–41

There are echoes here of the earlier eighteenth-century poetic turn against visuality, though the senses themselves are not rejected as irreligiously corporeal; rather, they are presented as working in a kind of harmonious opposition or tension (Potkay 2011), and "subservient" to "Liberty and Power." That these political abstractions, rather than religion, are the framework for understanding the senses, indicates poetry's shifting ethical impulse in this period; however, the final emphasis on pleasure is consistent with many of the earlier texts discussed in this chapter (Boyson 2012).

Another characteristic aspect of Wordsworth's treatment of the "senses" is their expansion into the broader term "sensation," as in the "Preface" passage quoted above. Numerous examples of this broader notion of corporeal sense appear in Wordsworth's writing: "Those hallowed and pure motions of the sense" (*Prelude* I.551); "those obstinate questionings / Of sense and outward things" in the "Immortality Ode" (see Empson [1951] 1995: 289–385).

Looking back in 1832, Coleridge stressed the humanist nature of Wordsworth's sensuous poetics: "He was to treat man as man, a subject of eye, ear, touch and taste in contact with external nature, and inferring the senses from the mind, and not compounding a mind out of the senses" (Coleridge [1835] 1990, II: 177). Coleridge's view of the senses was on guard against materialism and skepticism, yet, as a great Romantic-era polymath, he was nonetheless enormously interested in the science of perception. He conducted numerous sensory self-experiments, noting carefully around 1801: "A dunghill at a distance sometimes smells like musk, & a dead dog like elder-flowers"; a shade of green "actually *grew* to my eye in a beautiful moss, the same that is on the mantle-piece in Grasmere" (Coleridge [1801] 1957, i: 223, 925). Wordsworth entreated Coleridge to stop "the multitude of minute experiments with Light & Figure" which was making him "nervous & feverish" (Vickers 2004: 109). Such self-experimentation is one context for the exquisite complaint in "Dejection: An Ode" (1802):

> All this long eve, so balmy and serene,
> Have I been gazing on the western sky,
> And its peculiar tint of yellow green:
> And still I gaze—and with how blank an eye!

His deadly lack of emotional response is coded in terms of tactility: the clouds, stars, and moon do not touch him: "I see, not feel, how beautiful they are!" The revelation of the failed experiment, and the route to Coleridge's recovery of "joy," is that perception is not merely objective or material but comes from "within": "We in ourselves rejoice! / And thence flows all that charms our ear or sight."

Numerous contemporary philosophical arguments for the internality or subjectivity of perception lend support to an interpretation of Coleridge's poem as aiming to recover sense perception as active rather than mechanical or passive (Crary 1990). Kant's critical project of the 1780s re-emphasized the individual perceiving *subject* and his or her cognitive faculties as the conditions of possibility for all experience. The French sensualist philosopher Maine de Biran, writing at the turn of the century, argued for the active, attentive dimension of perception. In Germany, the poet, novelist, and philosopher J. W. Goethe emphasized the emotional and sensual importance

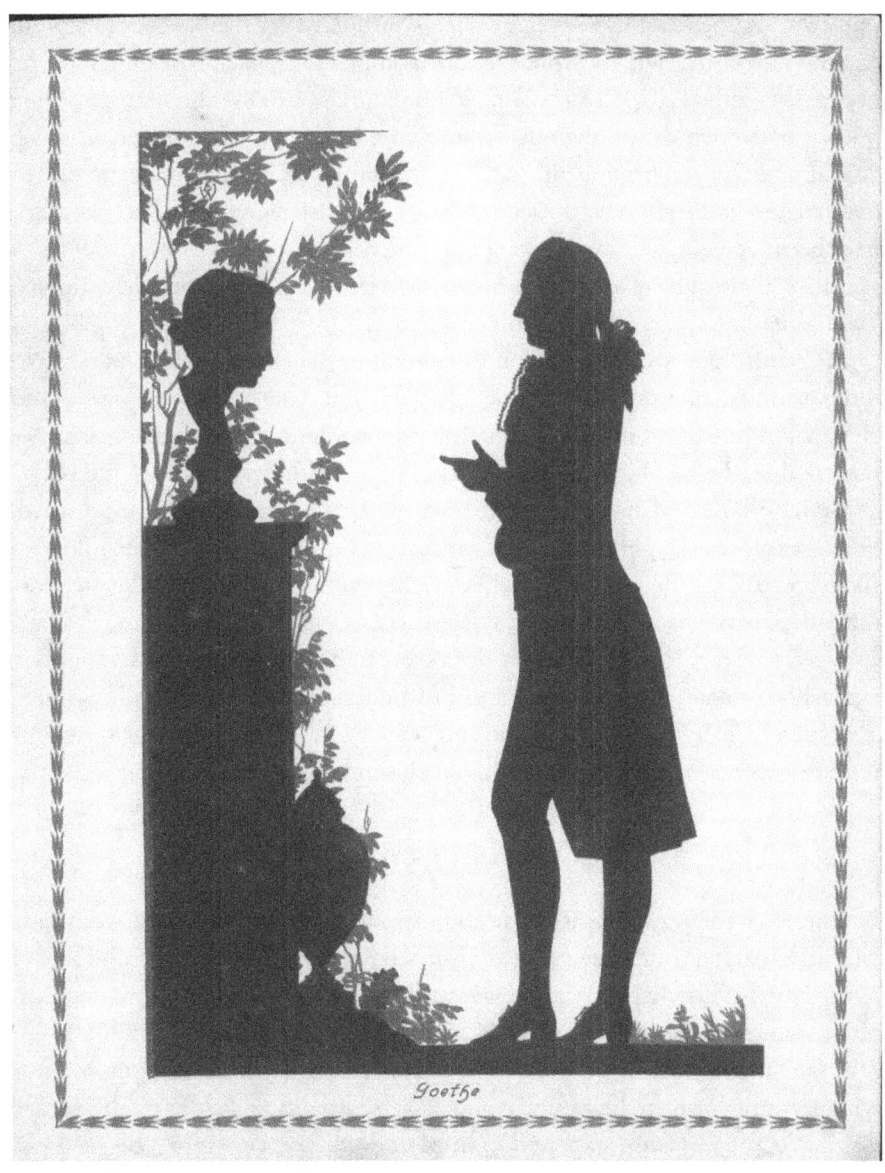

FIGURE 7.4: Silhouette of Goethe in Tieburg (26cm × 20.3cm), *c.* 1780. Harry Beard Collection. Credit: Victoria and Albert Museum.

of polarity, loosely echoing Blake's demands for firm lines and precise differentiation. Goethe's *Theory of Colours* (1810) argued that the experience of color was not a mathematical absolute; rather, it was something that unfolded inwardly. Contrasting the tacit knowledge of painters and dyers with the abstraction of Newton's prismatics, Goethe re-evaluated color from the perspective of everyday experience, giving examples of waking sensations in our eyes, or the shadow and light effects produced by the lovely sight of "a well-favoured girl, with a brilliantly fair complexion, black hair and a scarlet bodice" (Goethe [1810] 1840: 22). Goethe's attempt to use the senses to bring science and poetry into alignment represented a historical moment in which "disciplines" were firming up, and at the same time found new modes of overlap and connection. The focus on *color* was also significant, because color had been categorized by Locke (and other philosophers previously) as a sensational or subjective aspect of the object secondary to its the primary, "real" qualities, extension, motion and figure.

Romantic poets of the "second" generation, such as Shelley and Keats, often showed interest in the new experimental sciences of chemistry and electricity, and drew on the history of philosophies of perception. Shelley's remarkable poem "Ode to the West Wind" (1820) describes colors and scents as having shape and agency of their own (ll. 9–12), whilst his "The Sensitive-Plant" explores the philosophical connotations of the scent of garden flowers (Boyson 2013). In both poems, Shelley's richly punning verse technique suggests that all sensation is in some sense synaesthetic (Classen 1998). Although it is a conventional tag, Romantic poetry does seem to display a marked "sensuality," especially evident in its representation of non-visual senses of tactility, smell, and sound, in its blend of science and poetry, and in its politicized view of sensation as essentially common, crossing boundaries of property and location.

CONCLUSION

Literature of the Age of Reason, or "our age of prose and reason" as Matthew Arnold had it, has often been seen as abstract, dry, or unsensuous in comparison to the bawdy, bloody poetry and plays of the seventeenth century, and the vivid object-world of the Victorian novel which came after (Arnold [1880] 1903: 30). One might however question the very terms of such an account and ask whether any form of literature *could* lack sensuality, given that all literary writing captures sense experience. And indeed, we can find "the senses" somewhere in any text from the long eighteenth century, whether in a description of the shades on a dove's neck (Young) or of a young woman inhaling the fresh air of freedom (Wollstonecraft). Yet the "age of reason" framework still retains a great significance for thinking about the senses. What we now call "literature" was throughout the Enlightenment engaged in a complex dance with modes of rationality and empiricism. By turns literature was enchanted by, and virulently reactive against, the discoveries of the Scientific Revolution, and simultaneously shaping those empirical discourses and practices. The senses were the ground over which these affinities were made and contested.

The Enlightenment's traditional association with one sense—vision—and vision's own ancient history as a metaphor for knowledge and rationality, played a crucial role in the way that "literature" was conceptualized in this period, and in shaping its descriptive tendencies or habits. As literature as a printed, mass-circulation medium came into existence, linking previously disparate practices of theater and elite manuscript poetry and engendering the essay and the novel, so too emerged new notions of the written word's ability to describe and evoke sensual experience. Taking the broadest possible view, one might observe that as "literature" became more self-conscious and more clearly defined in its own right against the domains of natural and moral philosophy, there was a slow devaluation of sight. At the beginning of the eighteenth century, the most "perfect" sense of sight was something held in common and celebrated by both aesthetic and epistemological writing; as it went on, literature gradually came to be characterized as offering obscurity, sublimity, or "counteracting" senses of sound, touch, and scent (cf. Potkay 2011).

Looking historically at the literary senses, one finds a pattern of slow-growing intellectual tensions that produce fertile new oppositions. Dryden's and Addison's claims about the pleasurable-imaginative work of literary description helped form aesthetics and the cult of sensibility, which themselves gave birth to the modern novel as the "vehicle" of feeling. But sensibility, that notion of general, merged sensitivity, prioritizing the ineffable, looks quite different from the aspiration to separate out and define the senses, the desire to pick out the distinctive musicality of a rhyme or the pungent precision of a scent. Perhaps the novel tended to stress a merged sensibility, and poetry to stress particular senses, though counter-examples could be adduced. We should also remember the extent to which the growth of "lyric," at its height in Romanticism, conditions our modern attitudes towards the senses as something worthy of "celebration," legitimate theme for expression, and perhaps enhancement. And equally influential upon modern attitudes, though on the surface very different to the lyric impulse, are the Enlightenment materialist and utilitarian arguments that helped generate the view that the senses and the body are the individual's "own," rather than God's, to be "enjoyed." Acknowledging and identifying modern prejudices about the senses helps us see other paths that have or might have been taken. The satirical treatment of the senses in the period is a useful reminder that they might also be dangerous, grotesque, or reductive. Such a critical view might be religious, moral, or political in origin: sensual "ambience" could be seen (and still is sometimes seen) as an evasion of clear philosophical and political commitments. From another point of view, one also with roots in the Enlightenment, literature's power might not lie in sensuality but in its power of abstraction; its ability to transcend sensual immediacy and privacy, and to enter us into a realm of communicability and shared imagination (cf. Stewart 2002).

CHAPTER EIGHT

Art and the Senses: Experiencing the Arts in the Age of Sensibility

SARAH COHEN AND DOWNING A. THOMAS

THE VISUAL ARTS

Sarah Cohen

Too impatient to wait for the guitarist to finish tuning his instrument, an ardent male lover yanks his partner's arm upwards and rolls her around and off her seat. As she plunges downward, the woman twists her torso and extends her other arm to complete a long diagonal of intertwined limbs and heads. The man's face, dark and beaked like a raptor's, looms menacingly above her light, swiveled head, while his long fingers splay across her back and catch a diaphanous piece of fabric that trails from her hair and winds sensuously around her body. The guitarist, who is dressed in the costume of the stock *Commedia dell'arte* character known in France as Mezzetin, watches the grappling pair with interest as he tunes his instrument, turning his head and shifting his leg and torso to present a neatly counteractive diagonal. We viewers are led into this three-person "dance" by a dwarf spaniel, neatly decked out in a belled collar, that turns to gaze and, perhaps, yap at the human action from the grassy foreground. The

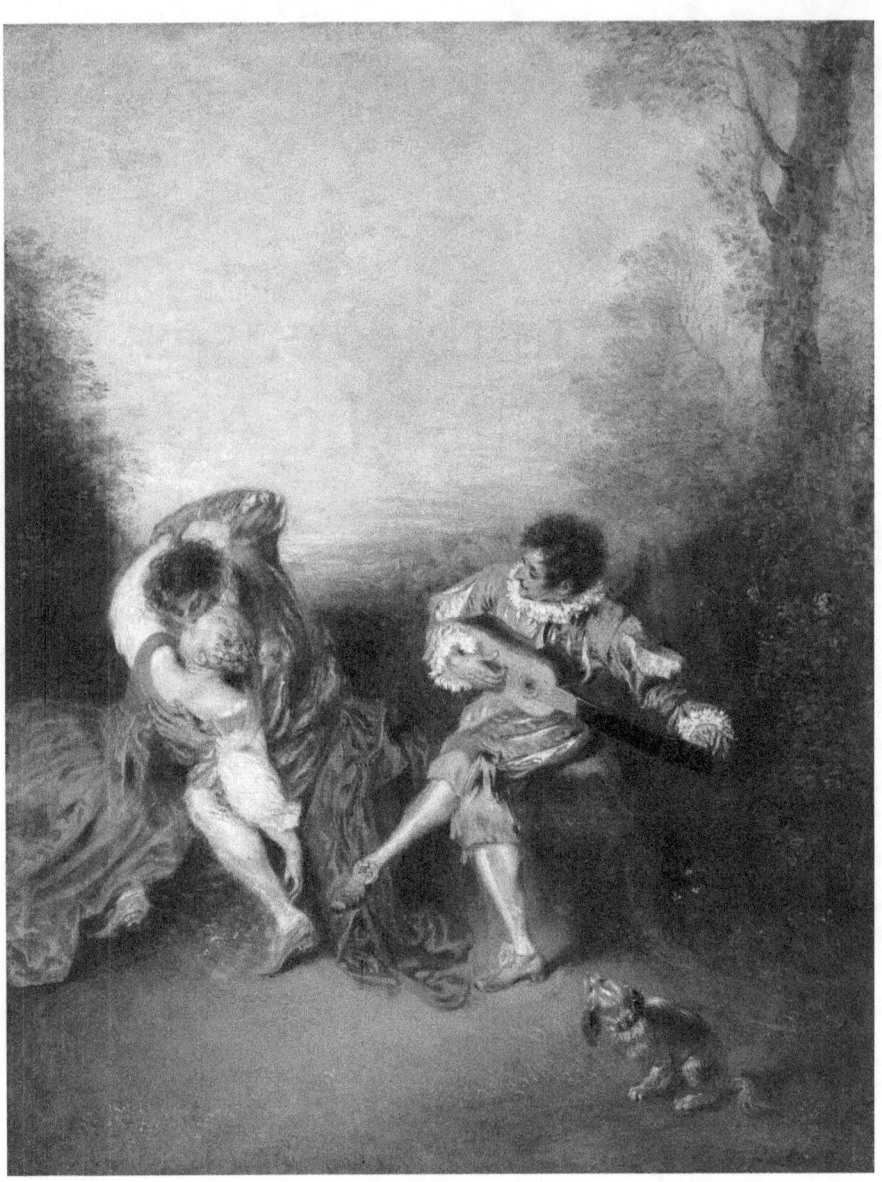

FIGURE 8.1: Antoine Watteau, *La Surprise*, c. 1718–19, oil on canvas, private collection. Photo: Michael Bobycomb.

scene is set within a park composed of cool greens, blues, and mottled pink; but hot, saturated reds and golds slash through the costumes of the human group, underscoring the shock of breakout passion that captures everyone's attention.

Antoine Watteau's painting known as *La Surprise*, painted in about 1716 and only recently brought to public light,[1] in many ways exemplifies the emphasis upon sensory awareness and understanding that dominated artistic themes and styles all over Western Europe in the first two-thirds of the eighteenth century. Its theme of love (or lust) made manifest; its inclusion of touch and sound within the visual attractions of paint, color, light, and brushwork; its intimate scale; and its use of a sensitive animal to engage the viewer physically with the scene, all privilege that which one takes in through the senses as a primary tool. Visible brushwork, rich color, and subtle glazes of paint materially exemplify the artist's process in building and elaborating the work. One could go so far as to say that the "story" of this painting is itself the mobilization of the senses, as experienced by the characters depicted within the scene, by the artist who so tangibly painted them, and by a viewer drawn in by sight to experience all these feelings vicariously. We are, like the guitarist and even the spaniel, at once witnesses and subjects of sensory action, so tactile, material, and emotive are the paint, color, and bodily movement on display.

In my contribution to this chapter I shall argue that in so highlighting sensory experience, eighteenth-century art offers a visual counterpart to the sensationalist and materialist theories of human understanding that pervaded philosophy during this era, especially in France and England. Although made mostly to please and seduce rather than to argue and prove, the visual arts demonstrate through their sensory embodiment the primary value of seeing, touching, hearing, and—through the unprecedented ascendance of portable arts of the table and the home—tasting and smelling as well. While all art, of course, is perceived through the senses, what distinguished the art of the eighteenth century was its elevation of sensory action to the status of subject. Featured prominently as a representational theme, sensory experience also worked as a tool to draw the viewer or user into the work vicariously, with a direct appeal to the bodily experiences of touch, rhythm, vibration, and kinesthetic movement. Watteau's guitarist, who at once attracts our notice, implies sound through his gestures, and watches, with us, a passionate dance, could stand as the ineffable emblem of his age.

Configuring the Senses

Art theory of the first half of the eighteenth century promoted the role of the senses, and backed its case more through empirical cause and effect than through the imposition of external ideals. Roger de Piles was the first art theorist to study at length the fundamental role of color in pulling spectators into a work and holding their attention through sensory force. His *Cours de peinture par principes* of 1708, in which he summarized the arguments he had been building in previous decades, features extensive discussion of color and other sensual effects such as richly painted fabric and variegated light and shadow. The primary goal of painting, de Piles argued, is to take us by surprise and to "seduce our eyes ... as if it had something to say to us" (Piles 1708: 2–3). Throughout his treatise he reinforced the principle of a painting's direct appeal to feeling through sight, and he often used music as an analogy for the experiential basis of art. Our physical organs of ears and eyes "are the doors through which our judgments of musical concerts and works of art enter. The primary concern of the Painter as well as the Musician thus ought to be to make the entry through these doors free and pleasant through the force of their harmony, the one through color accompanied by light and shadow, and the other through its *accords*" (7; see also 104–5, 204). Compelling visual representation on its own can mobilize the other senses in the viewer's imagination, as when a landscape painter recreates water so convincingly that viewers can hear its gentle murmuring, or feel the texture of trees and the coolness of a depicted forest (157–8).

De Piles was a strong partisan of "Rubenism" in the French academic debate between the followers of the Flemish painter Peter Paul Rubens, known for his color and sensual form, and the followers of the French painter Nicolas Poussin, who was thought to favor linear structure and cerebral themes (Lichtenstein 1993; Puttfarken 1985; Tessèdre 1957). In the "scale of painters" that closes the *Cours de peinture par principes,* de Piles gave Rubens the highest grades in color, expression, and composition, and the Flemish master appears throughout the text as a model for aspiring artists, not just in his figural works but in his landscapes as well (Piles 1708: 390–2, 170). De Piles indeed promoted the expressive capacity of landscape in his art theoretical writings, thus relaxing the traditional academic hierarchy of subjects that placed landscape lower than figurative art.[2] Landscape, he argued, allowed special creativity on the part of the artist, for nature contained the greatest variety of tangible objects and effects that could stimulate a viewer's sensual response (157–8).[3]

Watteau, who early in his Parisian career gained special access to the series of paintings in the Luxembourg Palace that Rubens had made for Marie de Médicis, adapted from Rubens' example both his rich, painterly coloristic effects and his emphasis upon tactile physicality. In composing *La Surprise,* Watteau borrowed from paintings by Rubens both the interlocked "dance" of his lunging couple and the startled spaniel in the foreground. The Flemish master's earthy village *Kermesse*, a work purchased by Louis XIV for the royal collection in 1685, features a peasant dance sprawling across a verdant landscape, from which Watteau plucked one furiously engaged pair as the object of a red chalk drawing (Paris, Musée des arts décoratifs). Rounding the man's arms to encircle his partner's upper body and forcefully crossing arms and legs, Watteau also worked out in this drawing the hawk-like eyes and "beak" of the man who usurps the action of *La Surprise*. The spaniel that registers in its tiny body the first "surprise" at the sudden sight of Watteau's Rubensian dance was taken from a similar canine surrogate for the viewer in a painting from Rubens' Médicis cycle, the *Marriage by Proxy* (Paris, Louvre).[4] Perhaps even more deeply inspired by Rubens are Watteau's thick, tactile use of paint and his reliance upon color and reflected light to instigate visual drama. The hot, saturated red that flows back and forth from the costume of the guitarist, through the abandoned drapery, to the woman's bodice sensually "calls" the viewer, as de Piles would put it, to respond (Piles 1708: 15).

For Watteau as for de Piles, the sense of sight conspires with the sense of touch to make the process of viewing a painting into an experience that is corporeally felt. The French painter François Boucher would develop this relationship in the succeeding decades, to make bodily experience the very essence of his artistic practice. Although Boucher was not a theoretically oriented painter, he shared with eighteenth-century empirical philosophy a preoccupation with how one perceives matter through the senses, as evidenced both in his themes and in his artistic style. For example, Boucher's drawing in red, black, and white chalk of a recumbent female nude evinces not just the sensuality of a woman's body as an object of sight, but a quality of subjective touch that we vicariously share *with* the figure.[5] Embracing with both arms and legs the drapery upon which she lies, the depicted woman appears already to be feeling the sensuous contact of matter on matter. Boucher subtly enhances this effect by periodically breaking off the red contour lines that define the woman's body, and substituting white strokes that compose the surrounding fabric. We can discern this "visible touch" along the woman's proper left shin; behind her proper right knee; along the left side of her waist; and, most remarkably, in the proper right hand that floats on its own beside a thick layering of white. Skin, flesh, and fabric together construct a physiology of sensuous experience.

Recent scholarship on Boucher's relationship with his most important patron, the Marquise de Pompadour, has called attention to the quality of vicarious touch that pervades the artist's depictions of female subjects. Having achieved her special position in the court of Louis XV through the sensuous

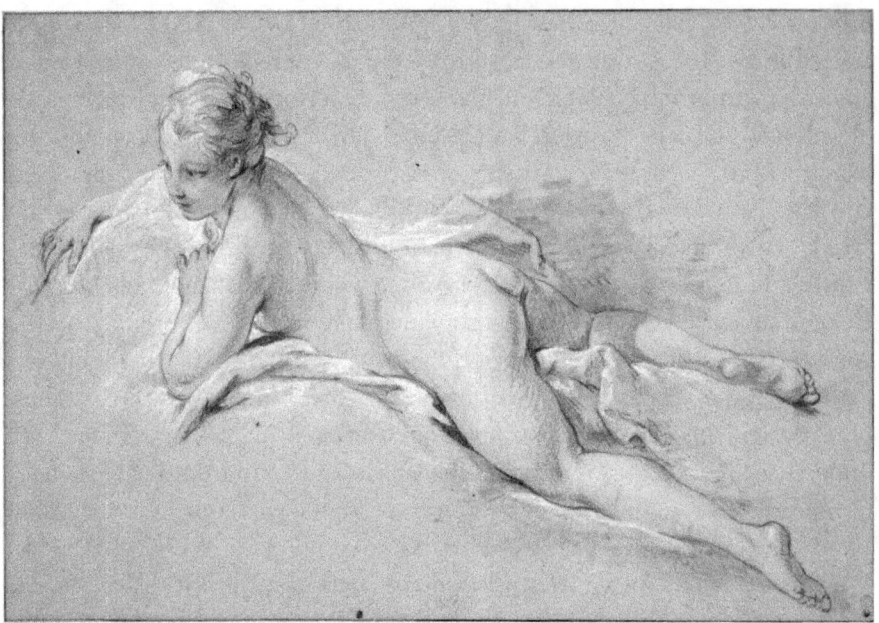

FIGURE 8.2: François Boucher, *Recumbent Female Nude*, c. 1742–3, black, white, and red chalk on cream antique laid paper. The Horvitz Collection, Boston inv. no. D-F-800.

capacities of her own body as mistress to the king, Pompadour appears to have favored the tactile appeal of Boucher's art and in turn inspired some of his most intricate expressions of subjective sensuality (Hyde 2006; Lajer-Burcharth 2001). Whereas in Watteau's painting we are invited to study the physical contact of the lunging couple through the surrogates of the musician and the spaniel, Boucher urges us to put ourselves in the position of his feeling subjects, even as we admire them visually.

Art and Empiricism

Boucher's long working career, which extended from the 1720s through 1770, coincided with an intense philosophical debate over the varieties of sensory experience initiated by John Locke's empiricist treatise *An Essay Concerning Human Understanding* of 1689. Locke's *Essay* helped to establish the experiential approach to studies of perception amongst the *philosophes* of the French Enlightenment (Locke [1690] 1975: xiv–xvii). The "Molyneux Question," which Locke raised in the second edition of the *Essay*, specifically paralleled sight and touch as dual means of understanding the material world (Rée 1999: 334–6). If a man born blind, who literally grasped the material world through his expert sense of touch, were suddenly awarded sight, would he be able visually to recognize the objects he knew through his hands? Locke argued that he would not, since he had not yet *experienced* sight and would thus not know how to process what his eyes could see (Locke [1690] 1975, ii: IX, Sections 8–12).

If touch were directly comparable to sight, as the Molyneux Question implies, then perception itself could be relocated from the mind to the body (Bermingham 2005: 13–14). The French philosopher Étienne Bonnot, Abbé de Condillac, argued in his *Traité des sensations* (1754) that touch was the primary sense among the five because it is through touching oneself that a person (or, in Condillac's story, a statue gaining life) recognizes her own subjectivity (Condillac 1947: II).[6] In his *Letter on the Blind* of 1749, Denis Diderot likewise emphasized the importance of touch to subjectivity; press your finger to your thumb, he instructed his reader, and then let go: "While the compression lasts, does not your self seem to be less in your head than at the extremity of your fingers?" Fascinated with touch as a direct counterpart to sight, Diderot proposed that ". . . The blind could thus have their own kind of painting, in which the skin would serve as their canvas" (Diderot [1749] 1977: 40, 48).

In delineating his sensuous female figure, Boucher acted as if he were quite literally feeling his surfaces, which alternated between smooth, soft skin and equally smooth and soft white drapery. A viewer at once appreciates the visual appeal of intertwined flesh and fabric and imaginatively experiences, with the woman, the luxurious folds of the weightless bed. We respond to this reciprocal touch almost unconsciously, familiar as we are with processing the nuances of what we see. So intermingled are the senses of touch and vision in Boucher's drawing we might almost interpret it as a refutation of Locke's position on the Molyneux Question: perhaps the blind man *could,* after all, use his experience of touch to help him see. Diderot is well known today for castigating Boucher's sensually laden figures in his *Salons*—perhaps precisely because they pulled the viewer too far into the physical experience of the depicted subject.[7] Sharing, through sight, a plump young woman's personal sensation of fabric against skin may have seemed, to the *philosophe*, illegitimate as art.

The depiction of pure matter, however, allowed for a closer fit between Diderot's materialist valuation of nature and artistic content. His enthusiastic response to the still lives of Jean-Siméon Chardin are a striking case in point. Of Chardin's *Bottle of Olives*, exhibited in the Salon of 1763, Diderot wrote:

> The porcelain vase is truly of porcelain; those olives are really separated from the eye by the water in which they float; you have only to take those biscuits and eat them, to cut and squeeze that orange, to drink that glass of wine, peel those fruits and put the knife to the pie ... Oh, Chardin! What you mix on your palette is not white, red, or black pigment, but the very substance of things; it is the air and light itself which you take on the tip of your brush and place on the canvas.
>
> Diderot [1763] 1970: 58

Air, light, porcelain, food to be eaten, wine to be drunk, and a pie to cut open with a knife: Chardin's gathering of consumable substances recalls the life cycle of matter that Diderot would subsequently put forth in the first dialogue of his tripartite *Rêve de d'Alembert* of 1769 (Diderot [1769] 1965). At the outset of this philosophical fantasy the author asserts to his colleague d'Alembert that all matter, regardless of how inert it appears, has the potential to become reanimated by passing into another state, and he points out that such a transformation happens every time a person eats. For in eating, one assimilates

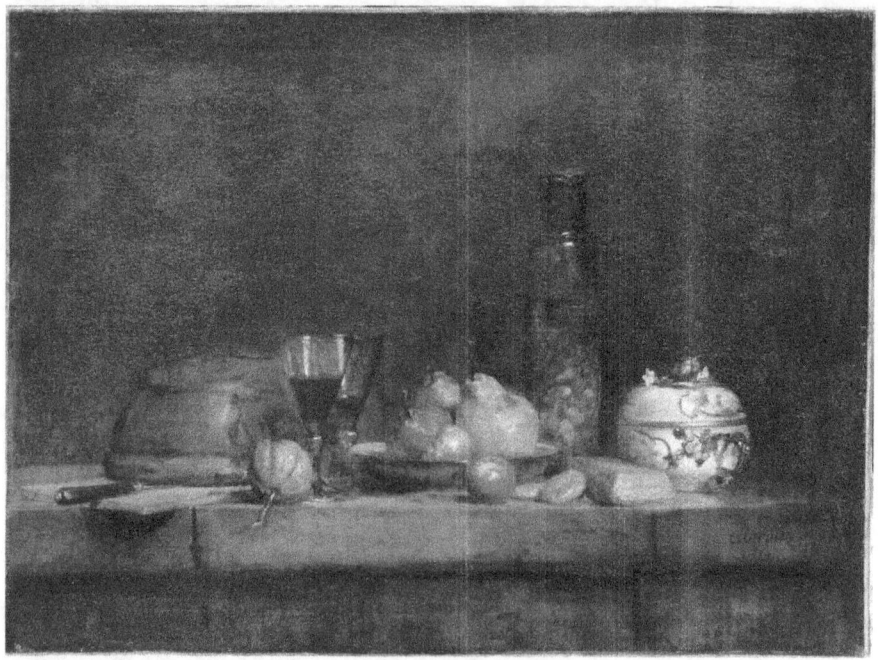

FIGURE 8.3: Jean-Siméon Chardin, *Still Life with Bottle of Olives*, 1763, oil on canvas. Musée du Louvre, Paris; © RMN-Grand Palais/Art Resource, NY.

matter into oneself, making it fully sensible. Even a finely crafted marble statue, Diderot claims, can become living flesh when it is ground into powder, mixed with earth, and used to raise the vegetables one eats (Diderot [1769] 1965: 35–41).[8] Chardin's attention to the feel, texture, and quality of his objects—his sculptural valuation of matter through paint—could serve as a kind of pictorial confirmation of Diderot's sensationalist life cycle.

Hogarth's Tangible Beauty

The sensual appeal of artworks such as those by Boucher and Chardin did not lend itself to extensive theorizing by artists and *amateurs*, but one book stands as a kind of empirical manifesto of eighteenth-century visual aesthetics: William Hogarth's The Analysis of Beauty of 1753 (Hogarth [1753] 1973). Promoting the double-curved, serpentine line as the essence of "beauty and grace," Hogarth proved his points by appealing to a reader's sensory experience of the world, and by citing the propensity of nature itself to favor the winding and the intricate over the straight and the static. Today we generally call the style Hogarth promoted "rococo," but in the eighteenth century it was most often characterized as the "modern," or "graceful" style (Clements 1992), and Hogarth emphasized its relation to the here and now by situating artistic response directly in the material realm. Evidently observing the saturation of the "modern" style in rococo interior design, Hogarth noted with approval that "there is scarce a room in any house whatever, where one does not see the waving-line employ'd in some way or other" (Hogarth [1753] 1973: 48). To demonstrate how such taste works on an experiential level, Hogarth asked his readers to consider how much the mind loves pursuit, whether it be physically enacted or taken in through the senses. Hunters and their dogs chasing a cunning hare; cats playing with their prey; people taking winding walks or enjoying a country dance—all appeal to us for their ability to "lead . . . the eye a wanton kind of chace" (24–5, 27; quotation from 25). In his chapter entitled "Of Compositions with the Serpentine Line," Hogarth explained how our natural preference for curving structures that "give . . . a sort of spring to the mind" reverberates literally to our bones, every one of which is gently curved or serpentine, some (such as the hip bone) quite gorgeously so (24, 54–7; quotation from 24).

Scholars have recently argued that both Hogarth's art and his theories of beauty owe much to the philosophical methods of Locke: as the British philosopher had grounded human knowledge and thought in sensory experience, so Hogarth used the objects and actions that we perceive in the everyday world as evidence for his artistic theory of grace (Baridon 2001: 85–101; Ogée 2001: 81–2, n. 8). Michel Baridon has shown that Hogarth even developed the main argument of the *Analysis of Beauty* in a manner comparable Locke's "Historical, plain Method," whereby the mind is characterized as "a processor of sense impressions" and can be dissected by proceeding from the simplest elements of sensory awareness to the most complex ideas (Baridon 2001: 90). Hogarth indeed began his treatise with the fundamental visual aspects of works of art—variety, simplicity, lines—and proceeded to the more complex, such as compositions with waving and serpentine lines (Hogarth [1753] 1973). According to Baridon, Locke was himself following the experimental methods of the scientists at the Royal Society, who wrote "histories" of their experiments, progressing "from data to theory." By using the "data" of what we perceive and respond to in the world to present his own theory of artistic beauty, Hogarth marshaled "what was then a modern method of investigation" (Baridon 2001: 90).

Long before he published *The Analysis of Beauty* Hogarth had indeed been building his theoretical case through the subjects and style of his own art (Ogée 2001: 78). In the *Enraged Musician*, an engraving that he published in 1741, a classical violinist, hands pressed to his ears beneath a formal powdered wig, yells angrily at the parade of noisy street life below him, where bodies make "music" through their voices, their hands, their bellowing breath, and even through forceful urination (Barlow 2005). The proliferation of sound is matched visually by Hogarth's crowded composition, in which a range of body types, postures, and actions intricately vie for space in the shallow "stage" of an urban thoroughfare. Spontaneity, rather than careful planning, appears to be the operative force in the street, a fiction underscored by the boy who summarily relieves himself beneath the iron rail that stakes out, quite literally, the angry musician's indoor fortress.

A notice plastered on the wall of this fortress announces a production of John Gay's *Beggar's Opera*, a contemporary theatrical production in which the daily life of the street served equally as subject and as primary author of musical sound. Hogarth's own gang in the street create a cacophony of noises—singing, crying, tinkling, pounding, grinding, blaring, beating, barking—and the lines of his graphic composition correspondingly lead the viewer's eye chasing up, down, in and out within each noise-making subject and from one to another. In the person of the tall milkmaid calling out her wares Hogarth demonstrated the grace which emanates from the world as we experience it. He would subsequently explain in *The Analysis of Beauty* that women ultimately exceed men in their physical attractiveness, for they manifest "all the varieties . . . of

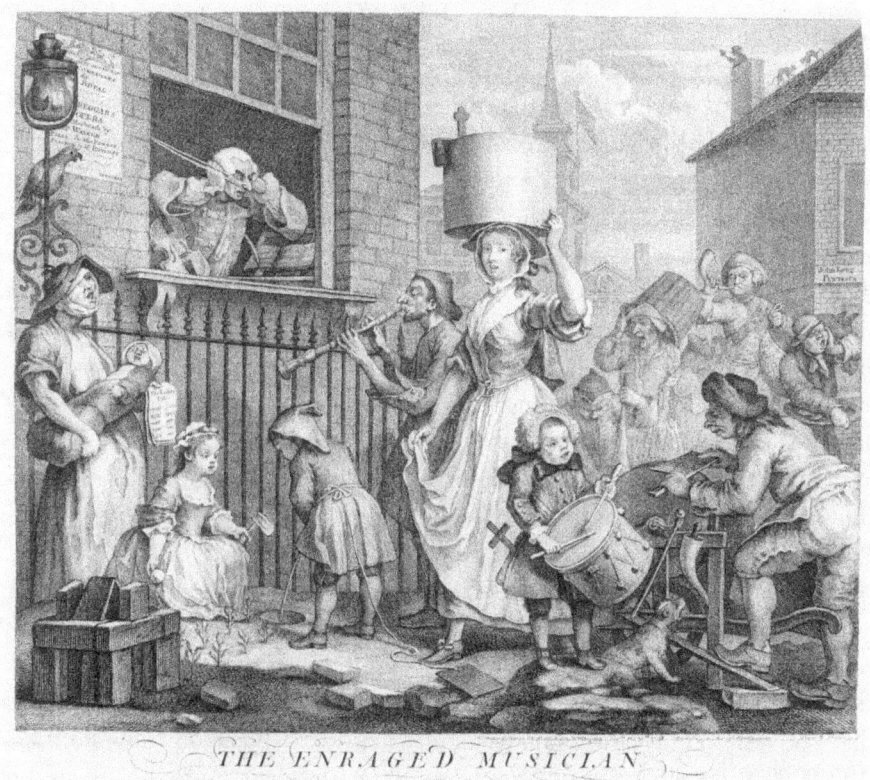

FIGURE 8.4: William Hogarth, *The Enraged Musician*, 1741, engraving. © Victoria and Albert Museum, London.

the body . . . more sweetly connected together" (Hogarth [1753] 1973: 65–6; cf. Ogée 2001: 79–80; Paulson 1997: xxv, xxxii).

As if to underscore the interconnection between the fundamental sensory "data" that we perceive in the world and the beauty that an artist seeks, Hogarth placed a small dog in the lower right corner who gazes raptly and barks at a serpentine horn that catches the shavings produced by the knife grinder. Just such a horn would reappear as an emblem of beauty in the second plate of *The Analysis of Beauty*; Hogarth characterized it in his text as a form that "gives play to the imagination, and delights the eye, on that account" (Hogarth [1753] 1973: 52; see also 51–3). So fundamentally attractive that an attentive dog can recognize its importance, the serpentine form is shown gracing the artist's own palette in his *Self-Portrait with Pug* of 1745 (London, Tate Gallery), where it is once again attended by a watchful canine. Like Watteau's startled spaniel in *La Surprise*, Hogarth's street dog, who gives the impression of knowing beauty when he sees it, could stand in for the perfect human spectator.

Material Culture

For Hogarth, as for the empirical British philosophers who preceded him, the material world, taken in through the senses, formed the groundwork for all subsequent knowledge, regardless of whether one's subject were lofty or mundane. Having begun his career as an apprentice to a silversmith, Hogarth was well aware of the centrality of tangible, material *things* to his culture's engagement with high art. A demand for artfully crafted objects of daily use skyrocketed in eighteenth-century Europe, as men and women both of the elite and of the middle class practiced intimate yet studied forms of social interaction in the home. Dining, in particular, became an opportunity for talk as well as taste, while trade with Asia and Africa and colonization in the New World introduced new foods and beverages into the realm of urban fashion. Artisans produced "modern" wares to accommodate the new demand for coffee, tea, and chocolate, as well as a host of other kinds of objects designed to serve an increasingly sophisticated consumer market.

Porcelain, long imported from China and Japan, finally became a European product with the discovery of its kaolin "recipe" in the early eighteenth-century Saxon court, and by the middle of the century both the true, hard-paste porcelain and its soft-paste, imitative cousin were flourishing in manufactories all over western Europe (Cavanaugh and Yonan 2010; Emerson 2000; Richards 1999). The porcelain soup tureen featured in Chardin's *Bottle of Olives* (see Figure 8.3), produced in the Saxon manufactory of Meissen (Rochebrune 2000: 44), reflects not only the mid-eighteenth-century European taste for porcelain, but also the prevailing fashion for soups and stews—thus adding suggested warmth, liquidity, and savor to Chardin's glowing objects.

Other porcelain serving vessels were created for the use of foods imported into Europe from colonies and trading partners overseas. A covered bowl modeled by Franz Anton Bustelli for the Nymphenburg porcelain factory in Bavaria was probably used for sugar, and would have appeared together with other such ornamental porcelains as part of a dessert service for elite dining (see Introduction, Figure I.2). The bowl is offered by a "Moor" whose African attributes referenced the slaves who actually labored for the production of sugar cane in the colonized Caribbean and Brazil. As Adrienne Childs has shown in her important study of these objects, dessert service porcelains such as the figurative sugar bowls replaced illusionistic sugar confections that had once graced elite European tables (Childs 2010: 159–77).[9] Their scintillating visual appeal and smoothness to the touch when handled would have sensually enhanced the sweet taste of their contents.

The Moor's feathered headdress and skirt, however incongruous, would have reminded diners of the New World origins of sugar, even as they tasted it. For eighteenth-century Europeans, both the dark-skinned body of the Moor and the "Indian" flavor of his feathered costume would have coalesced into a single characterization of an exotic Other.[10] His elegant porcelain body, meanwhile, curves and spirals into a shining s-shape that obligingly masks the real slaves' physical suffering. Profits from the slave trade fueled the economy of luxury objects in eighteenth-century Europe, and confections such as the "Moorish" sugar bowls obliquely acknowledged this fact through what Childs calls the "ornamentality' of black servitude" (Childs 2010: 167).

Sensibility

While the intricate, physically tactile art of the "modern" style prevailed in the first half of the century, the latter half was dominated by the "sensibility" movement, whose appeal to feeling lay above all in the process of "touching" a viewer emotionally. Certain painters continued to privilege the material qualities of paint and a direct appeal to the viewer's physical sense of touch, as seen in Chardin's late still lives, as well as in the landscapes and portraits of the English painter Thomas Gainsborough (Bermingham 2005: 1–34; Cohen 2004; cf. Sheriff 1990). In contrast, many other later eighteenth-century artists emphasized sentimental narrative content that was intended to attract the vicarious response of the viewer on a sensible, "moral" level, through identification with painted characters' inner emotions (see, e.g., Barker 2005; Sheriff 2004). Diderot, as well as academic theorists such as Sir Joshua Reynolds, called for art that would in some way elevate its subject and inspire particular emotional responses in its viewers. In the *Discourses* that Reynolds presented before the Royal Academy between 1769 and 1790, he argued that all art should aim to address "the imagination and its sensibility" (Reynolds 1966: 202). While Reynolds followed de Piles in noting that pictures should "please at first sight, and appear to invite the spectator's attention" (113), ultimately they should eschew "mere gratification of the sight" in favor of worthy content (64). The spectator will, in consequence, "feel the result in his bosom" (57).

In shifting the discourse on artistic response from the sensual, tangible realm to the internal movements of the emotions, Reynolds was promoting the moral value of sensate experience as "felt" within the body. He could have found justification for this stance in the writings of eighteenth-century British philosophers who likewise argued that moral action proceeds from sensate experience as opposed to rational thought.

As Ann Bermingham has shown, mid-century British thinkers such as Lord Kames and David Hume theorized that morality lay in a person's basic capacity for sympathy with others (Bermingham 2005: 8). In his *Enquiry Concerning Human Understanding* of 1748 Hume asserted that "The feelings of our heart, the agitation of our passions, the vehemence of our affections, dissipate all its [i.e., the "abstruse philosophy's"] conclusions, and reduce the profound philosopher to a mere plebian." Artists have a particular role to play in exposing such universal sentiment: "An artist must be better qualified to succeed . . . who, besides a delicate taste and a quick apprehension, possesses an accurate knowledge of the internal fabric, the operations of the understanding, the workings of the passions, and the various species of sentiment which discriminate vice and virtue" (Hume [1748] 1974: 308, 310).

In visual art, precise figural definition and scenic renderings that could be easily read in the manner of staged dramas emerged as the principal vehicle for expressing emotional content and engaging the sympathy of the viewer. Such focused, dramatic scenes replaced the more embodied and vicarious appeal to the senses that had characterized the "modern" rococo taste.[11] Feeling was now channeled into stories and depicted situations, as in the tumultuous family scenarios and private displays of intense emotion fashioned by the French painter Jean-Baptiste Greuze, or the impassioned history painting promoted in the academies of France and England. A leading exemplar of sentimental history painting in Europe was Angelica Kauffman, originally from the Rhineland but prominent in the artistic communities of Rome and London, where she was a founding member of the Royal Academy (Rosenthal 2006). Kauffman's neoclassical style banished much of the overtly sensuous use of paint and ornamental configurations that characterized the work of her European predecessors. Her subjects, however, frequently focused upon stories that would stir the sentiments, perhaps in part because Kauffman knew that such themes would make the work of a woman artist publically acceptable.

Cornelia, Mother of the Gracchi, a painting that Kauffman made in 1785 for one of her British patrons, George Bowles (Baumgärtel 1998: 382), both thematizes sentiment and rejects sensuous surface allure. The painted drama literally and figuratively centers upon the Roman heroine Cornelia, virtuous widow of Tiberius Sempronius Gracchus. In response to another Roman matron's request that she display her valued jewels, Cornelia gestures toward her two young sons, who enter carrying a scroll and book that signify the life of the mind. Cornelia's daughter, however, eagerly fingers the neighbor's trinkets, as if to remind a viewer that Cornelia herself rises above the natural attraction of her own sex toward glittery, tangible rewards. Color reinforces

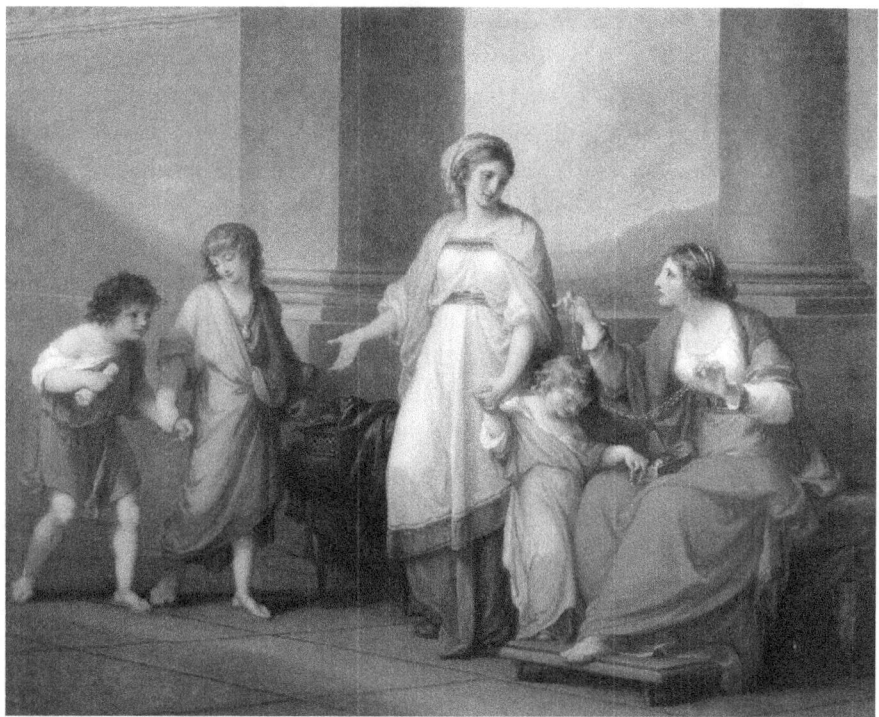

FIGURE 8.5: Angelica Kauffman, *Cornelia, Mother of the Gracchi*, 1785, oil on canvas. Virginia Museum of Fine Arts, Richmond; Adolph D. and Wilkins C. Williams Fund. Photo: Katherine Wetzel.

the contrast between the woman who clings to surfaces and the woman who values internal sentiment and family bonds: while the neighbor's drapery pulsates with a deep, saturated red—echoed in the little girl's pink peplos—Cornelia's robes gleam pure white, softened with gentle earth tones. Kauffman's sentimental, even moral use of color contrasts strikingly with the sensual coloristic effects of Watteau's dancers, Boucher's nude, or Chardin's luscious foods.

Angela Rosenthal has argued that Kauffman herself cultivated a reputation for personal sensibility: a consummate singer and lover of spoken poetry, she impressed those who entered her domestic studio both with her pictures and with the affective power of her own personality. After visiting the painter in her studio, Luise van Göchhausen wrote, "This woman is such a beautiful soul the likes of which are only few, and through love toward her I think oneself becomes better" (Rosenthal 2006: 90–4; quotation from 93). A few years after she executed *Cornelia, Mother of the Gracchi* Kauffman would put herself in the role of the woman who chooses the virtuous path in her *Self-Portrait Hesitating Between the Arts of Music and Painting* (Yorkshire, Nostell Priory). Truly autobiographical at heart, since Kauffman did, early on, choose painting over music as her own profession (Rosenthal 2006: 272–3), the work also demonstrates a theory of art as sentimentally elevating, rather than sensually engaging. While Music, dressed in red, grasps the artist's hand to keep her with her on the ground, Painting, in blue, exhorts her to surmount the merely sensual by pointing upward in the direction of high mountain peaks. Kauffman, with eyes cast softly down upon the Music that she loves, turns toward Painting with a resolute gesture exactly echoing that which the virtuous mother uses to show her dedication to her sons in *Cornelia, Mother of the Gracchi*.

While Watteau, at the outset of the eighteenth century, had presented music and its attendant sensuality as the principal content of the artist's vision (see Figure 8.1), for Kauffman visual experience was essentially "felt in the bosom," as her friend Reynolds put it. Kauffman's reputation as a professional woman artist demanded that she depict her female subjects taking the elevated moral path. But her works also advocate through their very structure and style that the noblest feelings are those which are internally experienced.

MUSIC

Downing A. Thomas

Eighteenth-century writers and philosophers approached music from a dizzying set of perspectives, from observing it as a universal phenomenon to be studied through the lens of science, to exploring its anthropological dimensions as an element of cultures and societies around the world. Illustrating the latter approach, Jean-Jacques Rousseau often took an anthropological approach in his writings, noting that music had meanings that were imperceptible to those outside very specific subcultures. For Rousseau, the most significant effects of music were predicated on belonging to a particular cultural or national group. Citing the famous Swiss herdsman's melody, the "Ranz-des-vaches" (best known today from Gioachino Rossini's use of it in the overture to his opera, *Guillaume Tell*), Rousseau noted in his *Dictionnaire de musique* that "it was forbidden under penalty of death to play it among their troops [the Swiss] because it caused those who heard it to burst into tears, to desert, or to die, so much it aroused in them the ardent desire to see their homeland again" (Rousseau 1959–95, v: 924). Rousseau explained that these effects are completely lost on foreigners because they "come only from habit, memories, and a thousand circumstances which, brought back by this Air for those who hear it, and recalling their country, their former pleasures, their youth, and all their ways of living, awaken in them a bitter grief for having lost all that." In this case, music "does not act precisely as *Music*," in other words as a pleasing combination of sounds, but rather "as a commemorative sign" (924). In his *Lettre sur la musique française* (a highly polemical text, it must be noted), Rousseau argued that music is so culturally specific that Italian musicians are incapable of executing French operatic airs: "it was not for them music that had any meaning, but only a series of arbitrarily placed notes, as if by chance; they sung them precisely as you would read Arabic words written in French characters" (Rousseau 1959–95, v: 301).

The more scientific approach is evident in Jean-Philippe Rameau's *Observations sur notre instinct pour la musique* of 1754, a work that reveals Rameau's strong conviction that our response to music results from the effects that sounds have on us as physical vibrations, from the hard-wired response we have as physical beings to sound. Rameau went so far as to argue that the universal musical principles substantiated in the resonance of natural bodies such as pipes and reeds constitute the scientific basis of all the arts and sciences (Rameau 1968–9, 3: 265).

Stepping back to take a broader look, if one were to characterize the landscape of musical thought during the Enlightenment, it is above all symptomatic of a renewed interest in understanding the connections between human beings and the world in which we live through the senses. The attention to these connections resulted in approaches varying from Rousseau's insistence on the grasp culture has on music ("it is not in their physical existence that one will find the greatest effects of sounds on the human heart"), to Rameau's insight into the connections between musical sounds and the resonance of physical bodies, and to other writers who focused more on the pleasure we derive in the arts, the workings of sensation, and the aesthetic prominence given to the emotions evoked by works of art (Rousseau 1959–95, v: 924).

The Powers of Music

Eighteenth-century commentators expressed a fascination with the effects of music on the body and on the mind. Writers from antiquity left many references to the power of music; and almost all writers on the subject cite the biblical story of David using his harp to calm Saul.[12] Scholars from the Renaissance onward made reference to these writings from antiquity and attempted to expand on them. In his *The Anatomy of Melancholy* (1621), Robert Burton noted that music could treat a variety of disorders: "besides that excellent power it hath to expell many other diseases, it is a sovereigne remedy against Despair and melancholy" (Burton 1800, 1: 451). Sounds were understood to have particular effects on the body through physical vibrations, and on the soul by engaging specific passions. Eighteenth-century commentators sought through music a better understanding of sensation, affect, and ultimately its connection to health.

Citing Plato in his *Dictionnaire de musique*, Rousseau noted that "he claims that one can determine the Sounds that can cause baseness, insolence, and the opposite virtues" (Rousseau 1959–95, v: 920–1). The absence of music seemed equally to have strong effects, not only on individuals but also with respect to the temperament of entire peoples. Rousseau went on to mention Polybius, the Greek historian, who claimed that the Cynetes, living on the Iberian Peninsula, did not practice music and, as a result, "surpassed all the Greeks in cruelty" (921). The ancients made use of music "to incite the heart to praiseworthy actions, & to become impassioned by the love of virtue" (921). He also referred to Timotheus, the musician from Thebes who is reported to have impelled Alexander the Great to arms by using the Phrygian mode and then immediately calming him with the use of the Lydian mode (921). While noting that one might doubt the powers ascribed to music in such accounts, Rousseau also cited similar incidents reported in recent history. During the reign of Henri III, for example, music played at the marriage of the Duc de Joyeuse is reported to have had such an effect on one of the members of the court that he suddenly, and as if mechanically, drew his sword. The musician quickly changed the musical key, which restored the man's calm—a story whose striking resemblance to that of Timotheus is noteworthy (922).

Drawing on this tradition of musical effects, a number of medical doctors and philosophers took particular interest in how music was used, or might be used in the future, to improve physical and mental health.[13] In Diderot's and Jean le Rond d'Alembert's *Encyclopédie*, the article "Ame," attributed to the Abbé Claude Yvon and to Diderot, recounts the story of a composer whose fever and delirium subsided after repeated doses of music, noting that the sense of hearing has a stronger effect than other senses:

> it is rather curious to note how in a man for whom *Music* had become, as it were, the soul through a long and continuous practice, musical concerts little by little returned his spirits to their natural course. It is not likely that a Painter could be cured in the same way by paintings; Painting does not have the same power over the spirits, it would not carry the same impression to the *soul*.
>
> Yvon and Diderot [1751] 2013, i: 343

Elsewhere in the *Encyclopédie*, Ménuret de Chambaud, a graduate of the Montpellier school of medicine, asserted that "the action of *Music* on men is so strong, & above all so *palpable*, that it appears absolutely superfluous to assemble evidence in order to verify the possibility" (Ménuret de Chambaud [1765] 2013, x: 903). Ménuret focused first on the action of sounds conveyed through the air on other objects, and then considered the effects of music on animals and human beings. He noted the effect musical sounds have on inanimate bodies through the vibrations they produce, which are capable of moving liquids and even large objects. This phenomenon serves as the natural explanation for biblical account of the fall of the walls of Jericho, which resulted from "the sounds of the instruments that Gideon had provided to the Israelites on God's orders" (904). One way in which music acts on the human body is through simple "mechanical" means: "considering the human body only as a collection of more or less taut fibers, and of fluids of various kinds, forgetting about their sensibility, life, and movement, one quickly realizes that Music must have the same effect on the fibers as it does on the strings of nearby instruments" (907). But when music passes through the ear, human sensibility brings in an array of complex responses, based on the individual's particular temperament, habits, and prior experience. Ménuret emphasized the difficulty of applying music in a systematic way to medical cases, remarking on the need to consider each case individually: "thus when seeking to apply music to medicine, the composer must create appropriate melodies for the state of the patient, choosing the tones most suited to arouse appropriate passions" (908). Reflecting on the use of music to cure scorpion or tarantula bites, he noted that "we are still reduced to blind empiricism" in understanding these kinds of treatments (908).

A number of writers agreed with the approach of Ménuret, arguing that music created sympathetic vibrations in the human organism, either through direct, physical impressions on the nerves as it does on other physical bodies, or through more indirect means, passing from the ear to the mind. Because music *moves* us, our emotions are characterized as the mental analogue of physical motion. For Daniel Webb, musical sounds and passions demonstrate a "coincidence of movements":

> we are then to take it for granted, that the mind, under particular affections, excites certain vibrations in the nerves, and impresses certain movements on the animal spirits. I shall suppose, that it is in the nature of music to excite similar vibrations, to communicate similar movements to the nerves and spirits. For, if music owes its being to motion, and, if

passion cannot well be conceived to exist without it, we have a right to conclude, that the agreement of music with passion can have no other origin than a coincidence of movements.

Webb [1769] 1970: 6–7

Leibniz came to a similar conclusion in a short text written in the 1690s where he explained that through our hearing the "uniform motion" that make up musical sounds "creates a sympathetic echo in us, to which our animal spirits respond. This is why music is so well adapted to move our minds" (Leibniz 1956, 2: 698).

Claude-Nicolas Le Cat, a surgeon and founding member of the Rouen Académie des sciences, took a more nuanced view. He was critical of "several physicians" who viewed nerves as "so many strings, analogous to those of musical instruments" (Le Cat 1765: 17). He felt that this model was much too simplistic: it could never explain the complexity of the contraction of the muscles, for example (18–19). Yet in his *Traité des sens*, Le Cat argued that hearing is superior to all other senses because it locks us into "commerce with other beings"; and whereas sight cannot refract colors, hearing can distinguish minute differences in sound and break chords down into their constituent notes (Le Cat 1744: 38). Moreover, men are more moved by hearing than by any other sense because of its effect on the "animal fluid," allowing for changes to this fluid in order to effectuate "healthy changes" in its course or character, regulating imbalances (65–6). Because of the way music affects listeners, it must be considered "very pertinent to health" (65).

Some medical minds clearly saw the need for more critical examination of accounts of music's therapeutic effects, and hoped to sort out the fantastic tales reported by previous generations from those treatments that seemed promising and could be studied further. The evidence of the effects that music had both on the mind and the body was indisputable; and a number of physicians and scholars regarded music as a new frontier in medicine, one to be explored systematically so that new treatments could be tried and proven.

Violent Sounds

The potential benefits doctors and philosophers saw in aligning music with medicine meant that most discussions of the matter focused on the soothing, indeed reparative, effect sounds can have on individuals. However, just as the ancient Greek word *pharmakon* can mean both remedy and poison, so eighteenth-century commentators noted that music could also be detrimental to the health and well-being of those who were exposed to it. Ménuret noted the physical effects that violent sounds could have on individuals:

> many people feel a malaise, a kind of tightening of the stomach, when canon are fired; and aside from the cases of deafness caused by unexpected loud noises, the same cause has been known to produce vertigo, convulsions, incidents of epilepsy, and can aggravate injuries; and army surgeons observe everyday how wounds take a turn for the worse when a battle is taking place nearby.
>
> Ménuret de Chambaud [1765] 2013, x: 907

And even less violent sounds, even music, could be irritating. William Hogarth's iconic 1741 engraving, *The Enraged Musician*, offers a window onto the noisy streets of eighteenth-century London, depicting every imaginable aural distraction: a parrot squawking, a ballad singer singing, a man sharpening a blade at a grindstone, a boy beating a drum, a young girl with a rattle, and more (see Figure 8.4).

Moving from the physical to the moral, Antoine Arnauld expressed concern that operatic verses, fueled by the music to which they were set, could convey "lewd morals" into the hearts and minds of spectators; "and what is worse," he writes, "is that the poison of these lascivious songs is not confined to the place where these performances are held but spread throughout France, where an infinite number of people try to learn them by heart and amuse themselves by singing them wherever they go" (Arnauld 1727, 7: 26). Even in the eighteenth century, tunes tended to go viral, leaving the opera house to proliferate throughout the country where listeners become "hosts," agents for the spread of the virus. While we use the term "viral" as a colorful metaphor, Pierre de Villiers was also quite serious about the ill effects musical sounds had in this form, referring to operatic songs as a moral "poison" that could spread from listener to listener (Villiers 1712: 359).

Writers who wished to criticize shifts in musical style, resist influences from abroad, and reject new instruments or musical practices, often resorted to characterizing music as noise. Doing so was both selective and systematic. It was quite common at the time, as is not surprising, to criticize a composer, performer, or style by labeling the music as mere babel. Parisian critics spoke of the meowing of cats, of the cacophony or babbling that French ears heard in Italian music, of the gibberish of excessive ornamentation (see Dill 2006: 70). The violinist Jean-Pierre Pagin so shocked the ears in attendance at the Concert Spirituel (a relatively subdued audience, compared with the opera-going crowd) that after a handful of performances he never again risked playing at the venue. The Concert Spirituel, a series devoted to religious vocal music and instrumental works, had hoped to revive lagging attendance by bringing in music in the Italian style (Pagin was a protégé of Guiseppe Tartini): yet, "listeners who had been hearing the grand motets of Lalande for the past quarter century had a hard time adapting" to the sounds that Pagin brought with him into the concert hall (Wilcox 2011: 112).

Music that was deemed too difficult, that featured rapid passagework and unusually high notes, was at least in part responsible for the audience's reaction. While Rameau was obviously not Italian, his music often challenged audiences in similar ways and was also rejected as noisy because of its unfamiliarity. Recalling the descriptions of music's violent physical effects cited above, Pierre-François Desfontaines characterized his experience of hearing instrumental passages from Rameau's opera *Les Indes galantes* as being "pulled about, flayed, dislocated" by the music (Desfontaines 1735: 238). Music could soothe; but it could also unsettle and "dislocate" listeners. For Claude-Carloman de Rulhière, a proponent of French music during the Querelle des bouffons which pitted the champions of French style against those who touted the Italian style, "to sing Italian one needs only the apparatus of the throat ... But French music requires feeling" (Rulhière 1992, 1: 441). The *Mercure de France* reported Christmas Day carols in 1746 that pitted the noise of Italian sonatas against the charms of French tunes: "One may feel disgust at the din of a sonata; one will always like pretty *vaudevilles* and graceful *brunettes*" (Charlton 2013: 186). Rousseau famously took the opposite stance in his *Lettre sur la musique française*, stating baldly that French singing "is nothing but a perpetual barking" (Rousseau 1959–95, v: 328).

Characterizing music as noise was also a *systematic* way of questioning the aesthetic position of music among the arts, where the metaphor of noise points to music's supposed lack of meaning in comparison to the other arts, in particular to poetry (Dill 2006). Eighteenth-century listeners expected music to function as a kind of language, claiming for it a position among the other fine arts as representing nature through musical means. The Abbé François Arnaud reflected a widely-held assumption when he stated that music functioned very much like eloquent language because it, too, uses "figures ... to please, to touch & to persuade" (Arnaud 1754: 33).[14] When it was not perceived to function as such—pleasing, touching, persuading—nothing remained for listeners other than raw sound, noise. D'Alembert argued that spoken theater was incontestably preferable to opera because "the first is an action whose truth depends only on those who perform it, [whereas] the second will never be anything other than a spectacle" (Alembert 1763, 4: 407). While here d'Alembert does not refer to music overtly, his characterization of opera as mere spectacle conveys the assumption that it is in part because music has such a large role in opera that the genre must be excluded from serious consideration as a form of theater. Spoken theater follows the poetic dictum by representing actions, whereas spectacle is merely the visual equivalent of pleasant noise. Opera presents colors, movement, and sounds, but conveys no meaning. As Charles Dill remarks, those who learned to appreciate the music that critics had lambasted as noise could do so by taking leave of the poetic framework in which music had been understood up to that point, by "taking pleasure in music's sensuous properties," enjoying complex harmonies, rich textures, unusual orchestrations (Dill 2006: 76).

The characterization of music as noise is not limited to the reception history of French music in the eighteenth century. The sounds made by Great Highland bagpipes were also reviled as "howling" because of the instrument's rustic origins, the immense volume it could produce, and its unusual tuning. Added to these characteristics, it was also used figuratively to designate the male genitalia and was a political symbol for Scottish insurgency after the Jacobite uprising of 1745 (Heyl 2011: 148). The early eighteenth-century aversion to and derision of bagpipes turned full circle towards the end of the century, when their sounds came to be associated with the noble savage and as expressive of an authentic and sublime simplicity (Heyl 2011: 159).

Our understanding of the ways in which eighteenth-century men and women heard musical sounds necessarily comes to us through the myriad cultural lenses, stylistic preferences, nationalistic proclivities, and aesthetic assumptions of the pamphlets, essays, treatises, and other commentaries to which we have access. In this sense, music is shaped and molded by the cultural framework in which it was written and appreciated, or on the contrary, reviled. Yet, it is also clear that the eighteenth century marked some of the first modern attempts to understand and harness sounds through the lens of medical and physical science. Musical sounds were ubiquitous in the eighteenth century, albeit in very different modes from today, in the refrains of street vendors, in the fair theaters, in churches, and at the opera. While music was a part of eighteenth-century everyday life, as Hogarth's noisy canvas depicts, it was also a central aspect in the aesthetic debates and scientific investigations of the time.

CHAPTER NINE

Sensory Media: Communication and the Enlightenment in the Atlantic World

RICHARD CULLEN RATH

In his 1784 essay "An Answer to the Question: What Is Enlightenment?" Immanuel Kant argued that enlightenment depended on a literate public and the ability of authors to write freely in that public, namely through the medium of print. He tied the emergence of this newly literate public to the rise of the Enlightenment, arguing that one could not have occurred without the other. This public was dependent on a steady stream of uniform ideas in the form of books and papers which could be critically read, discussed, and acted upon (Kant 1996). For Kant and many others since, print and an enlightened public constituted each other.

Print, with its strong visual bias, was indeed a leading factor in shaping the Enlightenment on many levels. The flow of printed materials from the presses increased exponentially during the Enlightenment. The changes this wrought are often overshadowed by the even more impressive growth of print culture in the nineteenth century, which dwarfed Enlightenment print production in much the same way as Enlightenment print production dwarfed that of the preceding two centuries. The Enlightenment changes are nonetheless important, for it is in the mid-eighteenth century that the point of inflection on the curve of production is to be found, marking a moment of what David Hackett Fischer calls "deep change" (Fischer 1999: xv). In this case, the inflection point signals the beginning of the move toward mass print culture, toward a market so saturated with print that it affected even those who did not read. The Enlightenment-era emergence of mass print culture is in itself sufficient to warrant increased attention, but there are other reasons too, especially once the senses are taken into consideration.

Combining Kant's definition of enlightenment as residing in a literate print-based public with a sensory understanding of print media helps us understand the role of the senses in the Enlightenment; such a perspective clarifies as well as complicates our understanding of how media worked in the process. Taking in massive amounts of information through the eyes (as in reading) probably did something to the ways Europeans and their colonist kin quite literally made sense of their worlds.[1] When scholars consider sense perception at all, it is

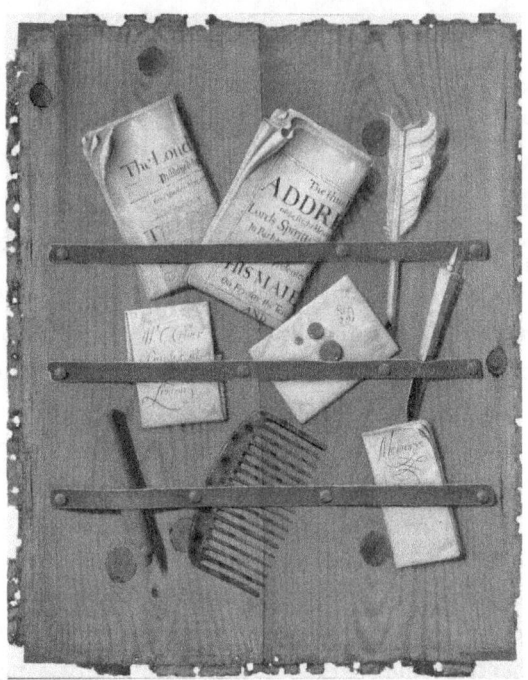

FIGURE 9.1: Edward Collier, *A Trompe l'Oeil of Newspapers, Letters and Writing*, c. 1699. Tate Gallery.

usually through vision alone, its dominance germinating in classical times to fully bloom in the Enlightenment (Jay 1993: 1–106). Another strand of thought has treated the printing press as an agent of change and attributed to it a massive societal shift in politics, religion, science, and the arts. Yet with the important exception of Marshall McLuhan's idiosyncratic work, print's ersatz agency or lack thereof has been debated with little or no reference to the senses (Eisenstein 1979; Johns 1998; McLuhan 1964, 2012). Print was no doubt a generative medium, though attributing agency to it moves us too far in the direction of technological determinism.[2] Its possibilities were unraveled slowly, over the course of centuries (rather than through the oft-proclaimed print revolution). As a result of this gradual unfolding, some of the most telling consequences of accelerating literacy rates and better access to printed goods emerge only in the Enlightenment rather than during the first two centuries of print.

Historical evidence tempers claims of vision's outright conquest of the senses. The other senses never go out of play, and when we begin to listen, touch, smell, and taste the past as well as look for it, a much more nuanced understanding of Enlightenment sensory milieus emerges, one in which all the senses both shape and are shaped by the various media of the eighteenth century (Classen 2012; Erlmann 2010; Schmidt 2000). When considering media, the most profound shifts can be seen in the ways that people worked sonic and visual media together to constitute complex communication networks in the eighteenth century. Sermons, reading aloud, tavern talk, town criers, gossip networks, emerging distribution networks of capitalist markets: all of these have important sensory elements beyond the visual which complicate and enrich our understanding of Enlightenment media as a society-wide phenomenon rather than a decontextualized, abstract vision based solely on print (Slaughter 1982).

In order to make sense (again, quite literally) of media in the Enlightenment, we need to consider media as process—mediation—as much as thing, attending carefully to how mediation shifted and flowed in time. Consider the etymology of the word "media": in the original Latin, it means roughly "the ways between." "Ways" always imply process and the passage of time. Remove the temporal and the passage becomes, of course, immediate. What, then, are these ways between? They allow the passage of thoughts, ideas, commands—in short, what we now call information—from the relational self or selves of their origin to one or many other such selves.

This invocation of relational selves is important for two reasons. First, they are not individualistic constructions. Relational selves are the paragon of social construction: each one is always in relation to other selves, with this web of relations constituting each. At the same time, relational selves sidestep the problem of scholars who reify the social as an unchanging thing in the same way the individualists do with the individual. The web of relations for each self will be different, but in order for it to work, some of the construction of self must align with how at least some others construct themselves for the possibility of communication to exist. The idea of the relational self is central to unpacking the Enlightenment sensorium and making sense of the rise of individualism.

Second, the senses play a key role in the construction of the relational self and by implication, to the construction of media, to the point that mediation can be thought of as having an internal or representational element—the senses that get extended and numbed to define a particular medium—and an external communicative element, the usual domain of the term "media." The communicative aspects of mediation are thus entirely external to the senses and the self, but reachable by no other means and therefore vitally connected to the sensory realm.

The senses are thus integral to our understanding of media and mediation, so it pays to attend not only to their historical and cultural construction but to their physical limits as well. Anyone who has ever jumped at a sudden sound while deeply engrossed in the visual realm of reading knows the limits of sensory attention intuitively. The senses act as filters as much as they do conduits, and the amount of sense data that can be "made sense of" at any one time is limited. This makes ratios between the different senses—which are central to McLuhan's argument that print played a central role in bringing about the Enlightenment—a zero-sum game. Using this common-sense notion of sensory attention it becomes easy to see how taking in ever-increasing amounts of information through the eyes would numb the other senses, particularly hearing.

While there probably is some validity to such sweeping statements that quantify the senses in a hierarchy, it is very difficult to get past anything more exact than "more or less" in describing changes in sensory ratios. A more productive approach is to return to our idea of ways and the process of mediation. Asking in what ways seeing and hearing shifted along with the great shifts in media during the Enlightenment yields more useful results than trying to quantify and order the importance of individual senses, implicitly or explicitly.

The approach taken here will be to focus on mediation and ways that the senses shifted, not only vision, but the other senses as well (hearing in particular). This chapter develops a complex relationship between the senses and the Enlightenment as that relationship shifted in the late seventeenth and early eighteenth centuries. That shift was intimately tied to the concurrent rise of cheap print, and the pressure exerted by the reading public—the enlightened public sphere—that led to the experiments with new kinds of government that marked either the culmination or the end of the Enlightenment.

While print made reading—consumption—cheaper, production required a press, which was a significant investment. Literacy became more common than the ability to write. By the beginning of the Enlightenment, vast media and commodity circuits emerged with complex mechanisms of feedback and feedforward that shaped what was written, sold, and read in ways that saturated Western society in the eighteenth century. This mass print culture transformed publication from its older meaning of "to make something public," which could be done through reading a manuscript aloud or by means of a town crier, into its Enlightenment meaning, which defaulted to "making public by means of print."

One approach to mass print culture would conceive of it as a chain, beginning with the author as creator staring silently at John Locke's blank slate proceeding through print and publication, and ending under the silent gaze of the reader. The conception of this process as silent and serial is itself perhaps the product of the internalization of literacy with its inexorable visual march from left to right and down the page (at least in the Latin script used in the Enlightenment). If we attend to other sensorial modalities, particularly hearing, the line gets complicated and becomes a circle or something more rhizomatic (Deleuze and Guattari 2004: 3–28), a circuit or more specifically for present purposes, a network of different but related media circuits.[3]

Applying this idea of a network of media circuits, this chapter follows the trail of print from authorship through the printing and distribution processes, to reading and then back to authorship. Along the way, it will consider all the senses in relation to the print circuit as well as other media circuits like oral communication, material culture, sermons, bells, and more.

THE AUTHORITY OF AUTHORS

Prior to print, publication depended on many people reading a single copy or hearing the same utterance made publicly. This was in fact the earlier meaning of "publication" and even written publications were announced vocally with the cry of "oyez oyez." In fact, town criers were able to remain gainfully employed as publishers throughout the eighteenth century. Announcements made via bells took on new roles combined with print. Sermons and manuscripts remained a first line of publication. In places like France, where the state tightly controlled print, the older methods of publication remained particularly important (Darnton 2000).

Sermons were of course read aloud, and (less obviously to a visually-oriented reader) already published in the older audible sense when they were spoken at the pulpit. Before reaching print, they might have circulated through hearsay or the sermon notes taken by an audience member, though the latter was probably more often for personal use and to bolster memory when discussing it. The point is that sermons had complex multimedia and multisensory lives prior to—and after—reaching print. Publication was a heard as well as seen phenomenon. Authors, whether of sermons or other titles, wrote not on a blank slate but from within a rich sensory and social context.

Authorship, that seemingly lonely and silent process, was often socially connected once we begin to listen to as well as visualize it. Consider the case of John Gyles, a nine-year-old Puritan boy who was captured late in 1689 and began eight years in captivity, first to the Micmac Indians, and toward the end, to the French. After his release, he parleyed his experience and new linguistic skills into a distinguished career as a translator, transforming the sounds of Algonquian languages into those of English and back. Apparently he was asked to tell the story of his captivity frequently, for his second wife, Hannah, asked him to set it to paper for posterity. Although Gyles was literate, his writing was limited to a signed paragraph at the end of the resulting manuscript that affirmed the truth of his story. The rest is in another hand (Gyles 1730). Perhaps one of his sons carefully wrote as his father spoke. Before it ever saw print publication, Gyles' narrative circulated out loud, and the process of creating the manuscript was in part a verbal one, not a voiceless scratching of words on the page.

Traces of Gyles' vocal delivery flavor the manuscript. It reads better aloud than silently, as if that were its purpose, not just its origin. Sentences run on indefinitely. Punctuation is minimal. Paragraphs are marked with infrequent hash marks hurriedly thrown down in the middle of a line so as not to miss the next spoken word. Snippets of other people's vocalizations—whether in the form of Algonquian language quotations, neighbors' dying sounds, or cries of alarm—are seamlessly woven in with no quotation marks to offset the voice of the narrator from the voice of other denizens of the story. Of course the narrator's tone functioned to do this in the telling, but that was lost in the dictation other than by inference or reading the resulting manuscript aloud to interpretively reconstitute it. It had no chapter breaks. The story flows out all at once, with tangents and repetitions.

Striking references to non-linguistic sounds pepper the manuscript, so that sound shaped not only the medium but the message. The boy's ordeal began around a series of sounds, with young Gyles first hearing the "great guns" from the fort, hoping it was good news. He and the other settlers quickly learned it was an Indian attack by "their yelling noise and the whistling of their shot." He heard his father "call to them what now, what now." "The noise of the Indians shots," disclosed Gyles, "terrified me," and he tried to run away but was captured unharmed. As the Indians silently marched the captive boy along, he noted the audible signs of the wreckage: here the dying departed saying "O Lord," there they died without a sound, or like his father, passed on "with a cheerful voice."

It would be tempting to listen for Algonquian features in the manuscript, passed on to Gyles as a youth, but any such influence was effaced (if it existed at all) by the purpose of this story, which belongs to the genre of the captivity narrative. Captivity narratives, whether spoken, written, or printed, were used by the returned captive to demonstrate the workings of providence and to ritually show a re-entrance to Puritan society. Micmac beliefs not run through the filter of Puritanism would have been a sign that Gyles had "gone wild" and had not made it back (Rath 2003: 147–8). Any Micmac names for the spirits Gyles said he encountered were translated either by his own Christian beliefs or pressure from the Christian society to which he returned into so many devils. He never grasped the Algonquian idea of the world as a set of relations, human and non-human kin. While he had a keen understanding of the Micmac people with whom he lived for several years, the quirks of the manuscript seem wholly attributable to Puritan oral culture rather than Algonquian.

As can be seen—and heard—from the manuscript, when we attend to the ways sound and vision worked together in creating authorship (and, not coincidentally, authority) we uncover a world much richer and more complex than can be captured by visual culture alone or a hierarchy of the senses. Vocal and scribal publication were alive and well throughout the colonies, and Europe, well into the eighteenth century (Darnton 2000; Hall 1996). The authority with which the author is invested came in part from the social processes that existed prior to the print shop, processes that had a crucial sonic context. Using the senses other than vision, particularly hearing, complicates the influential notion of print discourse as an abstract space (a hallmark of visual culture) where ideas freely competed on merit alone—the public sphere (Habermas 1991). But print's authority also came at least in part from the next stage of the circuit, when the manuscript was transformed into a book, pamphlet, or broadsheet.

Gyles provides one of the few examples we have of the process of transforming a manuscript into a book. Usually such manuscripts were ephemeral, used up by the process of circulation or in setting them to print. An editor, perhaps the minister and perhaps in verbal consultation with Gyles, as well as the compositor (about whom more below) massaged the document, reorganizing it and adding the visual hallmarks of print. The manuscript was divided and subdivided into chapters and sections, with some sections moved from their original order and others added to meet the demands of the book market. For example, Gyles' endorsement, narrating the trip to publication, appeared at the end of the manuscript. In the book it, along with a long quote from Homer and a somewhat reluctant homage to his father, comprised the introduction, which is completely absent in the manuscript. Whole sections on natural history (Gyles 1736: 24–7) and manners and customs (28–32) were added, probably at the behest of the publisher.

The book was virulent in its stance toward the Micmacs and all other Native Americans, especially when juxtaposed with the relatively respectful tone found in the manuscript. The book included marginal summaries of each section that allowed the reader to set it down and pick it up later, reading a section at a time, perhaps even at random, and then visually re-orienting herself later. Run-ons were chopped into neater sentences. Paragraphs and punctuation were introduced systematically, breaking up the spoken quality of the manuscript. Fonts were used to replace tones of voice, setting off emphasis, foreign words, names, and quotations. The Indians' yelling and the whistling of their shot during their attack was relegated to a footnote, literally marginalizing the auditory (Gyles 1736).

All of these changes were editorial gestures toward an imagined reader. Did the editor impose a visual-centered approach to text? Or was he responding to a market that demanded their books come with these features? Critically, neither way reflects changes in Gyles'—the author's—mindset. If the storied rise of visual culture in the Enlightenment was so thin on the ground in what the author actually wrote, who is to say what all the manuscripts that were used up in the publication process could tell? Any shift in the ratio of senses, while perhaps demonstrable at the level of the medium, the book, was never absolute, and involved both hearing and vision in a complex process of mediation.

Authors and readers have received much attention, perhaps because for scholars authorship and reading are the two most familiar facets of the medium. Two other circuits intervened between the author and the reader, often folded into the rather abstract notion of publication, the printing process itself and distribution. Studies of printers and booksellers have spent time on their business networks and social relations (Johns 1998), and on the content of the trade, tracking particular titles or shipments for example (e.g., Lyons 2003: 127–32), but not much on the physicality of the print shop and the emerging capitalist distribution network. The senses are inherently embodied, and to understand print it makes sense to explore the material culture of the printing process itself, in part to ground the ideal nature of the Enlightenment in the lived reality of those actually producing and moving in the medium.

THE MATERIAL CULTURE OF PRINTING

The process of printing began long before the pressman ever printed a sheet. Ink was made in-house, a difficult, dangerous, and putrid task. In 1683 Joseph Moxon wrote that the process was "as well laborious to the Body as noysom and ungrateful to the Sence" (1896: 79). Eight decades later, William Lewis noted that "the oil emits, during the whole time of boiling, very offensive penetrating fumes" (1763: 372). Different batches had different consistencies, and the journeyman printer had to gauge the viscosity by feeling its resistance when stirred in order to mix the inks to the right consistency.

The manufacture of type was a hellish process that required a combination of strength, endurance, and fine motor skills. The alloy for the type had to be prepared first. Lead was melted with iron and antimony, the latter of which gave off poisonous fumes when added. A single-use sealed furnace was built around the metal and fire outdoors to avoid poisoning the workers. They would "lay their Ears near the Ground and listen to hear a Bubling in the Pots" to measure when the metal was molten (Moxon 1896: 166). They then broke open the upwind side and two men, working directly over the flames and fumes, stirred in more lead. Once mixed, it was ladled out into smaller containers to cool until casting. Finished with the worst, the print shop owner gave each of the furnace crew a half pint of sack mixed with salad oil, "intended for an Antidote" (Moxon 1896: 168).

At the shop, the type caster reheated and ladled the alloy into the molds, typically producing about 4,000 characters per day. Apprentices broke out the characters and "rubbed" the type against a long grindstone to remove outer imperfections, using finger cots made of scrap leather to keep their skin from rubbing off (Moxon 1896: 176). More experienced workers then dressed the letters, removing the last imperfections with specialized tools for the task.

Next came the compositor. If the supply of characters was new, he filled his case with the proper letters in the proper slots. Usually, however, he had to recycle type from used plates which had been washed in lye to make the ink adhere. The compositor or an apprentice washed the characters by tumbling them in water bare-handed. With his cases filled, the compositor set the type. He and the press men, more than anyone else, made the manuscripts into the silent visible language of print. The compositor had to eye up and remember five or six words at a time and quickly spell them out in his composing stick, a small box which held a few lines of type. Here was the paragon of the typographical man, breaking language into letters and placing them on the page serially, right to left, on down the page, "so that his Thoughts run no faster than his Fingers" (Moxon 1896: 213). A good compositor's eye-hand coordination made it appear that he could work with preternatural speed, laying out the page and making aesthetic and practical decisions on the fly.

Running a press was hard physical work that shaped, even deformed, the bodies of the pressmen. Every motion was calculated and optimized. The machine required strenuous twists, always in the same direction, that wrought the bodies of the pressmen like trade winds shape the trees. The work was hard and the two pressmen traded jobs every few hours, with one pulling while the other inked the type.

McLuhan argued that movable type regimented the print shop and provided the impetus for the rationalization of labor into discrete, repetitive, interchangeable tasks that characterized industrialization. This much is evident in Moxon's carefully disaggregated recipes. What is not as clear is whether this

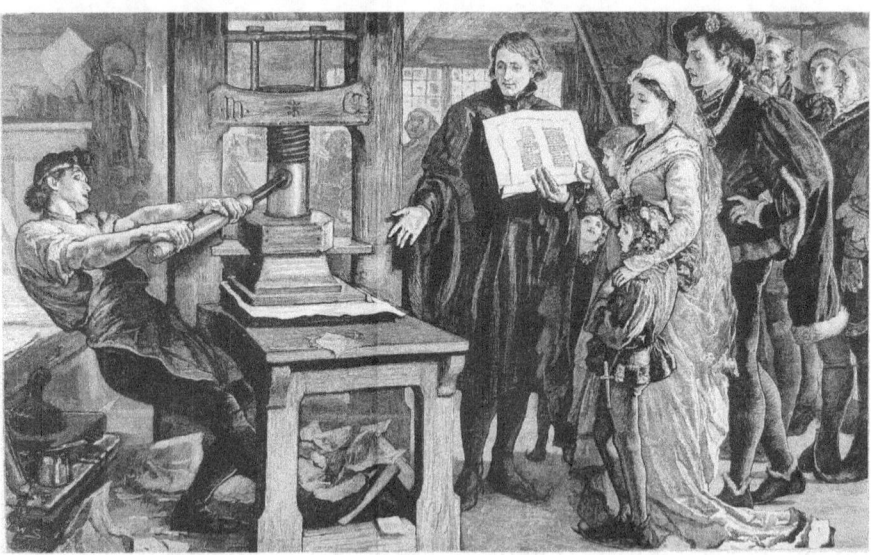

FIGURE 9.2: William Caxton showing specimens of his printing to King Edward IV and his queen. Wikimedia Commons.

rationalization came before or after the rise of the print shop. It seems to have co-occurred, with print being a generative medium that fed into a propensity for rationalization of labor that was then spreading through Europe (Sewell 1980). That propensity drove further rationalization of the work flow that would have made Frederick Winslow Taylor envious.

The idea of Moxon taking this multifaceted and extremely complex process and rendering it into discrete tasks right down to the placement of the body, hands, and feet speaks to an optimism combined with atomism that characterized the rise of Enlightenment individualism. The task for Moxon's imagined reader, and a highly difficult one, was to visualize each move from reading the text in his (or occasionally, her) mind's eye. The book was not for workers, there was no time in a properly run print shop for reading. Moxon's *Mechanick Exercises*, and others like it, provided a set of prescriptions so that the shop owner, the master printer, could make sure everyone was performing his job. In effect, the book provided an early version of the visual discourse of surveillance that Foucault (1977) and others have associated with the late Enlightenment. Moxon's status as a master printer both grounded his prescriptions in experience and granted him his authority on the topic.

DISTRIBUTION

Once the sheets were cut into pages and bound into books or folded into newspapers, the next phase of the print circuit took over. The distribution of books and newspapers, both as commodity and for their content, was part and parcel of the rise of modern capitalistic markets. London and continental printers found buyers for their products well beyond the doors of their shops, though those too remained an important factor during the eighteenth century. Particularly in North America, with its relatively high rates of literacy, wealthy and middling people yearned for a connection to the wider European world—and even beyond—that books and news from London and other colonial centers fulfilled. Without a medium of distribution, there could be no reading public, and thus, following Kant's logic, no Enlightenment. Without this vast system, print remained ever local.

In the Atlantic world, printed goods from the home country were carried through a multiracial, partly enslaved, partly free—and partly neither—network of human motion: the carters, stevedores, sailors, dockworkers, and laborers who moved printed goods from one place to the next. Their contribution to the history of print in the Enlightenment has been rendered mostly invisible and silent to us in the present, yet the commodities were moved, and a sensory approach to this portion of the circuit helps us to recover this key connection between the print shop and the reader.

Nothing moved without the touch of this human network, including all the information carried in print. It was a medium in its own right, perhaps what Lewis Mumford called a "container technology," one that carried another medium rather than its own information, much like the earliest books, called incunabula, contained the texts of older manuscripts (Febvre and Martin 1976; Mumford 1963: 12–14; Sofia 2000). But labeling it only as a container fails to capture the full picture, for this network also carried spoken information as an unintended but unavoidable consequence of putting people in touch with each other.

Here we need to pause for a moment to consider media as communication. During the Enlightenment and well into the nineteenth century, communication referred to routes, roads, and bodies of water in addition to the now-disembodied information we usually associate with the term. This made perfect sense in a world where information—with a few exceptions such as village bells or the drum languages of African American slave revolts—could travel no faster than the humans who carried it. Printed news was always late to the party. Printed goods traveled along the same networks as speech, but only revealed their information, their news, long after the human network had finished its dual work of conveying its messages and its commodities. The people on the far ends of the distribution networks, readers, were in effect the last to know.

This communicative aspect of the distribution medium was a marvel of speed and efficiency, a fact not lost on workers or their would-be betters. It relied on partial publics,[4] where news and knowledge traveled efficiently, but only in some circles, not others. In the case of enslaved laborers, they often knew of—and relayed to other working people both enslaved and free—news of (those drum-language led) revolts and uprisings throughout the Americas before their masters, a fact that the masters found supremely disconcerting.

For example, enslaved Africans in the southern United States knew about the revolt in Saint-Domingue before their masters because the enslaved worked on the docks and spoke with people in the ships who had spoken to people who were closer to the events (Scott 1986). By the time it arrived in print, that news was already old. This knowledge that their ersatz property knew more than they did, and sooner, kept planters in a constant state of anxiety. In another case, an African American man, Briton Hammon, with an ambiguous status as neither slave nor free, was both helped and hindered by the partial public. When he was in jail, he was unable to get a message out to his patron, an outsider to the network, as to his whereabouts, but later he was able to effect an escape to sea through conversations at one of the hubs of the maritime communication network, the "publicke House." And when by chance his former master was on board another voyage—on which he had also gotten work through a meeting at a tavern—Hammon knew of it first and was able to remain anonymous until a chance encounter (Hammon 1760). Peter Linebaugh and Marcus Rediker underscore the importance of these worker-led, multi-ethnic, oral (and thus sound-based) maritime networks in spreading a radical working people's revolutionary ideology throughout the Atlantic world (Linebaugh and Rediker 2000).

READING AND HEARING

Once printed goods made their way through the distribution system to consumption, the world of print looks familiar and well-trodden at first. Kant's enlightened public took shape from its literacy and reading habits. If we pay closer attention to the sounds as well as the sights of reading then new dimensions to our understanding of Enlightenment politics and governance open up. Whether through newspapers, bells, street poetry, or all of the above and more working in tandem, reading was a social activity and was often connected through sound in the form of heated discussions, to praxis, the place where thought and action meet and inform each other. Without readers, the Enlightenment was nothing more than the thoughts of a few dozen thinkers. When those readers began to take Enlightenment ideas into the world, particularly in the realm of governance, a great social shift was set into motion.

That process of readers taking ideas garnered from reading into the world both constituted and was made possible by the onset of mass print culture. At different times and places during the eighteenth century, the output of the presses, the extent of the market, and the consolidation of vernacular languages reached an inflection point at which print culture became a powerful force not just among the literate, but in the whole universe of the Enlightenment. The onset of mass print culture marked the point where print and literacy shaped the ideas and the senses of all members of a given society, regardless of their literacy or access to print. That shaping was not, however, unidirectional: in engaging with the ideas of the Enlightenment, people reshaped them to fit their realities, and to some degree the Enlightenment, if not all of its thinkers, took note. It is only once we move beyond the treatment of the era as only visual that the dynamism of this circuit, as well as some of its shortcomings, becomes apparent.

Visually soaking up information from news and books made for an informed citizen. With print, the message—at least of a particular press run of a particular item—remained the same across all copies, creating a community of readers who were all reading the same information. Benedict Anderson, in an analysis borrowed from McLuhan, dubbed this creation of large bodies of readers taking in the same message the "imagined community" and argued its centrality to the emergence of the modern liberal nation state, perhaps the central political development of the Enlightenment.[5]

McLuhan, riffing on Alexis de Tocqueville, further claimed that print's individuation of language, breaking it into the base units of visible, interchangeable characters, was reflected in Enlightenment governance in the idea that the fundamental unit of society was the citizen, each of whom had the same rights as each and every other citizen. He argued that nationalism derives from this repeatability and from the "fixed point of view" that arrived with print, perspective, and visual quantification. Print culture had a homogenizing effect on language and even speech (McLuhan 2012: 218–25). As publishing centers arose, their dialects dominated the emerging standards, provincializing and to some extent replacing outlying dialects even as far away as the colonies.

Literacy, McLuhan argued, shifted the sensorium away from hearing and toward vision, and in the process changed the way Europeans and European Americans saw and made sense of their worlds. However, when we look and listen a little closer, this version of visual domination gets complicated. Europeans and Americans did not suddenly grow deaf, and even in the most literate places, sound and vision still worked together in interesting and changing ways. Nor was reading the lonely exercise it has become today. One particular form of print, one of the most ephemeral, helps to show how vision and hearing were part and parcel of each other.

Newspapers, which really came into their own in the eighteenth century, were an integral part of the creation of the enlightened public about which Kant wrote, at least in the countries where newspapers were allowed. While news of major events such as slave uprisings or revolution might travel faster through the North American commodity distribution network than the papers, other less drastic events tied the Americas to the rest of the world, and increasingly across the eighteenth century, tied one colony to another.

The earliest newspapers often focused extensively on what was being shipped as well as what news came in with the ships. The shipping news often drifted imperceptibly across the border into the advertisements. Here was the heart of what made a colonial newspaper useful, often comprising nothing more than column-length lists of the contents of this or that ship and how

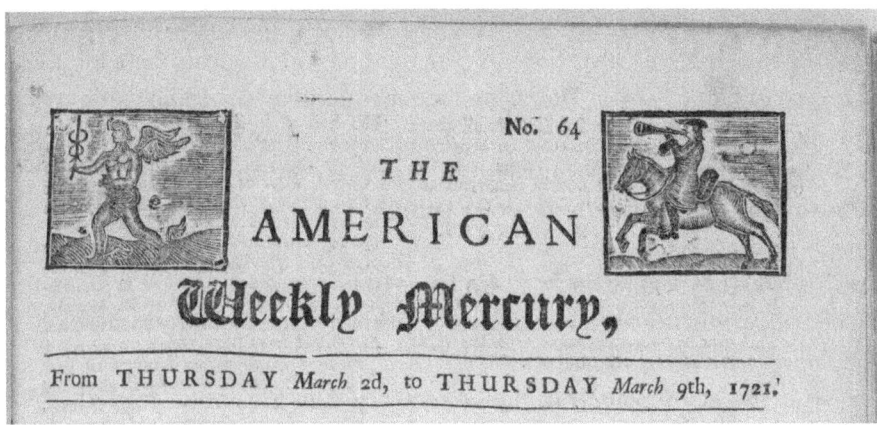

FIGURE 9.3: Post horn. The *American Weekly Mercury* used this image of a courier blowing a post horn as one of its masthead images for over twenty years. The post horn announced the arrival of the paper among other things. *American Weekly Mercury*, no. 64, March 9, 1721. American Antiquarian Society.

those goods were to be sold. Lists are, of course, another of the visual hallmarks of print culture. The interspersed advertisements often sold books, but might also seek the return of human commodities who had used the distribution network for their own own ends—runaway servants and slaves. The news itself was seldom local except to editorialize early on. Everyone knew what happened locally already. Instead the early papers told the stories collected from where the ships had been, especially England.

In the wake of the Seven Years War, a shift took place in American newspaper content. Local stories with an editorial slant proved popular, and as the colonies increasingly found themselves at loggerheads with the king and Parliament, local began to stretch out into something bigger, Anderson's imagined community, where people from Boston to Charleston began to consider themselves as Americans. The news from other parts of the continent was rendered visible at home, and people who would never meet face-to-face began thinking of themselves as belonging to the same entity, "America." All this seems to be a visually dominated process until we consider the intersection of print with another medium that played to a different sense, bells.

Bells had long been used locally as a coded medium, marking births, deaths, and marriages along with calls to worship, alarms, and other announcements (Corbin 1998; Rath 2003: 43–68; Lubken 2012). During the seventeenth and eighteenth centuries, the British royal family had sought to use them as a local-to-central tool for creating national unity and identity. Bells would be rung for the same life events as for local people, but all across the kingdom at the same time for the royals. Declarations of war, victories, and defeats were all tolled (Cressy 1989: 67–76). The simultaneous nationwide tolling for royal demographic moments rang the nation into being from the local rather than creating it authoritatively and having it trickle outward, as in theories of nationalism that focus only on print culture. For a century or so during the Enlightenment, bells and print, urban and rural, secular and religious, mingled creatively before coming apart at the seams to be reformulated yet again in the nineteenth century, a process that Alain Corbin maps beautifully in the case of the French countryside (Corbin 1998).

Nowhere was this mix so potent as in the American colonies during the eighteenth century, where the aural medium of bells worked in conjunction with print media, particularly newspapers. I have counted 1,724 examples of bell-ringing in a database of colonial newspapers (Corry et al. 1997). At first glance it looks like the newspapers silenced the bells to some extent by moving them from the immediate experience of sound to the realm of visual symbol, something to be read about rather than heard. The local tintinnabulations did not cease however. Early in the century, reports of bells ringing in London could set them off in Boston or New York as well. After the Seven Years War, reports of bells in Charleston might set them ringing in Boston. In fact, the bells, combined with the reports from other places, served as a powerful unifying force, first in a common experience of British monarchical nationalism, and then later as Americans. Thinking about the relationship of bells and print as they worked together this way complicates sensory hierarchies and narratives of substitution and replacement. The sound of a local bell could carry meaning generated elsewhere.

In particular, the protests against the Stamp Act in 1765 and 1766 generated at least 197 reports of bells being rung in protest or at the repeal of the act. Only twenty-eight of those events were in England, the remaining 169 were in the British colonies. One hundred twenty-six of those articles reported bells rung in cities different from the location of the paper, a broadening of continental concerns from the earlier pattern of localism combined with Anglophilia. None of the bells being rung were in the newly acquired British Canadian colonies, and only two were reported from the Caribbean, aligning almost perfectly with the colonies that would revolt a decade later, which shows the beginnings of an emerging American national identity before the Revolution.[6]

The range of the bells was extended by newspapers, echoing McLuhan's construction of media as extensions of the senses. In this case the effects were two layers thick at least. Even as their range grew from rendering them in print, their sounds were lost in the translation: extension combined with numbing. They became an absent presence (Gergen 2002) unless reconstituted by local peals.

Enlightened publics took many different forms, so it is impossible to simply extrapolate from print alone. In France, layers upon layers of traditional governance seemingly held fast in the mid-eighteenth century. Newspapers were banned, but in Paris and elsewhere, an informed and critical public still thrived—if indeed something that needed to be discrete to avoid police hounding could be called a public. But that very response indicated that the repressed or covert public, just by being repressed, was in fact at least effective in getting the word, or in many cases, the song, out (Darnton 2000, 2010a).

Understanding the covert publics of Old Regime Paris flounders if one stops with Kant at the reader. According to Robert Darnton, the tree of Cracow in Paris "attracted *nouvellistes de bouche*, or newsmongers, who spread information about current events by word of mouth." Other informal locations for "public noises" (*bruits publics*) existed in Paris: certain street corners, cafés, and boulevards developed reputations for news. Facetious broadsides caught one's visual attention while hurdy-gurdy players fought for the ears with songs known to all for their double meanings, with imaginary farces about far-off places masking critiques of the king and court, often in bawdy terms (Darnton 2000: 2). Scraps of verse and stories were carried about and exchanged as well, many captured for posterity when their bearers were caught and sent to the Bastille. Salons catered to the better off, who had servants gather gossip which was used as the basis for comparing notes. Transcriptions of the salon gatherings were sometimes sold by subscription, often far into the countryside. Some of these newsletters were printed as the banned but widely circulated *Mémoires secrets pour servir à l'histoire de la république des lettres en France*. The media of the Old Regime were thus, as Darnton shows, mixed: "They transmitted an amalgam of overlapping, interpenetrating messages, spoken, written, printed, pictured, and sung" (2000: 9).

The lesson of the bells and the French newsmongers is that without understanding at least hearing as well as visual culture, we miss the moments of praxis, the times when thought and action met, putting words and ideas into deeds, which then informed and reformed the words and ideas. Reading was a socially situated act. It was often done aloud, sometimes with an audience of family members, sometimes in public, and sometimes for practice alone.

Once purchased, a book, pamphlet, or newspaper may have been taken home and silently read, but if it was a good one, that was the beginning of its life rather than the end. In the American colonies, texts could be passed around to multiple readers. Many came to be located in the libraries of coffeehouses and public houses (taverns) where they might be read aloud, discussed, and perhaps if the ideas were compelling enough, put into action in some form or another. Bernard Bailyn made the case that pre-revolutionary pamphlets reflected the commonwealth strand of Enlightenment political thought that shaped the ideological underpinnings of the American Revolution (Bailyn 1968). Public houses almost always had reading material on hand, some even holding enough to qualify as having a library of sorts (Conroy 1995). No doubt some of the commonwealth pamphlet ideas were worked into actions over a mug of beer. Tavern talk could result in praxis heading in the other direction too, with "many pamphlets and newspapers mirroring tavern speech" (Thompson 1999: 10). This social reading space constituted Kant's enlightened

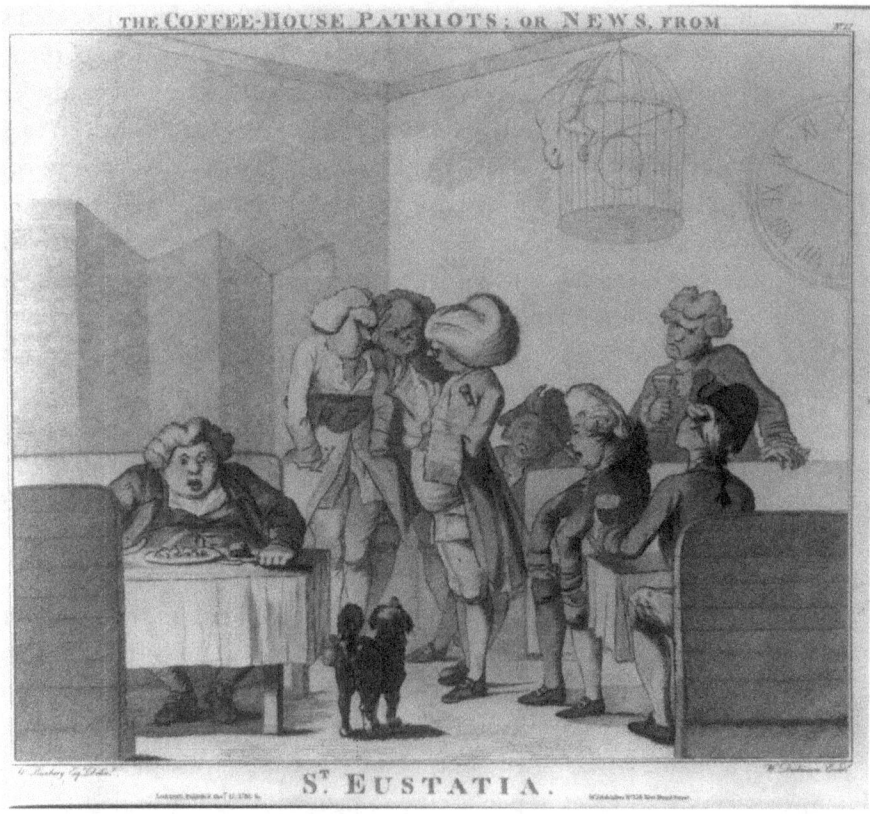

FIGURE 9.4: William Dickinson (engraver), "The Coffee-House Patriots, or News, from St. Eustatia" (London: W. Dickinson, 1781). Courtesy US Library of Congress.

public as well as the idea of the public sphere, but, as in Paris, it played out in many scenarios beyond the genteel salons of those authors' theories. Here the affect- and status-free theorized world where nothing mattered beyond the merit of an author's ideas met with the cantankerous realities of the pub. It was in these and other social reading spaces, some public, some private, that the ideas of the Enlightenment began to take shape as actions in the world.

In 1749, Ben Franklin, the leading figure of the Enlightenment in North America, argued that in ancient times, the best oratory by itself had "wonderful Effects" in "governing, turning and leading great Bodies of Mankind, Armies, Cities, Nations." But, he continued, "Modern Political Oratory being chiefly performed by the Pen and Press" was superior in the task of governing and leading because its effects were "more extensive, more lasting" (Franklin 2002b). This did not mean, however, that "Pen and Press" were sufficient. In a letter to Richard Price late in his life and as the revolution was winding down, Franklin wrote:

> The ancient Roman and Greek Orators could only speak to the Number of Citizens capable of being assembled within the Reach of their Voice: Their Writings had little Effect because the Bulk of the People could not read. Now by the Press we can speak to Nations; and good Books & well written Pamphlets have great and general Influence. The Facility with which the same Truths may be repeatedly enforc'd by placing them daily in different Lights, in Newspapers which are every where read, gives a great Chance of establishing them.
>
> Franklin 2002c

The reading he had in mind was not today's lone individual silently perusing *The Times*. Franklin knew that in order for the publication process to be effective, the news had to be published a second time by voice for two reasons: first, to spur discussion and then action, and second, to reach those without the paper or who could not read.

Widely available cheap print in the form of newspapers, books, and pamphlets had become the chief location of modern oratory according to B. Franklin, printer. These works were printed with an eye, and an ear, to a neighborhood reader finishing the job of publication by reading it aloud. Franklin thought this art of public reading had fallen on hard times because students learned to read aloud "as Parrots speak" and thus lacked the understanding of what they read necessary for the right intonation to get a point across. "For want of good Reading [aloud]," he wrote in 1751, "Pieces publish'd with a View to influence the Minds of Men for their own or the publick Benefit, lose Half their Force. Were there but one good Reader in a Neighbourhood, a publick Orator might be heard throughout a Nation with the same Advantages, and have the same Effect on his Audience, as if they stood within the Reach of his Voice" (Franklin 2002a).

Franklin was making the opposite case from McLuhan, that voice extended the reach of print, rather than vice versa. The print author/orator could literally be heard because of secondary publication, the reading aloud of the paper in public. Thus print alone was not enough to get national ideas across. They had to be read well and heard to get them into circulation as ideas that people talked about and acted upon. Without the discussion and the impetus to act, print was nothing but ideas rendered visually. It was still in the realm of the voice and hearing that ideas began to turn into actions. Thus, theories of the public sphere and nationalism need to be grounded by Franklin's praxis.

Franklin was not, however, calling for a return to oral culture. The goal of teaching people to read aloud well was to allow them to reproduce the effect of a printed text for those with no access to it, either through illiteracy or through lack of resources to obtain the printed version. Franklin wanted not a parrot, but a person who had completely learned and internalized the ideas of the author, a somewhat perturbing fantasy of control and homogeneity. Tellingly, what Franklin the printer wanted was the mass-production of language, just like in print, but by voice. A simple invocation of oral culture fails here, where Franklin hoped that the printed word's repeatability could be instilled in auditory readers to achieve national political ends at the level of the neighborhood.

The last segment of the circuit of print mediation sketched here is also the first, the socially embedded author/reader. Reading spurred new writing, creating a feedback loop. Following generic principles of marketing, printers were on the lookout for writing that would sell, a predictive process of feedforward. Discussions shaped by both experience and reading incubated ideas and caused new manuscripts to be written to be transformed yet again by the multisensorial alchemy of print as mediation rather than medium. Here we return to the circuit that led to the writing and publication of Gyles' narrative.

If we focus all our attention on the medium or even the printer in our media history, we lose half the story. By following the process of mediation all the way through from authorship through print, reading aloud, discussion, and action, and then, crucially, connecting those actions back to authorship and publication, we get a much richer explanation of how media, the senses, and the rise of nationalism were all tied together.

CONCLUSION

In the discussion of media, the senses, and enlightenment, the proximal senses—smell, taste, and touch—necessarily take a back seat to the distal senses. On the one hand, handshakes, kisses, or perfumes could all add layers of meaning to spoken and sung (if not so much to the printed) media. For example, the French king's touch served as a medium of royal power.[7] On the other hand, pushing the proximal senses too far as media in their own right shades into metaphor because the sources of touch, taste, and smell sensations were often not intentional acts meant to carry information: they did so only indirectly and often accidentally.

The place where the proximal senses do come into play is in their repression along with that of their association with the body, which we can tentatively explore as a response to increasing reliance on the distal senses. Alain Corbin's seminal work on smell in France attributes the increased sensitivity to and repression of smell to the rise of science (Corbin 1986). Perhaps the abstraction that the visual medium of print represented could have played a role in changing the written response to smell, repressing it in the medium rather than in the world. This in turn may have fostered desires for the removal of odors, the refinement of taste, and the repression of touch that scholars have found in the later years of the Enlightenment (Classen 2012).

In conclusion, to get to the relationship of the senses to mass print culture, and from there, to an enlightened public, we need to develop the analysis beyond the eyes. By taking the focus off the media themselves and their enabling technologies, and attending more to mediation, the actual lived processes by which the spread of ideas, knowledge, and information moved from creation to consumption and back again, we arrive at a much richer understanding of the forces at play in creating and maintaining the Enlightenment. When we consider mediation as processes rather than media as things, we uncover the central role played by the senses in the dynamism and revolutionary changes set in motion by the Enlightenment. In particular, the sense of hearing comes back into the foreground as the location of praxis: for the ideas conveyed in print to effect change in the world, people had to discuss them with each other and decide how and whether to implement them, not just assent or dissent to printed authority.

NOTES

Introduction

1. Some of the discussion in the second part of this chapter is adapted from Vila (1998).
2. These metaphors, borrowed from the formerly dominant discourse of theology, were both naturalized and secularized by the French *philosophes* (Mortier 1969). On the Enlightenment's "scopic regimen" and other ocularcentrist aspects, see Jay (1993: 83–147) and Riskin (2011).
3. Medical texts frequently referred to pain as useful, "a sort of sixth sense, a vigilant inner sense, which may sometimes even indicate to the physician how he should proceed" (Rey 1995: 92). This notion underpinned the therapeutics of sensory perturbation which many physicians recommended.
4. "There are no deep thinkers, no ardent imaginations that are not subject to momentary catalepsies. A singular idea comes to mind, a strange connection distracts us, and our heads are lost. We come back from that state as from a dream, asking those around us, 'where was I? What was I saying?'" (Diderot [1778a] 1975–, xvii: 328–9).

Chapter One

1. See Freedman (2012: 235). Freedman, however, also cites Erich Schön (1987: 118–19) to the effect that in the course of the eighteenth century, at least in Germany, the experience of reading was gradually reduced to the dimension of sight alone.
2. Louis Bollioud-Mermet, *De la corruption du goust dans la musique française* (1746), cited in Tsien (2012: 40).
3. Voltaire, "Goût" ([1757] 2013), cited in Tsien (2012: 56).
4. [Mathieu François Pidanzat de Mairobert?], *L'Observateur anglois, ou correspondance secrete entre Milord All'Eye and Milord All'Ear* (London

[Amersterdam?], 1777–8), no. 1 (December 1, 1775). The second edition appeared under the title *L'Espion anglois, ou correspondance secrete . . .* (1779) and this title was used for further, unattributed continuations of the series into the mid-1780s.
5. Hans-Jürgen Lusebrink, in Popkin and Fort (1998), stresses the emphasis in these periodicals on conveying just how words sounded when they were originally heard. Darnton (2010b) points to efforts in similar kinds of "news" publications to place the reader in the vantage point of a first-hand observer.
6. Ludwig Wekhrlin, *Chronologen* 7: 184 (1780), cited in Freedman (2012: 35).
7. Edme-Michel Petit, *Entendons-nous* (1794), quoted in Rosenfeld (2001: 170).
8. Montesquieu, *The Spirit of the Laws* ([1749] 1989, Bk. 2, Ch. 2: 11).
9. The Constitution of Year III is reprinted in Aberdam *et al.* (1999: 250).
10. Delacroix (1815: 252, 256). This text is briefly mentioned by Crook and Crook (2007, 2011); but neither considers the context—political and/or sensory—in which this suggestion for increased secrecy was made.

Chapter Two

1. Eliz Montagu, February 1778, see http://www.henrycort.net/hulondon.htm.

Chapter Three

1. In recent decades, an important body of work has been published on the history of Western consumer culture. Most authors identify the long eighteenth century as the key moment in the birth of a modern consumer culture. Readers interested in exploring this scholarship might begin with two classic studies: Berg, Brewer, and Plumb (1982) and Berg (2005). The majority of this work has focused on eighteenth-century England.
2. In France, coffee consumption was immediately seen as such an exceptional development that various aspects of its history began to be recorded almost as soon as that history began. Important early works include de La Roque (1716), Blégny (1687), and Mailly (1702). Recent studies include Leclant (1951) and Spary (2012).
3. Jean-Baptiste Rousseau's comedy *Le Caffé* demonstrates that the name "café" was clearly in active use by 1694. The usage must therefore have begun some years before.
4. Joachim Christoph Nemeitz, author of the first guidebook to Paris designed for a German-speaking audience, commented at length on the differences between cafés and the coffeehouses of Holland and England—the fact that *tabac à fumer*, smoking tobacco, was, for example, banned in cafés but a staple of coffeehouses (Nemeitz 1719, 1: 110–14). Nemeitz's guidebook has a publication history that is more than unusually strange. It first appeared in English as an anonymous publication (*The Present State of the Court of France*, 1712). It was then published in German, see Nemeitz (1718). The earliest French edition appeared in 1719; see Nemeitz (1719).
5. On the history of the Café Procope, see Moura and Louvet (1929).

6. In 1715, Louis Liger, self-described German visitor to Paris, published an account of his experiences (see Liger 1715). He was surprised when, on his first visit to a café, a waiter came to ask what he wanted to drink. Recent attempts to attribute this work to its publisher, Ribou, are not convincing.
7. "Almost all Parisian cafés are magnificently decorated," Jacques Savary des Bruslons declared. His *Dictionnaire universel du commerce* is the best early source of information on the commercialization of luxury goods in Europe. See Savary des Bruslons (1723–30).
8. On the role of coffeehouses in English political culture at the turn of the eighteenth century, see Pincus (1995). For an early account of the Café Laurent, see Nemeitz (1719, 1: 114). For an early account of the role cafés played in the circulation of news, see Liger (1715: 35–7).
9. There is an important recent body of work on the marketing of Indian cotton in early modern Europe. The classic study remains Irwin and Brett (1970). Among recent studies two stand out: Crill (2008) and Lemire (2003). See also DeJean (2009: Ch. 13).
10. For these examples of the French wearing Indian textiles and using them as upholstery fabrics, see DeJean (2009: Chs. 12 and 13).
11. The *Ordonnance rendue par Monsieur Hérault* from 1728 describes "plusieurs particuliers" seen wearing "étoffes des indes" in the streets of Paris, among them, the concierge of the Hôtel de Vendôme, rue de Varenne.
12. For information on the place of cotton textiles in the wardrobes of non-elite women in London in the eighteenth century, see Styles (2010).
13. The best introduction to the history of different kinds of furniture remains Havard (1890). On the evolution of the same models in England see Bowett (2002). On upholstery techniques, see Deville (1878–80) and also Thornton (1978).
14. Horace Mann wrote to Horace Walpole about "a Windsor chair, a double one, without a division" in November 1743 (Walpole 1954, 18: 332).
15. When they were first used, these engravings did not have a specific name. The 1732 edition of the *Dictionnaire universel français et latin* (generally known as the *Dictionnaire de Trévoux*) appears to be the first to include the new name, "modes," for engravings of fashionable items (entry *mode*).
16. On the history of shopping and shops, see Davis (1966). On the display of goods in eighteenth-century English shops, see Walsh (1995). On the variety of shops in eighteenth-century Paris, see Coquery (2011).
17. For more on the Princesse Palatine's views on sofa manners at the French court, and for other body language created in the late seventeenth century under the influence of the new luxury goods, see DeJean (2009: Ch. 14).

Chapter Four

1. Portions of this chapter are reprinted from Mack (2008).
2. These reforms were not always appealing to the rural peasantry of Catholic Europe, however: "In 1707 Bishop Gaston de Noailles ... was visiting ... in Chalons when

he opened the reliquary in front of a multitude of worshippers. Finding the revered relics to be three small pieces of stone wrapped in red cloth, the bishop took them away. The alarmed sacristan rang the parish bell to summon resistance. Even the notables of the town joined in the petition, beseeching the bishop to return the relic "because the townspeople had been deprived of a 400-year-old object of veneration . . . which has often been the remedy of the ills that afflict them" (Po-chia Hsia 2005: 220). Michael Printy writes that in the early eighteenth century, "[Catholic] missionaries in Europe shifted their efforts away from trying to force peasants to completely abandon their so-called superstitious beliefs . . . this shift in pastoral practice should be seen in concert with the revolution in moral theology that—while not abandoning the concept of original sin—downplayed the strongly negative Augustinian condemnation of human nature and embraced a generally more optimistic view of human moral capability" (Printy 2005: 439).

3. "As the apple tree among the trees of the wood, so is my beloved among the sons. I sat down under his shadow with great delight, and his fruit was sweet to my taste. He brought me to the banqueting house, and his banner over me was love . . . His left hand is under my head, and his right hand doth embrace me" (*Song of Songs* 2: 3–4, 6).
4. My thanks to David Wilson for this insight.
5. However, Peucker rejects Aaron Spencer Fogleman's thesis that Jesus himself was believed to be essentially female (Peucker 2007).
6. John Wesley, sermon no. 95, "On the Education of Children," *Works*, 3: 350.
7. Edmund Burke, *A Philosophical Enquiry into the Origin of Our Ideas of the Sublime and the Beautiful*, quoted in Hindmarsh (2009: 24).
8. Wesley, "An Earnest Appeal." For non-believers, the spiritual senses were interpreted not as an intense religious experience but as mere enthusiasm. There was a movement in Scottish philosophy to improve the operation of the ordinary senses without having recourse to a Christian concept of spiritual senses. Thus Benjamin Rush argued that one sense can be used to monitor other senses, ". . . with reason disciplined against superstitious judgments and unruly passions, and with hearsay held in check." You might see or hear a ghost, but you can't touch one (Schmidt 2000: 165).
9. John Wesley, *Queries Proposed to the Right Reverend and Right Honourable Count Zinzendorf* (1755), 27–8, quoted in Abelove (1990: 54).
10. Cennick to the *Gemeine*, Dublin [1998], July 25, 1746. Moravian Archive, London.
11. The linguist Jean-Pierre van Noppen writes, ". . . the imagery of blood . . . refers both to the canceling of sin and to the cleansing from sin. In most instances, 'blood' is . . . a shorthand term for redemption and atonement . . . without any sordid suggestions of physicality" (van Noppen 2005: 26).
12. John Fletcher, letter to Miss Hatton, Madeley, January 9, 1787 (Jeffrey 1987: 380). A rare Methodist hymn on Christ as a bridegroom says merely "Raise our hearts to things on high/To our Bridegroom in the sky . . ." (C. Wesley 1989: 322).
13. F/T MAM Fl 09/05, The John Rylands University Library.

Chapter Five

1. The title of this chapter was determined by the publishers. I employ the terms "science" and "philosophy" here in the most conventional way possible.
2. For chemistry, see Roberts (1995).
3. Calinger (2007: 17) claims that Euler only lost the use of his right eye in 1738.
4. Euler (1738) esp. pp. 345–6. English translation, available online: http://www.gss.ucsb.edu/Langton1.pdf.
5. On political arithmetic, see Poovey (2005).
6. For a non-dualist cognitive approach, see Hutchins (1995); Tribble (2005); Sutton *et al.* (2011).
7. See e.g. Linnaeus' condescending description of Lapp courting rituals. "In other parts of the world you must be wooed with coffee and chocolate, preserves and sweets, wines and dainties, jewels and pearls, gold and silver . . . [in Lapland] you are satisfied with [the scent of] a little withered fungus!" (Blunt 2001: 49).
8. Compare with Bourdieu (1984).
9. Susan Faye Cannon (1978) coined the term "Humboldtian science."
10. See e.g. Steller ([1793] 1988: 119).
11. Knowledge regarding indigo and its use accompanied slaves from West Africa to the western hemisphere, where it mixed with indigenous and European traditions (personal communication with Jenny Balfour-Paul).
12. Cañizares-Esguerra (2005) documents, however, the active involvement and lasting legacy of Nahua (Aztec) practitioners and the independent course taken by Creole naturalists in Latin America.
13. Hiraga (1763); Marcon (2007); Liss (2009) esp. pp. 17–31; Nappi (2009) esp. pp. 20–1, for comparison between *honzogaku* and its Chinese counterpart *bencao*.
14. For the pre-history of Europe's acquaintance with natural rubber see Reisz (2007).
15. On training the senses as investigative instruments, see Roberts (1995).
16. Compare Stafford (1991); Vila (1998).
17. Authors such as Charles Bonnet, Albrecht von Haller, and David Hartley used the language of vibrating strings or threads, especially to discuss the sensible action of nerves and how that was cognized (Glassman *et al.* 2007; Whitaker and Turgeon 2007). For Diderot's *horloge ambulante*, see Diderot (1751: 112); Vartanian (1983: 173–8). For Diderot's *tableau mouvant* see Diderot (1751b: 122–3). While often interpreted as a metaphorical expression composed by Diderot, *tableaux mouvants* were in fact popular contrivances that featured fast-moving scenes and figurines, first invented by Father Sébastien Truchet for the children of Louis XIV. I thank Anne Vila for pointing this out.
18. Diderot contrasted this with workers' intuitive ability to "smell out" (*subodorer*) the truths of nature (Diderot 1754).
19. For Europe see Schaffer (1999); Riskin (2003a); Voskuhl (2013); Metzner (1998). For China see Corbeiller (1960); Schaffer (2006). For Japan see Screech (2002).
20. See also Connor (2005).

Chapter Six

1. Some passages of this section are adapted from Singy (2006).
2. A note on Figure 6.2. This is one of several letters sent by this sufferer to Tissot. The other letters describe Lavergne's many symptoms, which included weakness, sweating, pains, coughs, etc. In this letter Lavergne relates the difficulties he has been encountering while trying to follow a prescription made by Tissot. For instance, Tissot prescribed asses' milk (a common prescription in the eighteenth century), and Lavergne complains that in the winter asses' milk is "suspect." He asks Tissot if it could be replaced with cow's milk or turtle broth.
3. *Consultations choisies de plusieurs médecins célèbres de l'Université de Montpellier sur des maladies aiguës et chroniques* (1748–50, 1: x).
4. Letter from Lavergne l'aîné to Tissot, Lyon, October 25 [1772], Tissot MSS, 3784/II/144.01.07.24, p. 1. Most of the letters to Tissot are located in the Bibliothèque Cantonale Universitaire in Lausanne, Switzerland, in the Fonds Tissot (hereafter referred to as "Tissot MSS"). A few others are in the Bibliothèque de Genève, Fonds Eynard (hereafter referred to as "Eynard MSS"). All the consultation letters sent to Tissot are available online and searchable with an elaborate database built by Séverine Pilloud, Micheline Louis-Courvoisier, and Vincent Barras. See www.chuv.ch/iuhmsp/ihm_bhms.
5. Letter from Birague de Brusque to Tissot, Turin, September 8, 1774, Tissot MSS, 3784/II/144.02.05.10, p. 1.
6. Letter from Bon to Tissot, Perpignan, April 16, 1790, Tissot MSS, 3784/II/144.05.02.35, p. 1.
7. Letter from de Barbazan to Tissot, Toulon, August 20, 1773, Tissot MSS, 3784/II/149.01.04.20, p. 1.
8. Letter from Thomassin to Tissot, Besançon, March 1775, Tissot MSS, 3784/II/144.02.08.13, p. 1.
9. Letter from Tronchin to Monsieur le Conseiller Fay in Lyon, September 15, 1756, Tronchin MSS, Ms. 204, pp. 9–10. The letters to and from Tronchin are located in the Bibliothèque de Genève, in the Fonds Tronchin (hereafter referred to as "Tronchin MSS").
10. Letter from Tronchin to Durin in Annonay, May 3, 1758, Tronchin MSS, Ms. 204, p. 166.
11. Letter from Savary père to Tissot, Fribourg, December 16, 1784, Tissot MSS, 3784/II/144.03.05.07, p. 2.
12. Since Corvisart reproduced the original Latin text of Auenbrugger, I refer to Corvisart's edition.
13. Some of Morgagni's cases of phthisis indeed do not mention tubercles. See, for instance, 1: 645–7 (§4 and §5), and 1: 655 (§16).
14. To this criticism, Morgagni replied that with enough practice the anatomist becomes able to see the relations between specific symptoms and specific lesions.

Chapter Eight

1. The painting, now in a private collection, was on public exhibition in The Frick Collection, New York City, in 2011–13. The authenticity of the work, and its attribution to Watteau are, in this author's opinion, unquestionable. See Bailey (2012).
2. For the seventeenth-century academic hierarchy, see André Félibien, *Conférences de l'Académie royale de peinture et de sculpture pendant l'année 1667* (1669), quoted and discussed in Duro (1997: 9–10).
3. Jacqueline Lichtenstein argues that de Piles consistently foregrounded the tangible realm through his advocacy of visual immediacy, sensuality, and surface effects. See, e.g., Lichtenstein (1993: 154–5).
4. Watteau reversed the position of the spaniel that in Rubens' painting draws the viewer's attention to the future queen by gazing up directly at her.
5. I would like to thank Alvin L. Clark, Jr., for helping me to acquire this image (Figure 8.2).
6. The section on touch is entitled: "Du Toucher, ou du seul sens qui juge par lui-même des objets extérieur"; see Condillac (1947: 251–74).
7. For Diderot's critique of Boucher in his *Salons*—book-length correspondences critiquing the biannual exhibitions of the Royal Academy of Painting and Sculpture held in the *Salon d'Apollon* of the Louvre—see Sahut *et al.* (1984: 101–7, 136–43) and Diderot (1995: 22–9). Melissa Hyde (2006: 56–8) has exposed the internal conflicts of Diderot's expressed opinions of Boucher, whom he praises for technical brilliance but opposes for his degraded, "feminized" taste.
8. See also Vila (1998: 75–7).
9. Childs' study focuses upon the first of these porcelain bowls that were made for the court of Augustus II in Saxony. Bustelli and other modelers employed by the Nymphenburg factory around the middle of the eighteenth century directly emulated the Meissen models, evidently to serve a growing taste for this type of ware in the eighteenth-century Germanic states and beyond.
10. For a subtle analysis of this conflation of the "Indian" and the African in eighteenth-century popular imagery in Europe, see Molineux (2007).
11. A stylistic and temperamental exception to this trend is the work of Thomas Gainsborough, whose paintings, as Bermingham (2005) and others have argued, are steeped in sensibility but also display the loose brushwork and emphasis upon color found in the works of the French rococo artists, as noted above. A similar combination of emotional sensibility and rococo-inspired tactility is found in the works of the French painter Jean-Honoré Fragonard (Sheriff 1990).
12. "And it came to pass, when the evil spirit from God was upon Saul, that David took an harp, and played with his hand: so Saul was refreshed, and was well, and the evil spirit departed from him" (1 Sam. 16:23 [King James Version]). For more on the effects of music, from occult properties attributed to it during the Renaissance to eighteenth-century discussions of sympathy, see Thomas (2002: 179–200).
13. For a detailed account of the eighteenth-century rise of sensibility in medical discourse, see Vila (1998: 13–107). See also Thomas (1995: 154–8) and Thomas (2002: 190–9).

14. On the rise and waning of the paradigm of music as a kind of language, see Thomas (1995: 20–33).

Chapter Nine

1. However, there is not agreement on whether this is true at all, much less on what that "something" is (Eisenstein 2002a; Johns 2002).
2. Jonathan Zittrain defines a generative technology as one with an "overall capacity to produce unprompted change driven by large, varied, and uncoordinated audiences" (Zittrain 2006). In the past as well as the present, generative media have often taken decades or even centuries to unfold (Rath 2008: 429). For social constructionism and its foil, see Daniel Chandler's *Technological or Media Determinism* (1996).
3. Robert Darnton (2000, 2010a) has tracked the visual and oral complexities of such networks for mid-eighteenth-century Paris.
4. A partial public is a concept related to but distinct from Michael Warner's (2002) notion of counterpublic. Whereas counterpublics seem always to be aimed at becoming full-blown publics with hegemonic if not universal claims to attentions, partial or covert publics were meant to be public only to some while remaining beyond the comprehension, even if not out of the sight or hearing, of others. An example would be African American uses of drum languages to organize revolts, which could be heard but not understood by planters (Rath 2003: 78–96).
5. Compare Anderson (1991: 1–47) with McLuhan (2012: 245–51).
6. Rather than in its aftermath (Breen 1997; Smith-Rosenberg 1992).
7. Darnton notes that its cessation in 1744 "signaled the end—or at least the beginning of the end—of the roi-mage, the sacred, thaumaturgic king . . . By mid-century, Louis XV had lost touch with his people, and he had lost the royal touch" (2000: 15).

BIBLIOGRAPHY

Abelove, H., 1990, *The Evangelist of Desire: John Wesley and the Methodists*, Stanford, CA: Stanford University Press.
Aberdam, S. et al. (eds), 1999, *Voter, élire pendant la Révolution française, 1789–1799. Guide pour la recherche*, Paris: CTHS.
Addison, J., [1711–14] 1965, *The Spectator*, 5 vols, ed. D. F. Bond, Oxford: Clarendon Press.
Addison, J., 1718, *Remarks on Several Parts of Italy &c., in the Years 1701, 1702, 1703*, London: J. Tonson.
Adorno, T. and Horkheimer, M., [1944] 1997, *Dialectic of Enlightenment*, trans. J. Cumming, London and New York: Verso.
Agrimi, J. and Crisciani, C., 1994, *Les Consilia médicaux*, Turnhout: Brepols.
Akenside, M., [1744] 1857, *The Poetical Works of Mark Akenside*, ed. G. Gilfillan, Edinburgh: James Nichol.
Alembert, J. L. R. d', [1751] 1929, *Discours préliminaire de l'Encyclopédie*, Paris: Bureaux de la publication.
Alembert, J. L. R. d', 1763, *Mélanges de littérature, d'histoire, et de philosophie*, Amsterdam: Zacharie Chatelain & Fils.
Allen, M., 2006, *An English Lady in Paris: the diary of Frances Anne Crewe* [1786], St. Leonards: Oxford-Stockley Publications.
Alpers, S., 1983, *The Art of Describing: Dutch art in the seventeenth century*, Chicago: University of Chicago Press.
An Account of the Earthquake Which Destroyed the City of Lisbon on the First of November, 1755, and the Appearance of the City previous to that Calamity: Illustrative of the Great Picture of the Earthquake at Lisbon, c. 1800, Now Exhibiting at the Lyceum, Strand, London: printed by W. Glendinning.
Anderson, B. R. O'G., 1991, *Imagined Communities: reflections on the origin and spread of nationalism*, London and New York: Verso.

Arasse, D., 1996, *Le Détail. Pour une histoire rapprochée de la peinture*, Paris: Flammarion.
Arendt, H., 1958, *The Human Condition*, Chicago: University of Chicago Press.
Arnaud, F., 1754, *Lettre sur la musique à Monsieur le comte de Caylus*, n.p.: n.p.
Arnauld, A., 1727, *Lettres*, 9 vols, Nancy: Joseph Nicolai.
Arndt, A., 2007, "Touching London: contact, sensibility and the city," in A. Cowan and J. Seward (eds), *The City and The Senses: Urban Culture Since 1500*, Aldershot: Ashgate Press.
Arnold, M., [1880] 1903, "The study of poetry," in *Essays in Criticism: Second Series, Contributions to "The Pall Mall Gazette", and Discourses in America*, London: Macmillan.
Ashfield, A. and de Bolla, P., 1996, *The Sublime: a reader in British eighteenth-century aesthetic theory*, Cambridge: Cambridge University Press.
Atwood, C. D., 2004, *Community of the Cross: Moravian piety in colonial Bethlehem*, University Park, PA: Pennsylvania State University Press.
Auenbrugger, L., 1761, *Inventum Novum ex Percussione Thoracis Humani ut Signo Abstrusos Interni Pectoris Morbos Detegendi*, Vindobonae: Joannis Thomae Trattner.
Auenbrugger, L., 1808, *Nouvelle méthode pour reconnaître les maladies internes de la poitrine par la percussion de cette cavité*, trans J. N. Corvisart, Paris: De l'Imprimerie de Migneret.
Aymen, J. B., 1752, *Dissertation dans laquelle on examine si les jours critiques sont les mêmes en nos climats qu'ils étaient dans ceux où Hippocrate les a observés, & quels égards on doit y avoir dans la pratique*, Paris: Chez Prault fils.
Azouvi, F., 1991, "Le magnétisme animal: la sensation infinie," *Dix-huitième siècle*, 23, 107–18.
Babbitt, I., 1919, *Rousseau and Romanticism*, Boston, MA: Houghton Mifflin.
Baecque, A. de, 1997, *The Body Politic: corporeal metaphor in revolutionary France, 1770–1800*, trans. from French by C. Mandell, Stanford, CA: Stanford University Press.
Bailey, C. B., 2012, "Jean-Antoine Watteau's *La Surprise*: a newly discovered masterpiece comes to the Frick Collection," *The Frick Collections Members' Magazine*, spring/summer, 12–15.
Bailyn, B., 1968, *The Ideological Origins of the American Revolution*, Cambridge, MA: Belknap Press of Harvard University.
Baker, H. F., 1897, "Nicholas Saunderson," in *Dictionary of National Biography*, Oxford: Oxford University Press.
Baridon, M., 2001, "Hogarth's 'living machines of nature' and the theorisation of aesthetics," in D. Bindman, F. Ogée, and P. Wagner (eds), *Hogarth: Representing Nature's Machines*, Manchester: Manchester University Press.
Barker, E., 2005, *Greuze and the Painting of Sentiment*, Cambridge and New York: Cambridge University Press.
Barker-Benfield, G. J., 1992, *The Culture of Sensibility: sex and society in eighteenth-century Britain*, Chicago: University of Chicago Press.

Barles, S., 2005, *L'Invention des déchets urbains: France (1790–1970)*, Seyssel: Champ Vallon.
Barlow, J., 2005, *The Enraged Musician: Hogarth's Musical Imagery*, Aldershot and Burlington, VT: Ashgate.
Barrell, J., 1988, "Being is perceiving: James Thomson and John Clare," in *Poetry, Language and Politics*, Manchester: Manchester University Press.
Barrow, J., 1804, *Travels in China, Containing Descriptions, Observations and Comparison, Made and Collected in the Course of a Short Residence at the Imperial Palace of Yuen-Min-Yuen and on a Subsequent Journey Through the Country from Peking to Canton*, London.
Bart, J. et al. (eds), 1998, *La Constitution de l'an III, ou l'ordre républicain*, Dijon: EUD.
Batteux, C., 1746, *Les beaux arts réduits à un même principe*, Paris: Durand.
Baumgärtel, B. (ed.), 1998, *Angelika Kauffmann*, Ostfildern-Ruit: Gerd Hatje.
Bensaude-Vincent, B. and Blondel, C. (eds), 2008, *Science and Spectacle in the European Enlightenment*, Aldershot: Ashgate.
Berg, M., 2005, *Luxury and Pleasure in eighteenth-Century Britain*, Oxford: Oxford University Press.
Berg, M. and Clifford, H. (eds), 1999, *Consumers and Luxury: consumer culture in Europe, 1650–1850*, Manchester: Manchester University Press.
Berg, M. and Eger, E. (eds), 2001, *Luxury in the Eighteenth Century: debates, desires, and delectable goods*, Basingstoke: Palgrave.
Berg, M., Brewer, J. and Plumb, J. H. (eds), 1982, *The Birth of a Consumer Society: the commercialization of eighteenth-Century England*, London: Europa Publications.
Bermingham, A., 2005, "Introduction: Gainsborough's *Cottage Door*: sensation and sensibility," in A. Bermingham (ed.), *Sensation and Sensibility: viewing Gainsborough's Cottage Door*, New Haven, CT and London: Yale University Press.
Bertucci, P., 2013, "Enlightened secrets: silk, intelligent travel, and industrial espionage in eighteenth-century France," *Technology and Culture*, 54, 820–52.
Blake, W., 1966, *Complete Writings*, ed. G. Keynes, Oxford: Oxford University Press.
Blake, W., 1979, *Blake's Poetry and Designs*, ed. M. L. Johnson and J. E. Grant, New York: Norton.
Blumin, S. M., 2008, *The Encompassing City: streetscapes in early modern art and culture*, Manchester: Manchester University Press.
Blunt, W., 2001, *The Compleat Naturalist: A Life of Linnaeus*, London: Frances Lincoln Ltd.
Bödeker, H. E., 2001, "On the origins of the 'statistical gaze': modes of perception, forms of knowledge and ways of writing in the early social sciences," in P. Becker and W. Clark (eds), *Little Tools of Knowledge: historical essays on academic and bureaucratic practices*, Ann Arbor, MI: University of Michigan Press.
Boerhaave, H., 1743, *Consultationes medicae*, Hagae-Comitum: Alex Johnson.
Boerhaave, H., 1745, *Boerhaave's Medical Correspondence*, London: John Nourse.
Bollioud-Mermet, L., 1746, *De la corruption du goust dans la musique française*, Lyon: A. Delaroche.

Bordeu, T. de, [1754] 2013, "Crise," in *Encyclopédie, ou Dictionnaire raisonné des sciences, des arts et des métiers*, ed. D. Diderot and J. le Rond d'Alembert, University of Chicago ARTFL Encyclopédie Project (Spring 2013 Edition), ed. R. Morrissey, http://encyclopedie.uchicago.edu/, vol. 4.

Bordeu, T. de, [1756] 1818, "Recherches sur le pouls par rapport aux crises," in *Oeuvres complètes de Bordeu*, Paris: Caille et Ravier, vol. 1.

Boswell, J., [1762–3] 1950, *The London Journal*, ed. F. A. Pottle, New Haven, CT: Yale University Press.

Bourdieu, P., 1984, *Distinction: a social critique of the judgment of taste*, Cambridge, MA: Harvard University Press.

Bowett, A., 2002, *English Furniture: 1660–1714*, London: Antique Collectors' Club.

Boyson, R., 2012, *Wordsworth and the Enlightenment Idea of Pleasure*, Cambridge: Cambridge University Press.

Boyson, R. 2013, "Shelley's Republic of Odours: aesthetic and political dimensions of scent in 'The Sensitive-Plant' ", *Keats-Shelley Review*, 27(2), 105–20.

Brant, C., 2004, "Fume and perfume: some eighteenth-century uses of smell," *The Journal of British Studies*, 43, 444–63.

Brant, C., 2011, " 'I will carry you with me on the wings of immagination': aerial letters and eighteenth-century ballooning," *Eighteenth-Century Life*, 35(1), 168–87.

Breen, T. H., 1997, "Ideology and nationalism on the eve of the American Revolution: revisions once more in need of revising," *Journal of American History*, 84(1), 13–39.

Bremer-David, C. (ed.), 2011, *Paris: Life and Luxury in the Eighteenth Century*, Los Angeles: Getty Museum.

Brewer, J., 1997, *The Pleasures of the Imagination: English Culture in the Eighteenth Century*, New York: Harper Collins.

Brewer, J. and Plumb, J. H. (eds), 1982, *The Birth of Consumer Society: the commercialization of 18th-century England*, Bloomington, IN: University of Indiana Press.

Brillat-Savarin, J-A., [1825] 1994, *The Physiology of Taste*, trans. from French by A. Dayton, Harmondsworth: Penguin.

Brocklesby, R., 1749, *Reflections on Antient and Modern Musick, with the Application to the Cure of Diseases*, London: M. Cooper.

Brockliss, L., 1994, "Consultation by letter in early eighteenth-century Paris: the medical practice of Etienne-François Geoffroy," in A. La Berge and M. Feingold (eds), *French Medical Culture in the Nineteenth Century*, Amsterdam: Rodopi.

Brockliss, L. and Jones, C., 1997, *The Medical World of Early Modern France*, Oxford: Clarendon Press.

Brown, E., 1923, *Journal of a Visit to Paris in the Year 1664*, ed. G. Keynes, London: J. Murray.

Brown, T., 1702, *Amusements Serious and Comical, Calculated for the Meridian of London*, 2nd edn, London: The Booksellers.

Buchan, W., 1774, *Domestic Medicine; Or, the Family Physician*, 2nd American edn, Philadelphia, PA: printed by Joseph Crukshank for R. Aitken.

Burke, E., [1757] 1968, *Philosophical Enquiry into the Origin of Our Ideas of the Sublime and Beautiful*, ed. J. Bolton, Notre Dame: Notre Dame University Press.
Burke, P., 1994, *The Fabrication of Louis XIV*, New Haven, CT: Yale University Press.
Burton, R., [1621] 1800, *The Anatomy of Melancholy*, 2 vols, London: J. Cundee.
Calinger, R., 1996, "Leonhard Euler: the first St. Petersburg years (1727–41)," *Historia Mathematica: International Journal of History of Mathematics*, 23, 121–66.
Calinger, R., 2007, "Leonhard Euler: life and thought," in R. Bradley and C. E. Sandifer (eds), *Leonhard Euler: life, work and legacy*, Amsterdam: Elsevier.
Camino, P., 1799, *Déterminer si les observations des modernes ont vérifié la doctrine des jours critiques, établie par les anciens*, Montpellier: De l'Imprimerie de F. Seran, Gras et Coucourdan.
Campbell, P. R., Kaiser, T. E. and Linton, M. (eds), 2007, *Conspiracy in the French Revolution*, Manchester: Manchester University Press.
Canetti, E., [1960] 1962, *Crowds and Power*, London: Victor Gollancz Ltd.
Canguilhem, G., [1943] 1998, *Le normal et le pathologique*, 7th edn, Paris: Presses Universitaires de France.
Cañizares-Esguerra, J., 2005, "Iberian colonial science," *Isis*, 96, 64–70.
Cannon, S. F., 1978, *Science in Culture: the early Victorian period*, New York: Dawson and Science History Publications.
Caraccioli, L-A. de, [1755] 1761, *La Jouissance de soi-même*, Frankfurt and Liège: chez Jean-François Bassompierre.
Carney, J., 2001, *Black Rice: the African origins of rice cultivation in the Americas*, Cambridge, MA: Harvard University Press.
Carr, J. L., 1960, "Pygmalion and the 'philosophes'," *Journal of the Warburg and Courtauld Institutes*, 23, 239–55.
Carrard, B., 1777, *Essai qui a remporté le prix de la Société Hollandoise des Sciences de Haarlem en 1770 sur cette question, Qu'est-ce qui est requis dans l'art d'observer; et jusqu'où cet Art contribue-t-il à perfectionner l'Entendement?* Amsterdam: Marc-Michel Rey.
Cavaillé, J-P., 1998, "De la construction des apparences au culte de la transparence: simulation et dissimulation entre le XVIe et le XVIIIe siècle," *Littératures classiques*, 34, 73–102.
Cavanaugh, A. and Yonan, M. E. (eds), 2010, *The Cultural Aesthetics of Eighteenth-Century Porcelain*, Farnham and Burlington, VT: Ashgate.
Cennick, J., 1754, *The Vision of dry Bones. Being the substance of a discourse delivered in Dublin, in the year 1754*, Dublin: S. Powell, for the author.
Chambers, N. (ed.), 2000, *The Letters of Sir Joseph Banks: a selection, 1768–1820*, London: Imperial College Press.
Chandler, D., 1996, *Technological or Media Determinism*, www.aber.ac.uk/media/Documents/tecdet/tecdet.html.
Charlton, D., 2013, *Opera in the Age of Rousseau: Music, Confrontation, Realism*, Cambridge: Cambridge University Press.
Charrière, I. de, [1784] 1993, *Letters of Mistress Henley Published by Her Friend*, trans. J. Hinde and P. Stewart, New York: Modern Language Association of America.

Chartier, R. (ed.), 1993, *A History of Private Life, vol. III: Passions of the Renaissance*, trans. A. Goldhammer, Cambridge, MA: Harvard University Press.

Childs, A., 2010, "Sugar boxes and blackamoors: ornamental blackness in early Meissen porcelain," in A. Cavanaugh and M. E. Yonan (eds), *Cultural Aesthetics of Eighteenth-Century Porcelain*, Farnham and Burlington, VT: Ashgate.

Clare, J., 2004, *Major Works*, ed. E. Robinson and D. Powell, Oxford: Oxford University Press.

Classen, C., 1998, *The Colour of Angels: cosmology, gender and the aesthetic imagination*, London: Routledge.

Classen, C., 2012, *The Deepest Sense: A Cultural History of Touch*, Urbana, IL: University of Illinois Press.

Clements, C., 1992, "The Academy and the Other: Les Graces et le Genre Galant," *Eighteenth-Century Studies*, 25 (summer), 469–94.

Cockayne, E., 2007, *Hubbub: filth, noise and stench in England, 1600–1770*, New Haven, CT: Yale University Press.

Cohen, S. R., 2004, "Chardin's fur: painting, materialism, and the question of animal soul," *Eighteenth-Century Studies*, 38, 39–61.

Coleridge, S. T., [c. 1801] 1957, *The Notebooks of Samuel Taylor Coleridge*, ed. K. Coburn, Princeton, NJ: Princeton University Press.

Coleridge, S. T., [1835] 1990, *Table Talk*, 2 vols, ed. C. Woodring, London: Routledge.

Colson, J., 1740, "Dr. Saunderson's palpable arithmetic decypher'd," in N. Saunderson, *The elements of algebra, in ten books; to which is prefixed an account of the author's life and character*, Cambridge.

Conac, G. and Machelon, J-P. (eds), 1999, *La Constitution de l'an III: Boissy d'Anglas et la naissance du libéralisme constitutionnel*, Paris: PUF.

Condillac, E. B. de, 1746, *Essai sur l'origine des connaissances humaines*, Paris.

Condillac, E. B. de, 1754, *Traité des sensations*, London.

Condillac, É. B. de, [1755] 1947, *Traité des animaux*, in *Oeuvres philosophiques* (q.v), 3 vols, Paris: Presses Universitaires de France, I.

Condillac, É B., de, [1754] 1947, *Traité des sensations*, in *Oeuvres philosophiques* (q.v), 3 vols, Paris: Presses Universitaires de France, I.

Condorcet, J. A. N. de Caritat, Marquis de, 1794, *Esquisse d'un tableau historique des progrès de l'esprit humain*, Paris.

Condorcet, J. A. N. de Caritat, Marquis de, 1785, "Eloge de M. de Vaucanson," *Histoire de l'Académie royale des sciences, année 1782*.

Connor, S., 2005, "Michel Serres' Les cinq sens," in N. Abbas (ed.), *Mapping Michel Serres*, Ann Arbor, MI: University of Michigan Press.

Conroy, D. W., 1995, *In Public Houses: drink and the revolution in authority in colonial Massachusetts*, Chapel Hill, NC and London: University of North Carolina Press for the Institute of Early American History and Culture, Williamsburg, Virginia.

Consultations choisies de plusieurs médecins célèbres de l'Université de Montpellier sur des maladies aiguës et chroniques, 1748–50, 8 vols, Paris: Chez Durand et Chez Pissot fils.

Coquery, N., 2011, *Tenir boutique à Paris au XVIIIe siècle: Luxe et demi-luxe*, Paris: Éditions du comité des travaux historiques et scientifiques.
Corbeiller, C. L., 1960, "James Cox and his Curious Toys," *The Metropolitan Museum of Art Bulletin*, 18, 318–24.
Corbin, A., 1986, *The Foul and the Fragrant: odor and the French social imagination*, trans. M. L. Kochan, R. Porter, and C. Prendergast, Cambridge, MA: Harvard University Press.
Corbin, A., 1994, *The Lure of the Sea: the discovery of the seaside in the western world, 1750–1840*, trans. from French by J. Phelps, Berkeley, CA: University of California Press.
Corbin, A., 1998, *Village Bells: sound and meaning in the nineteenth-century French countryside*, trans. M. Thom, New York: Columbia University Press.
Corfield, P. J., 1990, "Walking the city streets: the urban odyssey in 18th-century England," *Journal of Urban History*, 16(2), 132–74.
Corry, M. J., Van Winkle Keller, K., and Keller, R. M., 1997, *The Performing Arts in Colonial American Newspapers, 1690–1783. Text Data Base and Index*, New York: University Music Editions.
Corvisart, J. N., 1808, "[Commentaires]," in L. Auenbrugger, *Nouvelle méthode pour reconnaître les maladies internes de la poitrine par la percussion de cette cavité*, Paris: De l'Imprimerie de Migneret.
Cowan, A. and Steward, J. (eds), 2007, *The City and the Senses: urban culture since 1500*, Aldershot: Ashgate.
Cowan, B., 2005, *The Social Life of Coffee: the emergence of the British coffeehouse*, New Haven, CT: Yale University Press.
Coxe, W., 1779, *Sketches of the Natural, Civil, and Political state of Swisserland; in a series of letters to William Melmoth, Esq*, Dublin: George Bonham.
Coxe, W., 1784, *Travels into Poland, Russia, Sweden, and Denmark, interspersed with Historical Relations and Political Inquiries*, 3 vols, Dublin: printed for S. Price, R. Moncriefffe, W. Colles, T. Walker, C. Jenkin, W. Wilson, L. White, R. Burton, J. Cash, and P. Byrne.
Crary, J., 1990, *Techniques of the Observer: on vision and modernity in the nineteenth century*, Cambridge, MA: MIT Press.
Cressy, D., 1989, *Bonfires and Bells: national memory and the Protestant calendar in Elizabethan and Stuart England*, Berkeley, CA: University of California Press.
Crewe, F. A., [1786] 2006, *An English Lady in Paris: the diary of Frances Anne Crewe*, ed. M. Allen, St. Leonards: Oxford-Stockley Publications.
Crill, R., 2008, *Chintz: Indian Textiles for the West*, London: Victoria and Albert Publications.
Crook, M., 1996, *Elections in the French Revolution: an apprenticeship in democracy, 1789–1799*, Cambridge: Cambridge University Press.
Crook, M. and Crook, T., 2007, "The advent of the secret ballot in Britain and France, 1789–1914: from public assembly to private compartment," *History*, 92(308), 449–71.
Crook, M. and Crook, T., 2011, "Reforming voting practices in a Global Age: the

making and remaking of the modern secret ballot in Britain, France and the United States, c. 1600–c.1950," *Past and Present*, 212(1), 199–237.
Crowley, J. E., 2001, *The Invention of Comfort: sensibilities and design in early modern Britain and America*, Baltimore, MD: Johns Hopkins University Press.
Cruickshank, J., 2009, *Pain, Passion and Faith: revisiting the place of Charles Wesley in early Methodism*, Pietist and Wesleyan Studies, no. 31, Lanham, Toronto and Plymouth: Scarecrow Press, Inc.
Curl, J. S., 2010, *Spas, Wells, and Pleasure-Gardens of London*, London: Historical Publications Ltd.
d'Amador, R., 1837, "Influence de l'anatomie pathologique sur la médecine depuis Morgagni jusqu'à nos jours," *Mémoires de l'Académie Royale de Médecine*, 6, 313–493.
Damrosch, L., 2005, "Generality and particularity," in H. B. Nisbet and C. Rawson (eds), *The Cambridge History of Literary Criticism*, Vol. 4: *The Eighteenth Century*, Cambridge: Cambridge University Press.
Darnton, R., 1968, *Mesmerism and the End of the Enlightenment in France*, Cambridge, MA: Harvard University Press.
Darnton, R., 1995, *The Forbidden Bestsellers of Pre-Revolutionary France*, New York: Norton.
Darnton, R., 2000, "An early information society: news and the media in eighteenth-century Paris," *The American Historical Review*, 105(1), 1–35.
Darnton, R., 2010a, *Poetry and the Police: communication networks in eighteenth-century Paris*, Cambridge, MA: Belknap Press of Harvard University Press.
Darnton, R., 2010b, *The Devil in the Holy Water or the Art of Slander from Louis XIV to Napoleon*, Philadelphia, PA: University of Pennsylvania Press.
Daston, L., 2008, "Attention and the values of nature in the Enlightenment," in E. Edwards and K. Bhaumik (eds), *Visual Sense: a cultural reader*, Oxford: Berg.
Davis, D., 1966, *A History of Shopping*, London: Routledge & Kegan Paul.
De Blégny, N., 1687, *Le Bon usage du thé, du café, et du chocolat*, Paris: l'auteur.
De Bolla, P., 2003, *The Education of the Eye: painting, landscape, and architecture in eighteenth-century Britain*, Stanford, CA: Stanford University Press.
de la Chassagne, R., 1770, *Manuel des pulmoniques, ou Traité complet des maladies de la poitrine*, Paris: Chez Humaire.
De La Roque, J., 1716, *Voyage de l'Arabie heureuse* and "Traité de l'origine et du progrès du café" (supplément), Paris: André Cailleau.
De Mailly, L., 1702, *Les Entretiens des cafés de Paris*, Trévoux: E. Ganeau.
Degenaar, M., 1996, *Molyneux's Problem: three centuries of discussion on the perception of forms*, Dordrecht: Kluwer Academic Publishers.
DeJean, J., 2005, *The Essence of Style: how the French invented high fashion, fine food, chic cafés*, New York: Simon & Schuster.
DeJean, J., 2009, *The Age of Comfort: when Paris discovered casual and the modern home began*, New York: Bloomsbury.
Delacroix, J. V., 1815, *Le Spectateur françois pendant le gouvernement révolutionnaire*, new ed., Versailles: De l'Imprimerie de J. A. Lebel [Paris, an IV].

Delany, M. (Mrs. Mary Granville), [1900], *A Memoir: 1700–1788*, ed. G. Paston, London: G. Richards.
Delbourgo, J., 2006a, "Slavery in the cabinet of curiosities: Hans Sloane's Atlantic world," www.britishmuseum.org/PDF/Delbourgo%20essay.pdf.
Delbourgo, J., 2006b, *A Most Amazing Scene of Wonders: electricity and Enlightenment in early America*, Cambridge, MA: Harvard University Press.
Deleuze, G. and Guattari, F., 2004, *A Thousand Plateaus: capitalism and schizophrenia*, London and New York: Continuum.
Desan, S., 1990, *Reclaiming the Sacred: lay religion and popular politics in revolutionary France*, Ithaca, NY: Cornell University Press.
Desfontaines, P-F., 1735, *Observations sur les écrits modernes*, Vol. 2, Paris: chez Chaubert.
Deville, J., 1878–80, *Dictionnaire du tapissier*, 2 vols, Paris: Claegen.
Dickie, G., 1996, *The Century of Taste: the philosophical odyssey of taste in the eighteenth century*, Oxford: Oxford University Press.
Dictionnaire universel français et latin: vulgairement appelé le dictionnaire de Trévoux, 1732, Paris: J.-M. Grandouin.
Diderot, D., 1749, *Lettre sur les aveugles, Oeuvres complètes, éditées par J. Assézat*, Paris: Garnier.
Diderot, D., [1749] 1977, "Letter on the blind," in *Molyneux's Question: Vision Touch and the Philosophy of Perception*, excerpted and trans. M. J. Morgan, Cambridge and New York: Cambridge University Press.
Diderot, D., [1751a] 1975–, "Animal," in *Œuvres complètes*, ed. H. Dieckmann *et al.*, Paris: Hermann, vol. V.
Diderot, D., [1751b] 2000, *Lettre sur les sourds et muets*, ed. M. Hobson and S. Harvey, Paris: Garnier-Flammarion.
Diderot, D., 1754, *Pensées sur l'interpretation de la nature*, Paris.
Diderot, D., [1763] 1970, *Salon of 1763* in *Neoclassicism and Romanticism 1750–1850: Sources and Documents*, excerpted and trans. L. Eitner, 2 vols, Englewood Cliffs, NJ: Prentice-Hall.
Diderot, D., [1765] 2013, "Locke, Philosophie de," in *Encyclopédie* (q.v.), Vol. 9.
Diderot, D., [1765] 1995, *Salon of 1765*, in *Diderot on Art*, trans. and ed. J. Goodman, 2 vols, New Haven, CT and London: Yale University Press.
Diderot, D., [1769] 1965, *Entretien entre d'Alembert et Diderot; Le Rêve de d'Alembert; Suite de l'entretien*, introduction by J. Roger, Paris: Garnier-Flammarion.
Diderot, D. [1778a] 1975–, *Éléments de physiologie*, in *Œuvres complètes* (q.v.), vol. 17.
Diderot, D. [1778b] 1975–, *Essai sur Sénèque*, in *Œuvres complètes* (q.v.), vol. 25.
Diderot, D., 1975–, *Œuvres complètes*, 34 vols anticipated, ed. H. Dieckmann, J. Proust, J. Varloot *et al.*, Paris: Hermann.
Diderot, D. and d'Alembert, J. le R. (eds.) [1751–65] 2013, *Encyclopédie ou dictionnaire raisonné des arts et des métiers*, University of Chicago ARTFL Encyclopédie Project (Spring), ed. R. Morrissey, http://encyclopedie.uchicago.edu/.
Dill, C., 2006, "Ideological noises: opera criticism in early eighteenth-century France," in R. Montemorra Marvin and D. A. Thomas (eds), *Operatic Migrations: transforming works and crossing boundaries*, Aldershot: Ashgate.

Dinkin, R. J., 1977, *Voting in Provincial America: a study of elections in the thirteen colonies, 1689–1776*, Westport, CT: Greenwood Press.
Doddridge, P. D. D., 1776, *Hymns Founded on Various Texts in the Holy Scriptures*, London.
Double, F. J., 1811, *Séméïologie générale, ou Traité des signes et de leur valeur dans les maladies*, 3 vols, Paris: Croullebois.
Douthwaite, J. V., 2002, *The Wild Girl, Natural Man, and the Monster: dangerous experiments in the age of Enlightenment*, Chicago: University of Chicago Press.
Doyon, A. and Liaigre, L., 1995, *Jacques Vaucanson, mécanicien de génie*, Paris: Presses universitaires de France.
Dryden, J., 1971, *The Works of John Dryden: Prose 1668–1691: An essay of dramatick poesie, and shorter works*, Volume 17, ed. S. H. Monk, Berkeley, CA: University of California Press.
Du Bos, J-B., [1719] 1755, *Réflexions critiques sur la poésie et sur la peinture*, 6th edn, 2 vols, Paris: Pissot.
Dugan, H., 2011, *The Ephemeral History of Perfume: scent and sense in early modern England*, Baltimore, MD: Johns Hopkins University Press.
Duro, P., 1997, *The Academy and the Limits of Painting in Seventeenth-Century France*, New York and Cambridge: Cambridge University Press.
Eisenstein, E. L., 1979, *The Printing Press as an Agent of Change: communications and cultural transformations in early modern Europe*, Cambridge: Cambridge University Press.
Eisenstein, E. L., 2002a, "An unacknowledge revolution revisited," *The American Historical Review*, 107(1), 87–105.
Eisenstein, E. L., 2002b, "[How to acknowledge a revolution]: reply," *The American Historical Review*, 107(1), 126–8.
Elias, N., 1978, *The Civilizing Process*, trans. from German by E. Jephcott, New York: Urizen Books.
Elias, N., 1982, *Power and Civility*, trans. from German by E. Jephcott, New York: Pantheon Books.
Ellis, M., 2004, *The Coffee House: A Cultural History*, London: Weidenfeld & Nicolson.
"Éloge et utilité du café," 1696, *Le Mercure galant* (May), 15–55, Paris: G. de Luynes, T. Girard, M. Brunet.
Emch-Dériaz, A., 1987, "L'enseignement clinique au XVIIIe siècle: l'exemple de Tissot," *Canadian Bulletin of Medical History*, 4, 145–64.
Emerson, J. et al., 2000, *Porcelain Stories: from China to Europe*, Seattle, WA: University of Washington Press.
Empson, W., [1951] 1995, *The Structure of Complex Words*, London: Penguin.
Encyclopedia Britannica: or, A Dictionary of Arts and Sciences, 1771–3, Edinburgh.
Epstein, S., 1998, "Craft guilds, apprenticeship and technological change in preindustrial Europe," *Journal of Economic History*, 58, 684–713.
Equino, O., [1814] 1999, *The Life of Olaudah Equino, or Gustavus Vassa, the African*, New York: Dover Press.

Erlmann, V., 2010, *Reason and Resonance?: a history of modern aurality*, New York and Cambridge, MA: Zone Books.
Euler, L., 1738, "Von der Gestalt der Erden," *Opera Omnia*, 3(2), 325–46.
Euler, L., [1765] 1822, *Elements of Algebra*, London.
Fabre, P., [1758] 1773, *Traité des maladies vénériennes*, 3rd edn, Paris: Chez P. Fr. Didot le jeune.
Fan, F., 2004, *British Naturalists in Qing China: science, empire and cultural encounter*, Cambridge: Harvard University Press.
Fara, P., 2002, *An Entertainment for Angels: electricity in the Enlightenment*, New York: Columbia University Press.
Farge, A., 1979, *Vivre dans la rue au XVIIIe siècle*, Paris: Gallimard.
Farge, A., 2007, *Effusion et tourment, le récit des corps: histoire du peuple au XVIII siècle*, Paris: O. Jacob.
Farley, J., [1783] 1988, *The London Art of Cookery, and Housekeeper's Complete Assistant*, ed. A. Haly, Lewes: Southover Press.
Farr, E., 1996, *Before the Deluge: Parisian Society in the Reign of Louis XIV*, London: Peter Owen Press.
Febvre, L. and Martin, H-J., 1976, *The Coming of the Book: the impact of printing 1450–1800*, London: N.L.B.
Félibien, A., 1669, *Conférences de l'Académie royale de peinture et de sculpture pendant l'année 1667*, Paris: Chez Frédéric Léonard.
Ferry, L., 1990, *Homo aestheticus: l'invention du gout à l'âge classique*, Paris: Grasset.
Figlio, K. M., 1975, "Theories of perception and the physiology of mind in the late eighteenth century," *History of Science*, 12, 177–212.
Fischer, D. H., 1999, *The Great Wave: price revolutions and the rhythm of history*, Oxford: Oxford University Press.
Fletcher, J., 1830, "The reality of manifestations," in *Christ Manifested*, London: Jones & Co.
Fletcher, J., 2008, *Unexampled Labours: letters of the Reverend John Fletcher to leaders in the Evangelical revival*, ed. P. S. Forsaith, Peterborough: Epworth Press.
Fletcher, M. B., n.d., *Autobiography*, Fletcher/Tooth Collection, MAM Fl 23.
Floyer, J., 1687–1690, *ΦΑΡΜΑΚΟ–ΒΑΣΑΝΟΣ: Or, the Touche-Stone of Medicines. Discovering the Vertues of Vegetables, Minerals, & Animals, by Their Tastes and Smells*, 2 vols, London: Printed for Michael Johnson.
Fogel, M., 1989, *Les Cérémonies de l'information dans la France de XVIe au milieu du XVIIIe siècle*, Paris: Fayard.
Fogleman, A. S., 2007, *Jesus is Female: Moravians and the challenge of radical religion in early America*, Philadelphia, PA: University of Pennsylvania Press.
Fontenay, E. de., 1998, *Le Silence des bêtes: la philosophie à l'épreuve de l'animalité*, Paris: Fayard.
Fontenelle, B. L. B. de, 1719, *Histoire du renouvellement de l'Académie royale des sciences en M.DC.XCIX. et les éloges historiques*, Amsterdam.
Forsaith, P. S., 2008, *Unexampled Labours: letters of the Revd John Fletcher to leaders in the Evangelical revival*, Peterborough: The Epworth Press.
Foucault, M., [1961] 1972, *Histoire de la folie à l'âge classique*, Paris: Gallimard.

Foucault, M., 1966, *Les mots et les choses*, Paris: Gallimard.
Foucault, M., 1973, *The Order of Things: an archeology of the human sciences*, New York: Vintage Books.
Foucault, M., 1977, *Discipline and Punish: the birth of the prison*, trans. from French by A. Sheridan, London: Allen Lane.
Foucault, M., 1994, *Naissance de la clinique*, 4th edn, Paris: Presses Universitaires de France.
Fouquet, H., [1765] 2013, "Sensibilité, sentiment (*médecine*)," in *Encyclopédie* (q.v.), Vol. 15.
Fouquet, H., 1767, *Essai sur le pouls*, Montpellier: Chez la Veuve de Jean Martel.
Frängsmyr, T., Heilbron, J. L., and Rider, R. E. (eds), 1990, *The Quantifying Spirit of the Eighteenth Century*, Berkeley, CA: University of California Press.
Frank, J. P., 1790, *Plan d'école clinique, ou Méthode d'enseigner la pratique de la médecine dans un hôpital académique*, Vienna: Chez Chrêtien Frederic Wappler.
Franklin, B., 1986, *The Autobiography and Other Writings*, ed. O. Seavey, Harmondsworth: Penguin.
Franklin, B., 2002a, "Idea of the English school," in *The Papers of Benjamin Franklin*, New Haven, CT: Yale University, http://franklinpapers.org/franklin/framedMorgan.jsp.
Franklin, B., 2002b, "Proposals relating to the education of youth in Pennsylvania," in *The Papers of Benjamin Franklin*, New Haven, CT: Yale University, http://franklinpapers.org.
Franklin, B., 2002c, "To [Richard Price]," in *The Papers of Benjamin Franklin*, New Haven, CT: Yale University, http://franklinpapers.org.
Freedman, J., 2012, *Books without Borders: French cosmopolitanism and German literary markets*, Philadelphia, PA: University of Pennsylvania Press.
Frey, M., 1997, *Der reinliche Bürger: Entstehung und Verbreitung bürgerlicher Tugenden in Deutschland, 1760–1860*, Göttingen: Vandenhoeck & Ruprecht.
Fulop-Miller, R., 1956, *The Power and Secret of the Jesuits*, trans. from German by F. S. Flint and D. F. Tait, New York: George Braziller.
Fuss, N., 1786, *Eulogy of Leonhard Euler*, www.math.dartmouth.edu/~euler/tour/tour_21.html.
Garrioch, D., 2003, "Sounds of the city: the soundscape of early modern towns," *Urban History*, 30(1), 5–25.
Gaukroger, S., 2010, *The Collapse of Mechanism and the Rise of Sensibility: science and the shaping of modernity, 1680–1760*, Oxford: Oxford University Press.
Gay, J., 1716, *Trivia, or The Art of Walking the Streets of London*, London: Bernard Lintott.
Gergen, K. J., 2002, "The challenge of absent presence," in J. E. Katz and M. A. Aakhus (eds), *Perpetual Contact: mobile communication, private talk, public performance*, Cambridge: Cambridge University Press.
Gibbon, E., 1766, "Saunderson," in *Biographia Britannica*, London, printed for W. Innys *et al*.

Giesey, R., 1987, "The king imagined," in *The French Revolution and the Creation of Modern Political Culture, vol. 1: the political culture of the Old Regime*, ed. K. M. Baker, Oxford and New York: Pergamon.

Gigante, D., 2005, "The century of taste: Shaftesbury, Hume, Burke," in *Taste: a literary history*, New Haven, CT: Yale University Press.

Gigante, D., 2005, *Taste: A Literary History*, New Haven, CT: Yale University Press.

Girouard, M., 1993, *Life in the English Country House: a social and architectural history*, new edn, New Haven, CT: Yale University Press.

Gittinger, M., 1982, *Master Dyers to the World: technique and trade in early Indian dyed cotton textiles*, Washington, DC: Textile Museum.

Glassman, R. B. and Buckingham, H. W., 2007, "David Hartley's neural vibrations and psychological associations," in H. Whitaker, C. M. Smith, and S. Finger (eds), *Brain, Mind and Medicine: essays in eighteenth-century neuroscience*, New York: Springer.

Goehr, L., 1992, *The Imaginary Museum of Musical Works: An Essay in the Philosophy of Music*, Oxford: Clarendon Press.

Goethe, J. W., [1810] 1840, *Goethe's Theory of Colours*, trans. C. Lock Eastlake, London: John Murray.

Goldstein, C., 2008, *Vaux and Versailles: the appropriations, erasures, and accidents that made modern France*, Philadelphia, PA: University of Pennsylvania Press.

Goldstein, J., Bertrand, A-J-F., and Despine, C-H-A., 2010, *Hysteria Complicated by Ecstasy: the Case of Nanette Leroux*, Princeton, NJ: Princeton University Press.

Goodden, A., 2001, *Diderot and the Body*, Oxford: Legenda.

Goodman, K., 2004, *Georgic Modernity and British Romanticism: poetry and the mediation of history*, Cambridge: Cambridge University Press.

Gordon, D. and Krech III, S. (eds), 2012, *Indigenous Knowledge and the Environment in Africa and North America*, Athens, OH: Ohio University Press.

Goring, P., 2005, *The Rhetoric of Sensibility in Eighteenth-Century Culture*, Cambridge: Cambridge University Press.

Gough, J., 1805, "A description of a property of caoutchouc, or Indian rubber, with some reflections on the cause of the elasticity of this substance," *Memoirs of the Literary and Philosophical Society of Manchester*, Second Series, I, 288–95.

Grmek, M. D., 1991, "La réception du *De Sedibus* de Morgagni en France au 18e siècle," *Dix-Huitième Siècle*, 23, 59–73.

Grootenboer, H., 2012, *Treasuring the Gaze: intimate vision in late eighteenth-century eye miniatures*, Chicago: University of Chicago Press.

Gueniffey, P., 1993, *Le Nombre et la raison: la Révolution française et les élections*, Paris: EHESS.

Guyer, P., 1998, "Baumgarten, Alexandre Gottlieb," in M. Kelly (ed.), *Encyclopedia of Aesthetics*, Vol. 1, New York: Oxford University Press.

Gyles, J., 1730, *A Memorial of the Strange Adventures and Signal Deliverances of John Gyles of Pemaquid, Maine, 1689.*

Gyles, J., 1736, *Memoirs of the Odd Adventures and Strange Deliverances, etc., In the Captivity of John Gyles*, Boston: S. Kneeland & T. Green.

Habermas, J., 1989, *The Structural Transformation of the Public Sphere: an inquiry into a category of bourgeois society*, trans. from German by T. Burger and F. Lawrence, Cambridge, MA: MIT Press.
Habermas, J., 1991, *The Structural Transformation of the Public Sphere: an inquiry into a category of bourgeois society*, Cambridge, MA: MIT Press.
Hagstrum, J. H., 1958, *The Sisters Arts: the tradition of literary pictorialism and English poetry from Dryden to Gray*, Chicago: University of Chicago Press.
Hall, D. D., 1996, "The Chesapeake in the seventeenth century," in D. D. Hall (ed.), *Cultures of Print: essays in the history of the book*, Amherst, MA: University of Massachusetts Press.
Hall-Witt, J., 2007, *Fashionable Acts: opera and elite culture in London, 1780–1880*, Durham, NH: University of New Hampshire Press.
Hamerton, K. J., 2008, "Malebranche, taste, and sensibility: the origins of sensitive taste and a reconsideration of Cartesianism's feminist potential," *Journal of the History of Ideas*, 69(4), 533–58.
Hammon, B., 1760, *A Narrative of the Uncommon Sufferings, and Surprizing Deliverance of Briton Hammon, a Negro Man*, Boston, MA: Green & Russell.
Hatfield, G., 1995, "Remaking the science of mind: psychology as natural science," in C. Fox, R. Porter, and R. Wokler (eds), *Inventing Human Science: eighteenth-century domains*, Berkeley, CA: University of California Press.
Havard, H., 1890, *Dictionnaire de l'ameublement*, 4 vols, Paris: Maison Quantin.
Havenlange, C., 1999, "L'Institution du regard au XVIIIe siècle," in R. Mortier (ed.), *Visualisation*, Berlin: Arno Spitz.
Heidegger, M., 1977, "The question concerning technology," in *The Question Concerning Technology and Other Essays*, New York: Harper & Row.
Heller-Roazen, D., 2007, *The Inner Touch: archaeology of a sensation*, Harvard: Zone Books.
Hempton, D., 2005, *Methodism: empire of the spirit*, New Haven, CT and London: Yale University Press.
Heyl, C., 2011, "Horrid howling or sublime sensation? Primitivism, romanticism, gothic horror and the eighteenth-century taste in music: the case of the Great Highland Bagpipes," in P. Wagner and F. Ogée (eds), *Taste and the Senses in the Eighteenth Century*, Landau-Paris Studies on the Eighteenth Century (LAPASEC), Vol. 3, Trier: Wissenschaftlicher Verlag Trier.
Hildebrandt, F. and Bederlegge, O. A. (eds), 1983, *A Collection of Hymns for the Use of People Called Methodists: the works of John Wesley*, Vol. 7, Oxford: Clarendon Press.
Hindmarsh, D. B., 1996, *John Newton and the English Evangelical Tradition*, Grand Rapids, MI: Eerdmans Publishing Co.
Hindmarsh, D. B., 2009, "Wesley Agonistes and the Calvinist sublime: the spiritual ideals of the early English Evangelical school," the Fifth Annual Manchester Wesley Research Centre Lecture, June 19.
Hiraga, G., 1763, *Butsurui Hinshitsu (Classification of Various Materials)*, Osaka.
Hobhouse, S. (ed.), 1994, *William Law and Eighteenth-Century Quakerism*, London: George Allen & Unwin Ltd.

Hoffer, P. C., 2003, *Sensory Worlds in Early America*, Baltimore, MD: Johns Hopkins University Press.
Hoffmann, F., 1754–5, *Consultations de médecine*, 8 vols, Paris: Chez Briasson.
Hogarth, W., [1753] 1973, *The Analysis of Beauty. Written with a view of fixing the fluctuating IDEAS of TASTE*, New York: Garland.
Horner, F., 1822, "Memoire of the life and character of Euler," in L. Euler, *Elements of Algebra*, trans. F. Horner, London: Longman, Horst & Co.
Howes, D., 2009, *The Sixth Sense Reader*, New York: Berg.
Hsia, A. (ed.), 1998, *The Vision of China in the English Literature of the Seventeenth and Eighteenth Century*, Hong Kong: Chinese University Press.
Huber F., 1792, *Nouvelles observations sur les abeilles*, Geneva.
Hume, D., [1748] 1974, *An Enquiry Concerning Human Understanding*, in *The Empiricists*, New York: Anchor Books.
Hume, D., [1748] 1999, *An Enquiry Concerning Human Understanding*, ed. T. L. Beauchamp, Oxford: Oxford University Press.
Hunauld, P., [1756] 2009, *La philosophie des vapeurs: Suivi d'une Dissertation sur les vapeurs et les pertes de sang*, ed. S. Arnaud, Mercure de France.
Hunt, L., 1984, *Politics, Culture and Class in the French Revolution*, Berkeley, CA: University of California Press.
Hunt, L., 1992, *The Family Romance of the French Revolution*, Berkeley, CA: University of California Press.
Hutchins, E., 1995, *Cognition in the Wild*, Cambridge, MA: MIT Press.
Hutton, C., 1795, "Dr. Nicholas Saunderson," in *Mathematical and Philosophical Dictionary*, London.
Hyde, M., 2006, *Making Up the Rococo: François Boucher and his critics*, Los Angeles: Getty Research Institute.
Irwin, J. and Brett, K., 1970, *Origins of Chintz*, London: Her Majesty's Stationery Office.
Ives, R. J., 2003, "Political publicity and political economy in eighteenth-century France," *French History*, 17(1), 1–18.
Jacot Grapa, C., 2009, *Dans le vif du sujet: Diderot corps et âme*, Paris: Garnier.
Jacot Grapa, C., 2010, "Des huîtres aux grands animaux: Diderot, animal matérialiste," *Dix-huitième siècle*, 42, 99–118.
Jainchill, A., 2003, "The Constitution of the year III and the persistence of classical republicanism," *French Historical Studies*, 26(3), 399–435.
Janković, V., 2010, *Confronting the Climate: British airs and the making of environmental medicine*, Basingstoke: Palgrave Macmillan.
Jarvis, S., 2010, "The melodics of long poems," *Textual Practice*, 24(4), 607–21.
Jaucourt, L. de, [1765] 2013, "Sensibilité (*Morale*)," in *Encyclopédie* (q.v.), Vol. 15.
Jay, M., 1993, *Downcast Eyes: the denigration of vision in twentieth-century French thought*, Berkeley, CA: University of California Press.
Jeffrey, D. L. (ed.), 1987, *A Burning and a Shining Light: English spirituality in the age of Wesley*, Grand Rapids, MI: Eerdmans Publishing Co.
Jenner, M. S. R., 2010, "Tasting Lichfield, touching China: Sir John Floyer's senses," *The Historical Journal*, 53, 647–70.

Johannisson, K., 1990, "Society in numbers: the debate over quantification in eighteenth-century political economy," in T. Frängsmyr et al., *The Quantifying Spirit of the Eighteenth Century*, Berkeley, CA: University of California Press.

Johns, A., 1998, *The Nature of the Book: print and knowledge in the making*, Chicago: University of Chicago Press.

Johns, A., 2002, "How to acknowledge a revolution," *The American Historical Review*, 107(1), 106–25.

Johnson, J. H., 1991, "Beethoven and the Birth of Romantic Musical Experience in France," *19th-Century Music*, 15, 23–35.

Johnson, J. H., 1995, *Listening in Paris: a cultural history*, Berkeley, CA: University of California Press.

Johnson, J., 2011, *Venice Incognito: masks in the serene republic*, Berkeley, CA: University of California Press.

Jones, R., 2008, "Empire of extinction: nature and natural history in the Russian North Pacific, 1739–1799," PhD dissertation, Columbia University.

Jouanna, J., 1999, *Hippocrates*, trans. M. B. DeBevoise, Baltimore, MD and London: Johns Hopkins University Press.

Jütte, R., 2005, *A History of the Senses: From Antiquity to Cyberspace*, trans. from German by J. Lynn, Malden: Polity Press.

Kadane, M., 2012, *The Watchful Clothier: the life of an eighteenth-century Protestant capitalist*, New Haven, CT and London: Yale University Press.

Kant, I., [1781] 1855, *Critique of Pure Reason*, London: Henry G. Bohn.

Kant, I., 1996, "An answer to the question: what is Enlightenment?" in M. J. Gregor (ed.), *Practical Philosophy*, Cambridge and New York: Cambridge University Press, pp. 11–22.

Kantorowicz, E. H., 1955, "Mysteries of the State: An Absolutist Concept and its Late Medieval Origins," *Harvard Theological Review*, 48, 65–91.

Keach, W., 2005, "Poetry, after 1740," in H. B. Nisbet and C. Rawson (eds), *The Cambridge History of Literary Criticism*, Vol. 4, *The Eighteenth Century*, Cambridge: Cambridge University Press.

Keats, J., [1817] 1884, *Poetical Works*.

Keats, J. 1990, *The Major Works*, ed. E. Cook, Oxford: Oxford University Press.

Keel, O., 2001, *L'avènement de la médecine clinique moderne en Europe, 1750–1815*, Montréal and Geneva: Presses de l'Université de Montréal, Georg Editeur.

Kinzer, B. L., 1982, *The Ballot Question in Nineteenth-Century Britain*, New York: Garland.

Klueting, H., 2010, "The Catholic Enlightenment in Austria or the Hapsburg lands," in U. L. Lehner and M. Printy (eds), *A Companion to the Catholic Enlightenment in Europe*, Leiden and Boston, MA: Brill.

Knott, S., 2010, "The patient's case: sentimental empiricism and knowledge in the early American Republic," *The William and Mary Quarterly*, 67, 645–76.

Koepp, C., 1986, "The alphabetical order: work in Diderot's *Encyclopédie*," in S. Kaplan and C. Koepp (eds), *Work in France: Representations, Meaning, Organization, and Practice*, Ithaca, NY: Cornell University Press.

Koerner, L., 1999, *Linnaeus: Nature and Nation*, Cambridge, MA: Harvard University Press.
Koslofsky, C., 2011, *Evening's Empire: a history of the night in early modern Europe*, Cambridge: Cambridge University Press.
Kostroun, D., 2011, *Feminism, Absolutism, and Jansenism: Louis XIV and the Port-Royal nuns*, Cambridge: Cambridge University Press.
Kuehner, P., 1944, "Theories on the origins of language in the eighteenth century in France," PhD dissertation, University of Pennsylvania.
La Fayette, Comtesse de (Marie-Madeleine Pioche de La Vergne), 1942, *Correspondance*, ed. A. Beaunier, 2 vols, Paris: Gallimard.
Lafuente, A. and Valverde, N., 2005, "Linnaean botany and Spanish imperial biopolitics," in L. Schiebinger and C. Swan (eds), *Colonial Botany: science, commerce and politics in the early modern world*, Philadelphia, PA: University of Pennsylvania Press.
Lajer-Burcharth, E., 2001, "Pompadour's touch: difference in representation," *Representations*, 73 (winter), 54–88.
Lamb, J., 2005, "The sublime," in H. B. Nisbet and C. Rawson (eds), *The Cambridge History of Literary Criticism*, Vol. 4, *The Eighteenth Century*, Cambridge: Cambridge University Press.
Land, I., 2001, "Customs of the sea: flogging, empire and the 'true British seaman', 1770–1870," *Interventions: International Journal of Postcolonial Studies*, 3, 169–85.
Landré-Beauvais, A. J., 1809, *Séméiotique, ou Traité des signes des maladies*, Paris: chez J. A. Brosson.
Laven, M., 2006, "Encountering the Counter-Reformation," *Renaissance Quarterly*, 59(3), 706–20.
Law, W., [1729] 1994, *A Serious Call to a Devout and Holy Life 1729*, Grand Rapids, MI: Christian Classics Ethereal Library.
Lawrence, C., 1979, "The nervous system and society in the Scottish Enlightenment," in B. Barnes and S. Shapin (eds), *Natural Order: historical studies of scientific culture*, Beverly Hills, CA: Sage.
Lawrence, S. C., 1993, "Educating the senses: students, teachers and medical rhetoric in eighteenth-century London," in W. F. Bynum and R. Porter (eds), *Medicine and the Five Senses*, Cambridge: Cambridge University Press.
Le Bossu, R., [1675] 1981, *Traité du poème épique: Réimpression de l'édition de 1714 avec une introduction de Volker Kapp*, Hamburg: Helmut Buske Verlag.
Le Cat, C-N., 1744, *Traité des sens*, Amsterdam: J. Wetstein.
Le Cat, C-N., 1750, *A Physical Essay on the Senses*, trans. from the French, London: printed for R. Griffiths.
Le Cat, C-N., 1765, *Traité de l'existence, de la nature et des propriétés du fluide des nerfs, et principalement de son action dans le mouvement musculaire*, Berlin: n.p.
Le Dran, H-F., 1765, *Consultations sur la plupart des maladies qui sont du ressort de la chirurgie*, Paris: chez P. Fr. Didot.
Le Guérer, A., 1992, *Scent, the Mysterious and Essential Powers of Smell*, trans. from French by R. Miller, New York: Turtle Bay Books.

Le Thieullier, L-J., 1739–47, *Consultations de médecine*, 4 vols, Paris: chez Charles Osmont.

Leclant, J., 1951, "Le Café et les cafés à Paris (1644–1693)," *Annales: Économie, Société, Civilisation*, 6, 1–14.

Lehner, U. L., 2010, "The many faces of the Catholic Enlightenment," in U. L. Lehner and M. Printy (eds), *A Companion to the Catholic Enlightenment in Europe*, Leiden & Boston: Brill.

Leibniz, G. W., 1956, "On wisdom," *Philosophical Papers and Letters*, ed. and trans. L. E. Loemker, 2 vols, Chicago: University of Chicago Press.

Lemire, B., 1992, *Fashion's Favourite: the cotton trade and the consumer in Britain, 1660–1800*, Oxford: Oxford University Press.

Lemire, B., 2003, "Domesticating the exotic: floral culture and the East Indies calico trade with England, c. 1600–1800," *Textile: The Journal of Cloth and Culture*, 1(1), 65–85.

Lessing, G. E., [1766] 1985, "Laocoon: or on the limits of painting and poetry," in H. B. Nisbet (ed.), *German Aesthetic and Literary Criticism: Winckelmann, Lessing, Hamann, Herder, Schiller, Goethe*, Cambridge: Cambridge University Press.

Levey, M., 1985, *Rococo to Revolution: major trends in 18th-century painting*, London: Thames & Hudson.

Lewis, W., 1763, *Commercium Philosophico-Technicum; Or, The Philosophical Commerce of Arts: designed as an attempt to improve arts, trades, and manufactures*, London: H. Baldwin, http://archive.org/details/commerciumphilo00lewi.

Lichtenstein, J., 1993, *The Eloquence of Color: rhetoric and painting in the French classical age*, trans. E. McVarish, Berkeley, CA and Los Angeles: University of California Press.

Lichtenstein, J., 2008, *The Blind Spot: an essay on the relations between painting and sculpture in the modern age*, trans. C. Miller, Los Angeles: Getty Research Institute.

Lieutaud, J., [1742] 1766, *Essais anatomiques, contenant l'histoire exacte de toutes les parties qui composent le corps de l'Homme*, Paris: chez d'Houry, Guillyn, P. F. Didot.

Liger, L., 1715, *Le Voyageur fidèle, ou le Guide des étrangers dans la ville de Paris*, Paris: Pierre Ribou.

Lincoln, W. B., 2007, *The Conquest of a Continent: Siberia and the Russians*, Ithaca, NY: Cornell University Press.

Linebaugh, P. and Rediker, M. B., 2000, *The Many-headed Hydra: sailors, slaves, commoners, and the hidden history of the revolutionary Atlantic*, Boston, MA: Beacon Press.

Liss, R., 2009, "Frontier tales: Tokugawa Japan in translation," in S. Schaffer *et al.* (eds), *The Brokered World*, Sagamore Beach, MA: Science History Publications.

Lister, M., 1699, *A Journey to Paris in the Year 1698*, London: Jacob Tonson.

Locke, J., [1690] 1975, *An Essay Concerning Human Understanding*, ed. P. H. Nidditch, 4th edn, Oxford and New York: Oxford University Press.

Lordat, J., 1810, "Préface de l'éditeur," in J. Lordat, *Consultations de médecine, ouvrage posthume de P.-J. Barthez*, Paris: Chez Michaud Frères.

Lordat, J., 1818, *Exposition de la doctrine médicale de P.-J. Barthez, et Mémoires sur la vie de ce médecin*, Paris: Chez Gabon.

Lowe, D. M., 1982, *A History of Bourgeois Perception*, Chicago: University of Chicago Press.

Lowood, H., 1990, "The calculating forester: quantification, cameral science and the emergence of scientific forestry management in Germany," in T. Frängsmyr *et al.*, *The Quantifying Spirit of the Eighteenth Century*, Berkeley, CA: University of California Press.

Lubken, D., 2012, "Joyful ringing, solemn tolling: methods and meanings of early American tower bells," *William & Mary Quarterly* 69, no. 4 (October), 823–42.

Luhrmann, T. M., 2012, *When God Talks Back: Understanding the American Evangelical relationship with God*, New York: Alfred A. Knopf.

Lunardi, V., 1785, *An Account of the First Aerial Voyage over England*, London: John Bell.

Lynn, M., 2010, *The Sublime Invention: Ballooning in Europe, 1783–1820*, London: Pickering & Chatto.

Lyons, C. A., 2003, "Mapping an Atlantic sexual culture: homoeroticism in eighteenth-century Philadelphia," *William and Mary Quarterly*, 60(1), 119.

M.***, 1756, "Lettre adressée à l'auteur du journal, sur l'usage que l'on doit faire des observations en médecine," *Recueil périodique d'observations de médecine, chirurgie, pharmacie, etc.*, 4, 19–36.

Mack, P., 1992, *Visionary Women: ecstatic prophecy in seventeenth-century England*, Berkeley, CA: University of California Press.

Mack, P., 2008, *Heart Religion in the British Enlightenment: gender and emotion in early Methodism*, Cambridge: Cambridge University Press.

Madiment, B., 2007, *Dusty Bob: a cultural history of dustmen, 1780–1770*, Manchester: Manchester University Press.

Maire, C., 1985, *Les convulsionnaires de Saint-Médard: miracles, convulsions et prophéties à Paris au XVIIIe siècle*, Paris: Gallimard/Julliard.

Mairobert, M. F. P. de [?], 1777–8, *L'Observateur anglois, ou correspondance secrete entre Milord All'Eye and Milord All'Ear*, London: J. Adamson.

Manning, S., 1997, "Boswell's pleasures, the pleasures of Boswell," *British Journal for Eighteenth-Century Studies*, 20(1), 17–31.

Marana, G. P., 1714, *Lettre d'un Sicilien à un de ses amis*, Chambery: P. Maubal.

Marcon, F., 2007, "The names of nature: the development of natural history in Japan, 1600–1900," PhD dissertation, Columbia University.

Marivaux, P. C. de, [1734] 1965, *Le Paysan parvenu*, ed. M. Gilot, Paris: Garnier-Flammarion.

Marshall, D., 2005, *The Frame of Art: Fictions of Aesthetic Experience, 1750–1815*, Baltimore, MD: Johns Hopkins University Press.

Maslan, S., 2005, *Revolutionary Acts: theater, democracy and the French Revolution*, Baltimore, MD: Johns Hopkins University Press.

May, G., 1998, "Eighteenth-century French aesthetics," in *Encyclopedia of Aesthetics* (q.v.), Vol. 2.

McLuhan, M., 1964, *Understanding Media: the extensions of man*, 2nd edn, New York: New American Library.

McLuhan, M., 2012, *The Gutenberg Galaxy: the making of typographic man*, Toronto: University of Toronto Press.
Melchoir-Bonnet, S., 2001, *The Mirror: a history*, London: Routledge.
Melosi, M., 2000, *The Sanitary City: urban infrastructure in America from colonial times to the present*, Baltimore, MD: Johns Hopkins University Press.
Ménuret de Chambaud, J-J., [1765] 2013, "Musique, effets de la, (*Médecine, Diète, Gymnastique, Thérapeutique),*" in *Encyclopédie* (q.v.).
Metzner, P., 1998, *Crescendo of the Virtuoso: spectacle, skill, and self-promotion in Paris during the age of revolution*, Berkeley, CA: University of California Press.
Meyer, M., 2003, "Theatrical spectacles and the spectators' positions in Wordsworth's London," *The Literary London Journal*, 1(1), www.literarylondon.org/london-journal/march2003/meyer.html.
Molineux, C., 2007, "Pleasures of the smoke: 'Black Virginians' in Georgian London's tobacco shops," *William and Mary Quarterly*, 3rd series, LXIV (April), 327–76.
Montesquieu, C. de S. [1721] 1973, *Persian Letters*, trans. from French by C. J. Betts, Harmondsworth: Penguin.
Montesquieu, C. de S., [1749] 1989, *The Spirit of the Laws*, trans. from French and ed. A. M. Cohler *et al.*, Cambridge: Cambridge University Press.
Morand, S-F., 1768, *Opuscules de chirurgie*, 2 vols, Paris: Chez Guillaume Desprez.
Morgagni, G. B., 1769, *The Seats and Causes of Diseases Investigated by Anatomy*, trans. B. Alexander, 3 vols, London: A. Millar, T. Cadell, Johnson and Payne.
Morgagni, G. B., 1820–4, *Recherches anatomiques sur le siège et les causes des maladies*, trans. A. Desormeaux and J. P. Destouet, 10 vols, Paris: Caille et Ravier.
Morgan, M. J., 1977, *Molyneux's Question: vision touch and the philosophy of perception*, Cambridge and New York: Cambridge University Press.
Mortier, R., 1969, "'Lumière' et 'Lumières': histoire d'une image et d'une idée au XVIIe et au XVIIIe siècle," in *Clartés et ombres du siècle des Lumières: Etudes sur le XVIIIe siècle littéraire*, Geneva: Droz.
Moura, J. and Louvet, P., 1929, *Le Café Procope*, Paris: Librairie Académique Perrin et Cie.
Moxon, J., 1896, *Moxon's Mechanick exercises: or, The doctrine of handyworks applied to the art of printing*, ed. T. L. De Vinne, New York: Typothetæ of the City of New York.
Mumford, L., 1963, *Technics and Civilization*, New York: Harcourt, Brace & World.
Musschenbroek, P. van, 1769, *Cours de physique expérimentale et mathématique*, trans. S. de la Fond, 3 vols, Paris: Chez Delalain.
Musselman, E. G., 2009, "Indigenous knowledge and contact zones: The Case of the Cold Bokkevelt Meteorite, Cape Colony, 1838," *Itinerario*, 33, 31–44.
Nacquart, J-B., 1813, "Consultation," in *Dictionaire des sciences médicales*.
Nappi, C., 2009, *The Monkey and the Inkpot: natural history and its transformations in early-modern China*, Cambridge, MA: Harvard University Press.
Nemeitz, J. C., 1718, *Séjour de Paris*, Franckfurt am Main: F. W. Förster.
Nemeitz, J. C., 1719, *Séjour de Paris*, 2 vols, Leiden: Jean Van Abcoude.
Nicholson, C., 1861, *The Annals of Kendal*, London: Whitaker & Co.

Nicolson, M., 1992, "Giovanni Battista Morgagni and eighteenth-century physical examination," in C. Lawrence (ed.), *Medical Theory, Surgical Practice*, London and New York: Routledge.
Nicolson, M., 1993, "The art of diagnosis: medicine and the five senses," in W. F. Bynum and R. Porter (eds), *Companion Encyclopedia of the History of Medicine*, Vol. 2, London and New York: Routledge.
Norton, M., 2006, "Tasting empire: chocolate and the European internalization of Mesoamerican aesthetics," *The American Historical Review*, 111, 660–91.
Nowacki, H., 2008, "Leonhard Euler and the theory of ships," *Journal of Ship Research*, 52, 274–90.
Nussbaum, F., 1984, *The Brink of All We Hate: English satires on women, 1660–1750*, Lexington, KY: University of Kentucky Press.
O'Gorman, F., 1989, *Voters, Patrons and Parties: the unreformed electorate of Hanoverian England, 1734–1832*, Oxford: Oxford University Press.
O'Gorman, F., 1992, "Campaign rituals and ceremonies: the social meaning of elections in England, 1780–1860," *Past and Present*, 135, 72–115.
O'Neal, J. C., 1996, *The Authority of Experience: sensationalist theory in the French Enlightenment*, College Park, PA: Penn State University Press.
O'Neal, J. C., 1998, "Auenbrugger, Corvisart, and the perception of disease," *Eighteenth-Century Studies*, 31, 473–89.
Ogée, F., 2001, "Je-sais-quoi: William Hogarth and the representation of the forms of life," in D. Bindman, F. Ogée, and P. Wagner (eds), *Hogarth: representing nature's machines*, Manchester: Manchester University Press.
Ordonnance rendue par Monsieur Hérault, 1728, Archives, Mulhouse: Musée de l'Impression sur Étoffes.
Otto, P., 2011, *Multiplying Worlds: romanticism, modernity, and the emergence of virtual reality*, Oxford: Oxford University Press.
Outram, D., 1996, "New spaces in natural history," in N. Jardine, J. Secord, and E. Spary (eds), *Cultures of Natural History*, Cambridge: Cambridge University Press.
Ozouf, M., 1991, *Festivals of the French Revolution*, trans. from French by A. Sheridan, Cambridge, MA: Harvard University Press.
Parish, S. S., 2006, *American Curiosity: cultures of natural history in the colonial British Atlantic world*, Chapel Hill, NC: University of North Carolina Press.
Parry, G., 2007, "Education and the reproduction of the Enlightenment," in M. Fitzpatrick (ed.), *The Enlightenment World*, London: Routledge.
Paulson, R., 1997, *Introduction to William Hogarth, The Analysis of Beauty*, New Haven, CT and London: Yale University Press.
Pelleport, A. Gédéon Lafitte, Marquise de, [1790] 2010, *The Bohemians*, trans. from French by V. Folkenflik, Philadelphia, PA: University of Pennsylvania Press.
Pététin, J-H-D., 1787, *Mémoire sur la découverte des phénomènes que présentent la catalepsie et le somnambulisme, symptômes de l'affection hystérique essentielle*, n.p.
Petit, A., 1757, *Discours prononcé aux écoles de médecine pour l'ouverture solennelle du cours de chirurgie*, Paris: De l'imprimerie de la Veuve Quillau.

Petit, E.-M., 1794, *Entendons-nous, ouvrage périodique*, Paris: Imprimerie de la place de la Liberté.
Peucker, P., 2006, "'Inspired by flames of love': homosexuality, mysticism, and Moravian brothers around 1750," *Journal of the History of Sexuality*, 15(1), 30–64.
Peucker, P., 2007, H-Net review of Aaron S. Fogleman, *Jesus is Female: Moravians and the challenge of radical religion in early America*, www.h-net.org/reviews/showrev.php?id=13909.
Philip, E., 1994, *The Story of the Voyage: sea-narratives in eighteenth-century England*, Cambridge: Cambridge University Press.
Picon, A., 1992, "Gestes ouvriers, operations et processus techniques: La vision du travail des encyclopédistes," *Recherches sur Diderot et sur l'Encyclopédie*, 13, 131–47.
Piles, R. de, 1699, *Abrégé de la vie des peintres: avec des reflexions sur leurs ouvrages, et un traité du peintre parfait, de la connoissance des dessins, & de l'utilité des estampes*, Paris: François Muguet.
Piles, R. de, 1708, *Cours de peinture par principes*, Paris: Jacques Estienne.
Pincus, S., 1995, "'Coffee Politicians Does Create': coffeehouses and restoration political culture," *The Journal of Modern History*, 67 (December), 807–34.
Pinel, P., [1793] 1980, *The Clinical Training of Doctors: An Essay of 1793*, trans. D. B. Weiner, Baltimore, MD and London: Johns Hopkins University Press.
Pinel, P., 1797, *Nosographie Philosophique, Ou la méthode de l'analyse appliquée à la médecine*, 2 vols, Paris: Chez Maradan.
Pinel, P., 1802, *La Médecine clinique, rendue plus précise et plus exacte par l'application de l'analyse*, Paris: Chez Brosson, Gabon et Cie.
Po-Chia Hsia, R., [1998] 2005, *The World of Catholic Renewal, 1540–1770*, Cambridge: Cambridge University Press.
Podmore, C., 1998, *The Moravian Church in England 1728–1760*, Oxford: Clarendon Press.
Poovey, M., 2005, "Between politic arithmetic and political economy," in J. Bender and M. Marrinan (eds), *Regimes of Description: in the archive of the eighteenth century*, Stanford, CA: Stanford University Press.
Pope, A., 1968, *The Poems of Alexander Pope*, ed. J. Butt, London: Routledge.
Popkin, J. and Fort, B. (eds), 1998, *The Mémoires secrets and the Culture of Publicity in Eighteenth-Century France*, Oxford: Voltaire Foundation.
Porter, R., 1993, "The rise of physical examination," in W. F. Bynum and R. Porter (eds), *Medicine and the Five Senses*, Cambridge: Cambridge University Press.
Potkay, A., 2011, "Eye and ear: counteracting senses in loco-descriptive poetry," in C. Mahoney (ed.), *A Companion to Romantic Poetry*, Chichester: Wiley-Blackwell.
Potter, I. R., 1824, *The Life and Remarkable Adventures of Isaac R. Potter*, Providence, RI: Henry Trumbull.
Price, L., 2012, *How to do things with Books in Victorian Britain*, Princeton, NJ: Princeton University Press.
Printy, M., 2005, "The intellectual origins of popular Catholicism: Catholic moral theology in the Age of Enlightenment," *The Catholic Historical Review*, 91(3), 438–61.

Puttfarken, T., 1985, *Roger de Piles' Theory of Art*, New Haven, CT and London: Yale University Press.
Raj, K., 2000, "Eighteenth-century Pacific voyages of discovery, 'Big Science', and the shaping of a European scientific and technological culture," *History and Technology*, 17, 79–98.
Rameau, J-P., 1968–9, *Complete Theoretical Writings*, ed. E. R. Jacobi, 6 vols, n.p.: American Institute of Musicology.
Rath, R. C., 2003, *How Early America Sounded*, Ithaca, NY: Cornell University Press.
Rath, R. C., 2008, "Hearing American history," *The Journal of American History*, 95(2), 417–31.
Ratte, E.-H. de., 1771, *Eloge de M. de Sauvages*, in F. Boissier de Sauvages, *Nosologie méthodique*, Paris: chez Hérissant le fils.
Rée, J., 1999, *I See a Voice: a philosophical history of language, deafness and the senses*, London: HarperCollins.
Reichardt, R., 1998, "Light against darkness: the visual representations of a central Enlightenment concept," trans. from German by D. L. Cohen, *Representations*, 61, 95–148.
Reill, P. H., 2005, *Vitalizing Nature in the Enlightenment*, Berkeley, CA: University of California Press.
Reiser, S. J., 1978, *Medicine and the Reign of Technology*, Cambridge: Cambridge University Press.
Reisz, E., 2007, "Curiosity and rubber in the French Atlantic," *Atlantic Studies*, 4, 5–26.
Rendall, J., 2007, "Feminizing the Enlightenment: the problem of sensibility," in ed. M. Fitzpatrick, *The Enlightenment World*, London: Routledge.
Rey, R., 1993, "Diagnostic différentiel et espèces nosologiques. Le cas de la phtisie pulmonaire de Morgagni à Bayle," in F-O. Touati (ed.), *Maladies, médecines et sociétés*, Paris: L'Harmattan et Histoire du Présent.
"Review of *Nouvelle découverte de la percussion du thorax, comme moyen de reconnoître les maladies cachées dans l'intérieur de la poitrine*," 1761, *Journal étranger* (April), 108–11.
Rey, R., 1995, *The History of Pain*, trans. L. E. Wallace, J. A. Cadden, and S. W. Cadden, Cambridge: Harvard University Press.
Reynolds, J., 1966, *Discourses on Art* [1769–90], introduced by R. R. Wark, London: Collier-Macmillan.
Reynolds, Sir J., [1797] 1988, *Discourses on Art*, New Haven, CT and London: Yale University Press.
Richards, S., 1999, *Eighteenth-Century Ceramics: products for a civilised society*, Manchester and New York: Manchester University Press.
Richardson, S., [1740] 2011, *Pamela: or, Virtue Rewarded*, ed. A. J. Rivero, Cambridge: Cambridge University Press.
Riskin, J., 2002, *Science in the Age of Sensibility: the sentimental empiricists of the French Enlightenment*, Chicago: University of Chicago Press.
Riskin, J., 2003a, "Eighteenth-century Wetware," *Representations*, 83, 97–125.
Riskin, J., 2003b, "The defecating duck, or, the ambiguous origins of artificial life," *Critical Inquiry*, 29, 599–633.

Riskin, J., 2011, "The divine optician," *American Historical Review*, 116(2), 352–70.
Risse, G. B., 1997, "La synthèse entre l'anatomie et la clinique," in M. D. Grmek (ed.), *Histoire de la pensée médicale en Occident*, Paris: Seuil.
Rivers, I., 2008, "William Law and religious revival: the reception of 'A Serious Call'," *Huntington Library Quarterly*, 71(4), 633–49.
Roberts, L., 1985, "From natural theology to naturalism: Diderot and the perception of *Rapports*," PhD dissertation, UCLA.
Roberts, L., 1995, "The death of the sensuous chemist: the 'new' chemistry and the transformation of sensuous technology," *Studies in History and Philosophy of Science*, 26, 503–29.
Roberts, L., 2012, "The circulation of knowledge in early modern europe: embodiment, mobility, learning and knowing," *History of Technology*, 47–68.
Roberts, L., Schaffer, S., and Dear, P., 2007, *The Mindful Hand: inquiry and invention from the late Renaissance to early industrialisation*, Amsterdam: Koninklijke Nederlandse Akademie van Wetenschappen.
"Robots in Providence," n.d., *The Rhode Island Historical Society*, http://rihs.wordpress.com/tag/woodcuts/.
Roche, D., 1989, *La Culture des apparences: une histoire du vêtement (XVIe-XVIIIe siècles)*, Paris: Fayard.
Rochebrune, M-L. de, 2000, "Ceramics and glass in Chardin's paintings," in P. Rosenberg et al., *Chardin*, trans. C. Beamish, New York: Metropolitan Museum of Art.
Rosenfeld, S., 2001, *A Revolution in Language: the problem of signs in late eighteenth-century France*, Stanford, CA: Stanford University Press.
Rosenfeld, S., 2011a, "On being heard: a case for paying attention to the historical ear," *American Historical Review*, 116(2), 316–34.
Rosenfeld, S., 2011b, *Common Sense: a political history*, Cambridge: Harvard University Press.
Rosenthal, A., 2006, *Angelica Kauffman: art and sensibility*, New Haven, CT and London: Yale University Press.
Rousseau, J-B., 1694, *Le Caffé*, Paris: P. Aubouyn, P. Emery, C. Clouzier.
Rousseau, J-J., [1762] 1921, *Emile, ou De l'éducation*, trans. from French by B. Foxley, London: John Dent & Sons.
Rousseau, J-J., [1762] 1979, *Emile: Or, On Education*, trans. A. Bloom. New York: Basic Books.
Rousseau, J-J., 1959–95, *Oeuvres complètes*, ed. B. Gagnebin et al., 5 vols, Paris: Pléiade.
Roussel, P., [1775] 1820, *Système physique et moral de la femme, ou Tableau philosophique de la constitution, de l'état organique, du tempérament, des mœurs et des fonctions propres au sexe*, 7th edn, Paris: Caille et Ravier.
Rulhière, C-C. de, 1992, *Jugement de l'orchestre de l'Opéra*, in D. Launay (ed.), *La Querelle des bouffons: texte des pamphlets*, 3 vols, Geneva: Minkoff.
Safier, N., 2008, "Fruitless botany: Joseph de Jussieu's South American odyssey," in J. Delbourgo and N. Dew (eds), *Science and Empire in the Atlantic World*, London: Routledge.

Sahut, M-C. et al., 1984, *Diderot et l'art de Boucher à David: Les Salons, 1759–1781*, Paris: Réunion des musées nationaux.
Saint-Ursin, M. de, 1807, "Discours préliminaire," in *Consultations de médecine de M. Barthez*, Paris: Chez Léopold Collin.
Sambrook, J., 2005, "The psychology of literary creation and literary response," in H. B. Nisbet and C. Rawson (eds), *The Cambridge History of Literary Criticism*, vol. 4: *The Eighteenth Century*, Cambridge: Cambridge University Press.
Saunderson, N., 1740, *The elements of algebra, in ten books; to which is prefixed an account of the author's life and character*, Cambridge.
Sauvages, F. B. de, 1732, *Nouvelles classes de maladies, qui dans un ordre semblable à celui des botanistes, comprennent les genres et les espèces de toutes les maladies, avec leurs signes et leurs indications*, Avignon: B. d'Avanville.
Sauvages, F. B. de, 1771, *Nosologie méthodique*, 3 vols, Paris: chez Hérissant le fils.
Savary des Bruslons, J., 1723–30, *Dictionnaire universel du commerce*, 4 vols, Paris: J. Estienne.
Schaffer, S., 1999, "Enlightened Automata," in W. Clark, J. Golinski, and S. Schaffer (eds), *The Sciences in Enlightened Europe*, Chicago: University of Chicago Press.
Schaffer, S., 2006, "Instruments and cargo in the China trade," *History of Science*, 44, 217–46.
Schaffer, S., 2007, "'The Charter'd Thames': naval architecture and experimental spaces in Georgian Britain," in L. Roberts et al. (eds), *The Mindful Hand: inquiry and invention from the late Renaissance to early industrialisation*, Amsterdam: Koninklijke Nederlandse Akademie van Wetenschappen.
Schaffer, S. et al., 2009, *The Brokered World: go-betweens and global intelligence, 1770–1820*, Sagamore Beach, MA: Science History Publications.
Schama, S., 1989, *Citizens: a chronicle of the French Revolution*, New York: Viking Press.
Schivelbusch, W., 1993, *Tastes of Paradise: a social history of spices, stimulants, and intoxicants*, trans. from German by D. Jacobson, New York: Vintage Books.
Schmidt, L. E., 2000, *Hearing Things: religion, illusion, and the American Enlightenment*, Cambridge, MA: Harvard University Press.
Schneider, R., 2002, "Disclosing mysteries: the contradictions of reason of state in seventeenth-century France," in G. Engel et al. (eds), *Das Geheimnis am Beginn der europäischen Moderne*, Frankfurt: Klostermann.
Schön, E., 1987, *Der Verlust der Sinnlichkeit oder die Verwandlungen des Lesers: Mentalitätswandel um 1800*, Stuttgart: Klett-Cotta.
Schuchard, M. K., 2006, *William Blake's Sexual Path to Spiritual Vision*, Rochester, VT: Inner Traditions.
Schulz, A., 2005, *Goya's Caprichos: aesthetics, perception, and the body*, Cambridge: Cambridge University Press.
Scott, J. S., 1986, "The Common Wind: currents of Afro-American communication in the era of the Haitian Revolution," PhD disssertation, Duke University, http://proquest.umi.com/pqdweb?did=749581181&sid=1&Fmt=6&clientId=3748&RQT=309&VName=PQD.

Screech, T., 2002, *The Lens Within the Heart: the Western scientific gaze and popular imagery in later Edo Japan*, Honolulu, HI: University of Hawaii Press.
Seigel, J., 2005, *The Idea of the Self: thought and experience in Western Europe since the seventeenth century*, Cambridge: Cambridge University Press.
Seigel, J., 2012, *Modernity and Bourgeois Life: society, politics, and culture in England, France and Germany since 1750*, Cambridge: Cambridge University Press.
Senebier, J., 1775, *L'art d'observer*, 2 vols, Geneva: chez C. Philibert & B. Chirol.
Senebier, J., 1802, *Essai sur l'art d'observer et de faire des expériences*, 3 vols, Geneva: chez J. J. Paschoud.
Serres, M., 1985, *Les cinq sens*, Paris: Grasset.
Sévigné, M. de Rabutin Chantal, Marquise de, [1646–96] 1972, *Correspondance*, ed. R. Duchêne, 3 vols, Paris: Gallimard.
Sewell, W., 1986, "Visions of labor: illustrations of the mechanical arts before, in and after Diderot's *Encyclopédie*," in S. Kaplan and C. Koepp (eds), *Work in France: representations, meaning, organization, and practice*, Ithaca, NY: Cornell University Press.
Sewell, W. H., 1980, *Work and Revolution in France: the language of labor from the old regime to 1848*, Cambridge: Cambridge University Press.
Shapin, S., 1989, "The invisible technician," *American Scientist*, 77, 554–63.
Shapin, S., 1998, "The philosopher and the chicken: on the dietetics of disembodied knowledge," in C. Lawrence and S. Shapin (eds), *Science Incarnate: historical embodiments of natural knowledge*, Chicago: University of Chicago Press.
Shelley, P. B., 2002, *Shelley's Poetry and Prose*, ed. D. H. Reiman and N. Fraistat, New York: Norton.
Sheriff, M. D., 1990, *Fragonard: art and eroticism*, Chicago and London: Chicago University Press.
Sheriff, M. D., 2004, *Moved by Love: inspired artists and deviant women in eighteenth-century France*, Chicago and London: Chicago University Press.
Shorter, E., 1993, "The history of the doctor-patient relationship," in W. F. Bynum and R. Porter (eds), *Companion Encyclopedia of the History of Medicine*, London and New York: Routledge.
Singy, P., 2006, "Huber's Eyes: the art of scientific observation before the emergence of positivism," *Representations*, 95, 54–75.
Slaughter, M. M., 1982, *Universal Languages and Scientific Taxonomy in the Seventeenth Century*, Cambridge: Cambridge University Press.
Sloan, P., 1976, "The Buffon-Linnaeus controversy," *Isis*, 67, 356–75.
Smith, J. M., 1993, "Our sovereign's gaze: kings, nobles, and state formation in seventeenth-century France," *French Historical Studies*, 18(2), 396–415.
Smith-Rosenberg, C., 1992, "Dis-covering the subject of the 'Great Constitutional Discussion,' 1786–1789," *Journal of American History*, 79(3), 841–73.
Smollett, T., [1766] 1981, *Travels through France and Italy*, ed. F. Felsenstein, Oxford: World's Classics.
Smollett, T., [1771] 1982, *The Adventures of Humphry Clinker*, Harmondsworth: Penguin.

Snyder, J. R., 2009, *Dissimulation and the Culture of Secrecy in Early Modern Europe*, Berkeley, CA: University of California Press.
Sofia, Z., 2000, "Container technologies," *Hypatia*, 15(2), 181–201.
Sorkin, D., 2008, *The Religious Enlightenment: Protestants, Jews and Catholics from London to Vienna*, Princeton, NJ and Oxford: Princeton University Press.
Sörlin, S., 2000, "Ordering the world for Europe: science as intelligence and information as seen from the northern periphery," *Osiris*, 15, 65–7.
Sorrensen, R., 1996, "The ship as a scientific instrument in the eighteenth century," *Osiris*, 11, 221–36.
Spacks, P., 2009, *Reading Eighteenth Century Poetry*, Chichester: Wiley-Blackwell.
Spang, R., 2000, *The Invention of the Restaurant: Paris and modern gastronomic culture*, Cambridge, MA: Harvard University Press.
Spary, E. C., 2000, *Utopia's Garden: French natural history from Old Regime to Revolution*, Chicago: University of Chicago Press.
Spary, E. C., 2009, "Self-preservation: French travels between *cuisine* and *industrie*," in J. Delbourgo et al. (eds), *Brokered World: go-betweens and global intelligence, 1770–1820*, Sagamore Beach, MA: Science History Publications.
Spary, E. C., 2012, *Eating the Enlightenment: food and the sciences in Paris, 1670–1760*, Chicago: University of Chicago Press.
Stafford, B. M., Terpak, F., and Poggi, I., 2001, *Devices of Wonder: from the world in a box to images on a screen*, Los Angeles: Getty Research Institute.
Stafford, B. M., 1991, *Body Criticism: imaging the unseen in Enlightenment art and medicine*, Cambridge, MA: MIT Press.
Stalnaker, J., 2010, *The Unfinished Enlightenment: description in the age of the Encyclopédie*, Ithaca, NY: Cornell University Press.
Steinbrügge, L., 1995, *The Moral Sex: woman's nature in the French Enlightenment*. trans. from German by P. E. Selwyn, Oxford: Oxford University Press.
Steinke, H., 2005, *Irritating Experiments: Haller's concept and the European controversy on irritability and sensibility, 1750–90*, Amsterdam and New York: Rodopi.
Steller, G. W., [1793] 1988, *Journal of a Voyage with Bering, 1741–1742*, Palo Alto, CA: Stanford University Press.
Stewart, S., 2002, *Poetry and the Fate of the Senses*, Chicago: University of Chicago Press.
Stolberg, M., 2011, *Experiencing Illness and the Sick Body in Early Modern Europe*, trans. L. Unglaub and L. Kennedy, Basingstoke: Palgrave MacMillan.
Strauss, J., 2012, *Human Remains: medicine, death, and desire in nineteenth-century Paris*, New York: Fordham University Press.
Styles, J., 2010, *Threads of Feeling: the London Foundling Hospital's textile tokens, 1740–1770*, London: The Foundling Museum.
Subligny, A. P. de, [1666] 1882, *Muse de la cour*, in J. de Rothschild (ed.), *Les Continuateurs de Loret*, 2 vols, Paris: Damascène Morgand.
Sutton, J., McIlwain, D., Christensen, W., and Geeves, A., 2011, "Applying intelligence to the reflexes: embodied skills and habits between Dreyfus and Descartes," *Journal of British Society for Phenomenology*, 42, 78–103.

Swift, J., 1937, *The Poems of Jonathan Swift*, ed. H. Williams, Oxford: Clarendon Press.
Tackett, T., 2000, "Conspiracy obsession in a time of revolution: French elites and the origins of the terror, 1789–1792," *American Historical Review*, 105(3), 691–713.
Tadié, A., 2001, "From the ear to the eye: perceptions of language in the fictions of Laurence Sterne," in M. Syrotinski and I. MacLachlan (eds) *Sensual Reading: new approaches to reading in its relations to the senses*, Cranbury, NJ: Associated University Presses.
Tanchoux, P., 2004, *Les Procédures électorales en France de la fin de l'Ancien Régime à la Première Guerre Mondiale*, Paris: CTHS.
Taussig, M., 1998, "Transgression," in M. C. Taylor (ed.), *Critical Terms for Religious Studies*, Chicago and London: The University of Chicago Press.
Temkin, O., [1946] 2006, "The philosophical background of Magendie's Physiology," in O. Temkin (ed.), *The Double Face of Janus and Other Essays in the History of Medicine*, Baltimore, MD: Johns Hopkins University Press.
Terrall, M., 2006, "Mathematics in narratives of geodetic expeditions," *Isis*, 97, 683–99.
Tessèdre, B., 1957, *Roger de Piles et les débats sur loe coloris au siècle de Louis XIV*, Paris: Bibliothèque des arts.
Tessin, N., 1964, *Relations artistiques entre la France et la Suède: 1693–1718 (Correspondance entre Nicodème Tessin le jeune et Daniel Crownström)*, Stockholm: Egnellska Boktryckeriet.
The Amours and Adventures of Two English Gentlemen in Italy, 1795, Worcester, MA: Isaiah Thomas, Jun.
The Present State of the Court of France and City of Paris in a Letter from M. ***, to the Honourable Matthew Prior, 1712, London: E. Curll.
The Universal Magazine of Knowledge and Pleasure, 1747–93, London: John Hinton.
Thébaud-Sorger, M., 2009, *L'Aerostation au temps des Lumières*, Rennes: Presses Universitaires de Rennes.
Thomas, D. A., 1995, *Music and the Origins of Language: theories from the French Enlightenment*, Cambridge: Cambridge University Press.
Thomas, D. A., 2002, *Aesthetics of Opera in the Ancien Régime, 1647–1785*, Cambridge: Cambridge University Press.
Thompson, P., 1999, *Rum Punch and Revolution: taverngoing and public life in eighteenth-century Philadelphia*, Philadelphia, PA: University of Pennsylvania Press.
Thomson, J., [1727–30] 1972, *The Seasons and The Castle of Indolence*, ed. J. Sambrook, Oxford: Clarendon Press.
Thornton, P., 1978, *Interior Decoration in England, France, and Holland*, New Haven, CT and London: Yale University Press.
Thunberg, C. P., 1784, *Flora Japonicum*, Uppsala.
Thunberg, C. P., 1796, *Travels in Europe, Africa and Asia, Performed between the Years 1770 and 1779*, 3rd edn, London.
Tissot, S. A., [1761] 1993, *Avis au peuple sur sa santé*, Paris: Quai Voltaire.

Tissot, S-A., [1770] 1778, *Essai sur les maladies des gens du monde*, Vol. 4, *Œuvres de M. Tissot, Nouvelle édition augmentée et imprimée sous ses yeux*, Lausanne: Grasset,
Tissot, S. A., 1785, *Essai sur les moyens de perfectionner les études de médecine*, Lausanne: Chez Mourer, Cadet.
Tooth, M., 1796–7, *Mary Tooth's Account of her Life and Journal*, September 13, 1796–December 31, 1797, Fletcher/Tooth Collection MAM 14, John Rylands Library, Manchester.
Török, B. Z., 2011, "The ethnicity of knowledge: statistics and *Landskunde* in late eighteenth-century Hungary and Transylvania," in G. Abbattista (ed.), *Encountering Otherness, Diversities and Transcultural Experiences in Early Modern European Culture*, Trieste: University of Trieste Press.
Tribble, E. 2005, "Distributing cognition in the globe," *Shakespeare Quarterly*, 56, 135–55.
Tsien, J., 2012, *The Bad Taste of Others: judging literary value in eighteenth-century France*, Philadelphia, PA: University of Pennsylvania Press.
Tunstall, K. E. and Diderot, D., 2011, *Blindness and Enlightenment: an essay*, New York: Continuum.
Tyson, J. R., 1989, *A Reader*, ed. C. Wesley, Oxford and New York: Oxford University Press.
Ure, A., 1835, *The Philosophy of Manufactures: or an exposition of the scientific, moral and commercial economy of the factory system of Great Britain*, London.
Van Damme, S., 2007, "Farewell Habermas? Deux décennies d'études sur l'espace public au XVIIe et XVIIIe siècles," http://dossiersgrihl.revues.org/682?lang=en.
Van Horn Melton, J., 2001, *The Rise of the Public in Enlightenment Europe*, New York: Cambridge University Press.
van Noppen, J-P., 2005, "Hymns as literature, language and discourse: Wesleyan ymns as a case example," *The Hymn*, 56(3), 22–30.
Van Sant, J., 1993, *Eighteenth-Century Sensibility and the Novel: the senses in social context*, Cambridge: Cambridge University Press.
Varey, S., 1996, "The pleasures of table," in R. Porter and M. Mulvey Roberts (eds), *Pleasure in the Eighteenth Century*, Basingstoke: Macmillan.
Vartanian, A., 1983, "La Mettrie and Diderot Revisited: An Intertextual Encounter," *Diderot Studies*, 21, 155–197.
Vaucanson, J. D., 1749. "Construction d'un nouveau tour à filer la soie des cocoons," *Mémoires de l'Académie Royale des Sciences, Année 1749*, 142–54.
Venel, G., [1754] 2013, "Digestion" (*OEconom. anim*), in *Encyclopédie* (q.v.), Vol. 4.
Vicente, M., 2006, *Clothing the Spanish Empire*, Basingstoke: Palgrave Press.
Vickers, N., 2004, *Coleridge and the Doctors 1795–1806*, Oxford: Clarendon Press.
Vidal, F., 2011, *The Sciences of the Soul: the early modern origins of psychology*, Chicago: University of Chicago Press.
Vigarello, G., 1988, *Concepts of Cleanliness: changing attitudes in France since the Middle Ages*, trans. from French by J. Birrell, Cambridge: Cambridge University Press.
Vila, A. C., 1998, *Enlightenment and Pathology: Sensibility in the literature and medicine of eighteenth-century France*, Baltimore, MD: Johns Hopkins University Press.

Villiers, P. de, 1712, *Poëmes et autres poësies*, Paris: Jacques Collombat.
Vincent-Buffault, A., 1991, *The History of Tears: sensibility and sentimentality in France*, trans. from French by T. Bridgeman, New York: St. Martin's Press.
Vinge, L., 1975, *The Five Senses: studies in a literary tradition*, Lund: LiberLäromedel.
Voltaire, F. M. A. de, [1757] 2013, "Goût," in *Encyclopédie* (q.v.), Vol. 7.
Voltaire, F. M. A. de, 1953–65, *Voltaire's Correspondence*, ed. T. Besterman, 107 vols, Geneva: Institut et Musée Voltaire.
Voskuhl, A., 2013, *Androids in the Enlightenment: mechanics, artisans and cultures of the self*, Chicago: University of Chicago Press.
Wakefield, A., 2009, *The Disordered Police State*, Chicago: University of Chicago Press.
Wall, C., 2006, *The Prose of Things: transformations of description in the eighteenth century*, Chicago: University of Chicago Press.
Walpole, H., [1954], *Horace Walpole's Correspondence with Sir Horace Mann*, ed. W. S. Lewis *et al.*, 48 vols, New Haven, CT: Yale University Press.
Walsh, C., 1995, "Shop design and the display of goods in eighteenth-century London," *Journal of Design History*, 8(3), 157–76.
Walton, J. K., 1983, *The English Seaside Resort—A Social History 1750–1914*, Leicester: Leicester University Press.
Warner, M., 2002, "Publics and counterpublics," *Public Culture*, 14(1), 49–90.
Watts, I., n.d., *Psalms and Hymns of Isaac Watts*, Christian Classics Ethereal Library, www.ccel.org/ccel/watts/psalmshymns.html.
Webb, D., [1769] 1970, *Observations on the Correspondence Between Poetry and Music*, New York: Garland Publishing.
Wellek, R., [1965] 1983, *A History of Modern Criticism 1750–1950*, Volume 3, *The Age of Transition*, Cambridge: Cambridge University Press.
Wesley, C., 1746, *Funeral Hymns*, 2nd edn, London: n.p.
Wesley, C., [1767] 1825, *Hymns for the Use of Families, and on Various Occasions*, 2nd edn, London: J. Kershaw.
Wesley, C., 1989, *Charles Wesley: a reader*, ed. J. R. Tyson, Oxford and New York: Oxford University Press.
Wesley, J., [1746] 1825, "A letter to a friend, concerning tea," London: A. Macintosh.
Wesley, J., 1747, *Primitive Physic. Or, an Easy and Natural Method of Curing most Diseases*, London: s.n.
Wesley, J., 1771, "An earnest appeal to men of reason and religion," Bristol: W. Pine.
Wesley, J., [1777] 1960, *A Plain Account of Christian Perfection. As Believed and Taught by the Reverend Mr. John Wesley, from the Year 1725, to the Year 1777*, London: The Epworth Press.
Wesley, J., [1779] 1835, "Thoughts on the power of music," in J. Emory (ed.), *The Words of the Reverend John Wesley, A.M.*, Vol. 7, New York: B. Waugh & T. Mason.
Wesley, J., 1983, *A Collection of Hymns for the Use of the People called Methodists*, *The Works of John Wesley*, Vol. 7, ed. F. Hildebrandt and O. A. Beckerlegge, Oxford: Clarendon Press.

Whitaker, H. and Turgeon, Y., 2007, "Charles Bonnet's neurophilosophy," in H. Whitaker, C. M. Smith, and S. Finger (eds), *Brain, Mind and Medicine: essays in eighteenth-century neuroscience*, New York: Springer.

Whitehead, J., 2009, *French Interiors of the Eighteenth Century*, London: Laurence King Publishers.

Wilcox, B., 2011, "The hissing of Jean-Pierre Pagin: Diderot's violinist meets the Cabal at the Concert Spirituel," *Studies in Eighteenth Century Culture*, 40, 103–32.

Williams, E. A., 1994, *The Physical and the Moral: anthropology, physiology, and philosophical medicine in France, 1750–1850*, Cambridge: Cambridge University Press.

Williams, E. A., 2003, *A Cultural History of Medical Vitalism in Enlightenment Montpellier*, Burlington: Ashgate.

Wollstonecraft, M., [1792] 1995, *A Vindication of the Rights of Men with A Vindication of the Rights of Woman and Hints*, ed. S. Tomaselli, Cambridge: Cambridge University Press.

Wollstonecraft, M., [1796] 1987, *A Short Residence in Sweden, Norway and Denmark and Memoirs of the Author of A Vindication of the Rights of Woman*, ed. R. Holmes, New York: Penguin Books.

Wood, G., 1982, "Conspiracy and the paranoid style: causality and deceit in the 18th century," *William and Mary Quarterly*, 39(3), 402–41.

Wordsworth, W., [c. 1805] 1979, *The Prelude, 1799, 1805, 1850*, ed. J. Wordsworth, M. H. Abrams, and S. Gill, New York: Norton.

Wordsworth, W., [1805, 1850] 1996, *The Prelude*, ed. J. Wordsworth, Harmondsworth: Penguin.

Wordsworth, W., [1850] 1974, *The Prose Works of William Wordsworth*, Vol. I, ed. W. J. B. Owen and J. W. Smyser, Oxford: Clarendon Press.

Wortley Montagu, Lady M., 1763, *Letters of the Right Honourable Lady M---y W----y M------e: Written, During her Travels in Europe, Asia and Africa, to Persons of Distinction*, London: printed for T. Becket and P. A. De Hondt, in the Strand.

Wren, C., 1750, *Parentalia: or, Memoirs of the Family of the Wrens; viz. of Mathew Bishop of Ely, Christopher Dean of Windsor, &c. but chiefly of Sir Christopher . . .* London: printed for T. Osborn and R. Dodsley.

Wright, J., 1991, "Metaphysics and physiology: mind, body, and the animal economy in eighteenth-century Scotland," in M. A. Stewart (ed.), *Studies in the Philosophy of the Scottish Enlightenment*, Oxford: Oxford University Press.

Yolton, J., 1984, *Perceptual Acquaintance: from Descartes to Reid*, Minneapolis, MN: University of Minnesota Press.

Young, E., [1742–5] 2008, *Night Thoughts*, ed. S. Cornford, Cambridge: Cambridge University Press.

Yvon, C. and Diderot, D., [1751] 2013, "Ame," in *Encyclopédie* (q.v.), Vol. 1.

Zimmermann, J. G., [1764] 1778, *A Treatise on Experience in Physic*, 2 vols, London: J. Wilkie.

Zittrain, J., 2006, "The generative internet," *Harvard Law Review*, 119(7), 1974–2040.

Zoberman, P., 1981, "Voir, savoir, parler: la rhétorique de la vision au XVIIe et au début du XVIIIe siècles," *Dix-septième siècle*, 33(133/4), 409–28.

NOTES ON CONTRIBUTORS

Rowan Rose Boyson is Lecturer in Eighteenth-Century Literature at King's College London, author of *Wordsworth and the Enlightenment Idea of Pleasure* (2012), and editor, with Tom Jones, of *The Poetic Enlightenment: Poetry and Human Science 1650–1820* (2013). She has published articles on scent in Shelley and Wordsworth, and is working on a book on smell in the literature and philosophy of the Enlightenment and Romantic periods.

Clare Brant is Professor of Eighteenth-Century Literature and Culture at King's College London, where she also co-directs the Centre for Life-Writing Research. She is the author of *Eighteenth-Century Letters and British Culture* which won the ESSE Book Award in 2008, and has published numerous articles on literature, culture, and gender. She is the Project Director of Strandlines, a digital community project about lives on the Strand, past, present, and creative, www.strandlines.com, and a creative editor for the *European Journal of Life Writing*, http://ejlw.eu/. Her book on eighteenth-century ballooning, *Balloon Madness*, will be published shortly.

Sarah Cohen is Professor of Art History and Women's Studies at the University at Albany, SUNY. Her publications include *Art, Dance, and the Body in French Culture of the Ancien Régime* (2000), as well as articles on gender and gesture in the paintings of Rubens and several studies on representations of animals in French and Netherlandish art. She is completing a book entitled *Envisioning Animals in Early Modern Europe: Art and Soul*.

Joan DeJean is Trustee Professor at the University of Pennsylvania. She is the author most recently of *The Age of Comfort* (2009) and *The Essence of Style* (2005). She recently completed a book about the rebirth of the city of Paris in the seventeenth century, *How Paris Became Paris: Making the City Modern*. She works on the literature and material culture of seventeenth- and eighteenth-century France.

Phyllis Mack is Professor of History and Women's Studies at Rutgers University. Her most recent books include *Visionary Women: Ecstatic Prophecy in 17th-Century England* (1992; winner of the Berkshire Prize in History), *In God's Name: Genocide and Religion in the 20th Century* (edited with Omer Bartov, 2001) and *Heart Religion in the British Enlightenment: Gender and Emotion in Early Methodism* (2008). She is currently working on a history of dreams and religion in Enlightenment England.

Richard Cullen Rath is Associate Professor of History at the University of Hawaii at Mānoa. He is the author of *How Early America Sounded* and is currently working on two books, one an introduction to the history of hearing and the other comparing the rise of print culture in eighteenth-century North America to the rise of internet culture today. He has also written three award-winning articles on music, creolization, and African American culture.

Lissa Roberts is Professor of Long-Term Development of Science and Technology at the University of Twente, the Netherlands. A strong believer in collaboration, she has (co-) edited several publications including *Centres and Cycles of Accumulation in and Around the Netherlands* (2011), *The Brokered World: Go-Betweens and Global Intelligence, 1770–1820* (2009) and *The Mindful Hand: Inquiry and Invention from the Late Renaissance to Early Industrialization* (2007).

Sophia Rosenfeld is Professor of History at the University of Virginia. She is the author of *A Revolution in Language: the Problem of Signs in late Eighteenth-Century France* (2001) and *Common Sense: A Political History* (2011), which won the 2012 Mark Lynton History Prize and the 2011 SHEAR Book Prize. She is also a co-editor of the journal *Modern Intellectual History*. Currently she is writing a history of choice-making with the support of a Guggenheim Foundation fellowship.

Patrick Singy is Adjunct Professor at Union College in Schenectady, NY. His research interests include the history of medicine and sexuality, the historiography of science, and the history and philosophy of psychology and psychiatry. He has recently published *L'Usage du sexe: Lettres au Dr Tissot, auteur de L'Onanisme (1760)* (2014) and is co-editing, with Steeves Demazeux, a book on the recent *DSM-5*.

Downing A. Thomas is Professor of French at the University of Iowa. He has served as Chair of the Department of French and Italian and is currently Associate Provost and Dean of International Programs. In 2007, Thomas was elected President of the Association of Departments of Foreign Language (ADFL). His book-length publications include *Music and the Origins of Languages* (1995) and *Aesthetics of Opera in the Ancien Régime* (2002).

Anne C. Vila is Professor of French at the University of Wisconsin-Madison. She is the author of *Enlightenment and Pathology: Sensibility in the Literature and Medicine of Eighteenth-Century France* (1998), as well as many articles on the body in the culture of the Enlightenment. She is completing *Singular Beings: Passions and Pathologies of the Scholar in France, 1720–1840* and co-directing a re-edition of the works of Dr. Samuel-Auguste Tissot.

INDEX

Locators shown in *italics* refer to figures.

abstraction, mathematical
   role of senses in relation to 110–15, *114*
Addison, J. 9, 158–9, 162, 177
aesthetics 2, 9, 12, 26, 122, 135, 137
   and literary theory 155–65, 175, 177
   and music theory 194–201
   as a "science" of sensation 12, 26–7, 156
   spiritual 88–90, 99–100, 106
   theories on beauty in visual arts 187–9
   see also sublime, sublimity
Akenside, M. 163–4
air quality 11–12, 63, 172
anatomy 3–4, 127–8, 149–52
Anderson, B. 216, 217
animals, non-human
   role in debates on human senses and sensibility 2, 3, 16–18, 197
architecture and decorative arts
   impact on senses 7, 44–51, *47*, 83–4
   of churches 87
Arnaud, F. 200
Arnold, M. 176
art, visual
   and empiricism 184–7, *186*
   role in configuring the senses 181–4, *184*
   significance for material objects 190–1
   significance for Moravianism 99–102, *100*, *101*
   significance of "sensibility" movement in 191–202, *193*
Auenbrugger, L. 146, *146*, 147, 148–9
Austen, J. 156, 172
authors, authorship 168, 207–11, 222
automation and mechanisation
   and "philosophy of manufactures" 127–30, *130*
   of the printing process 211–13
automatons 127–8

Baillie, J. 165
Bailyn, B. 220
balloons, hot-air 12, 59
Baridon, M. 188
Barker, R. 7
Barker-Benfield, G. J. 3
Barrow, J. 123, 129
Barthez, P-J. 141–2
bathing 13, 24, 26, 56

INDEX

Baumgarten, A. 12
Bederlegge, O. 95
bells, bell-ringing 23, 87, 207, 214–19
Beresford, J. 2
Bermingham, A. 192
Bichat, X. 6
Blake, W. 47, 49, 51–2, 172, 176
blindness
  in philosophical debates 4, 109, 111–12, 125, 185
  in literary tropes 166
  significance in interpretation of mathematics 111–13
  significance in interpretation of natural history 116–18
Blumenbach, F. 5
Blumin, S. M. 45–6
body, bodies
  and health or disease 10–12, 92, 133–53, 196
  and mind-body relationship, 2–20, 5, 15, 54, 92, 185
  laboring 16, 59, 110–11, 125–31, 190, 211–15
  see also women and gender
Boerhaave, H. 141, 142
Boileau, N. 165
Boilly, L-L. 57
books and manuscripts
  role in shaping and describing Enlightenment 203–5
  see also elements e.g. authors; media, print circuits; reading; type and typesetting
Bonnet, C. 116, 118
Bordeu, T. de 4, 138–9
Bosse, A. 46
Boswell J. 52–3, 62–3
Boucher, F. 183, 184, 184, 185
Bowles, G. 192
Brillat-Savarin, J-A. 54–5
Brown, T. 61–2
Browne, E. 68
Buffon, G. L. 2, 17, 166
Burke, E. 13, 96, 165, 169

Burnens, F. 118
Burton, R. 195–6
Bustelli, F. A. 8, 190

Cabanis, P-J-G. 6, 16
cafés and coffeehouses 9, 26, 56–7, 57, 66–71, 69, 77, 220, 220
Canaletto (Giovanni Antonio Canal) 46
Canetti, E. 62
Caraccioli, L-A. de 18
Cartwright, J. 37
catastrophes, urban
  impact on the senses 43–4
Caxton, W. 212
cemeteries 12, 50–1
Cennick, J. 88, 102–3
Cennick, S. 102
Certeau, M. de 86
Chardin, J-S. 185, 186, 186, 187, 190
Charrière, I. 14
chest, human
  diagnosis using percussion of 140–5, 142, 143
Childs, A. 190, 191
Chiquet, 81
cities
  impact on senses of development of 41–64, 47–9, 57
clothing
  history of development of 65–6
  marketization of 80–2, 81
Cockayne, E. 23
coffee and coffee consumption 11, 23, 24, 65–71, 69, 80, 83, 190, 220
Coleridge S. T. 172–4
Collier, E. 204
Collins, W. 165–6
color 5, 13, 15, 27, 66–76, 122–4, 129, 134, 164, 176, 181–2, 183, 192–3, 198, 201
  color-blindness 124
Combe, W. 89
commercialization
  of luxury goods 80–2, 81

common sense 18, 98
Condillac, E. B. de 6, 13, 126, 127, 138, 183, 185
Corbin, A. 218, 223
Corfield, P. J. 41
Corvisart, J. N. 146, 147, 148
cotton
  history of development and tastes in Europe 72–6, *73*
Cowper, W. 45
Crewe, F. A. 59, 60
Cronström, D. 77–8, 80, 82
crowds 12, 22, 57–8, 59, 87
Cruikshank, J. 95–6
corruption
  and the senses 12, 31, 87, 91
Curl, J. S. 50, 56
Cuvier, G. 121

d'Alembert, J. L. R. 26, 111, 126–7, 196, 199, 200–1
Dalton, J. 124
Darnton, R. 219
Darwin, E. 170
Daston, L. 116
David, J-L. *33*
deafness 14–15
de Piles, R. 181–2, 183
Dei Coltelli, F. 68
Delacroix, J-V. 38
Delille, J. 166
Desfontaines, P-F. 200
diagnosis, medical 135–52, *142*, *143*, *146*, *150*
Dickinson, W. *220*
Diderot, D. 2, 6, 17–18, 26, 111, 112, 125, 166, 169, 185–7, 196, 199
Dieu de Saint-Jean, J. 78, *79*
Dill, C. 201
Dillon, H-L. 75
dirt 22–23, 45, 51, 52
disgust 27, 42, 51, 120, 156–60, 200
Doddridge, P. D. 103–4
drums, drumming 33, 99, 214
Dryden, J. 156–7, 177

Du Bos, J-B. 12, 157, 158
Dunker, E. 42

education
  and the senses 13–16, 30, 34, 89–96, 138, 170
electricity 18, *93*, 170, 176
emotions
  and the senses 12, 30, 92, 96, 191, 195, 197
Empson, W. 156
Enlightenment
  as "age of reason" 1, 109–11, 131, 176–7
  and notions of modernity, progress 16, 43, 110, 113, 131, 139, 146, 170, 192
  political milestones marking age of 2–3, 21–39
  role of print culture in shaping 203–5
  role of senses in definitions of 1–3, 30, 169, 177, 205–6
entertainments engaging the senses
  concerts, opera, theater 27, 155, 156–7, 169, 177, 199–201
  courtly entertainments 7, 23, 25, 27, 44
  see also balloons; fireworks; fountains; gardens
Epée, A. C. M. de l' 14
eroticism 11, 55, 90–1, 98–9, 102–4, 163, 165, 170–1, *171*
Euler, L. 112–13
exotic, exoticism 7, 26, 65–7, 68, 69, 71–3, 76, 84, 111, 118, 120, 121, 191
exploration, global 3, 113, 115–23, 162

fabric, cotton
  history of development and tastes in Europe 72–6, *73*
Fabre, P. 141
fairs and tourism
  impact on senses in urban areas 58–9
Farley, J. 52–3

Ferguson, A. 127
Fielding, H. 169
fires, urban
 impact on senses 43–4
fireworks 7, 25, *25*
Fisher, D. H. 204
Fletcher, J. 97–8, 105
Fletcher, M. 92, 97, 106
Floyer, J. 15, 134
Fontenelle, B. L. B. de 111
food
 cuisine, gastronomy 52–4, 67–70, 190
 invention of the sandwich 53
 see also cafés and coffeehouses;
  hygiene, diet and exercise;
  restaurants and taverns
Forsaith, P. S. 97
Foucault, M. 10, 27, 115, 116, 135, 136, 148, 213
fountains 7, 26, 56
Fouquet, H. 9–10, *140*
Frederick the Great 28
Frank, J. P. 152
Franklin, B. 60–1, 221–2
furniture
 history of development and tastes in Europe 76–80, *79*
 marketiszation of 80–2, *81*
Fuss, N. 112

Gainsborough, T. 191
Galen 140
gardens and green space 7, 15, 24–5, *24*, 44, 55–8, 102, 122, 123, 157, 170, 176
 impact on senses in urban areas 55–8
 see also parks
Göchausen, L. von 193
Gay, J. 58, 159, 188
gender *see* women and gender
Gerard, A. 169
Gillray, J. *161*
Goethe, J. W. 175–6
goods, luxury
 history of development of 65–6

 impact on domestic senses and sensibility 82–4
 marketisation of 80–2, *81*
 see also specific e.g. cafes and coffeehouses; clothing; furniture; textiles
Gough, J. 123, 124
Goya, D. F. 18, *19*
Gray, T. 58
Greuze, J-B. 192
Gyles, J. 208–10, 222

Habermas, J. 29–31, 209
Haidt, J. V. *100, 101*
Haller, A. von 3–4
Hammon, B. 214–15
Harris, J. 158
Hartley, D. 6
hearing and listening
 in cities 22–3, 46–50, *48, 49*
 role of reading in 215–22, *217, 220*
 roles accorded to in socio-political life 22–39, *24, 25*
 significance of music for 7, 194–201
 significance of visual arts in depicting sense of 188–9, *189*
 spiritual 2, 88–9, 96–7, *99*
 see also bells, bellringing; deafness; drums, drumming; language theories; media; noise; sermons; silence
"heavenly city"
 in relation to senses 51–2
Helvétius, C-A. 13
Hempton, D. 86
Herder, J. G. 2
Herz, M. 5
Hildebrandt, F. 95
Hindmarsh, D. B. 96
Hoffmann, F. 141
Hogarth, W. 187–90, *189*, 199
Hohenberg, P. 45
Home, H. (Lord Kames) 192
Horace 158
Horner, F. 112

Howes, D. 6
Huber, F. 116, 118
Humboldt, A. von 121
Hume, D. 158, 169, 192
Hunauld, P. 10
Hunt, L. 34
Hutcheson, F. 169
hygiene, personal and public
   diet and exercise 10–11, 14, 92
   sanitation 12, 23 *see also* cemeteries

insight, spiritual 89, 90, 94
imagination
   and the senses 2, 7, 9, 11, 43, 46, 51, 96, 157–9, 162–4, 169–70, 178, 182, 189, 191
irritability 3–4

Jancović, V. 63
Jansen, C. 87
Jansenism 9, 87
Jaucourt, L. de 9
Jefferys, T. *114*
Joule, J. P. 123
Judaism 87–8, 165
Jussieu, J. de 121

Kant, I. 12, 109, 111, 126, 131, 159, 174–5, 203, 204, 215, 216, 219
Kauffman, A. 192–4, *193*

Laclos, P. C. 170
La Fayette, M. M. P. de L. V. 72
La Mettrie, J. O. de 4, 169
Lamotte, C. 158
Lancret, N. 24–5, *24*
language theories
   role of senses in 2, 14, 87–8, 125–6, 200, 208, 216
Laroon, M. 46–8, *48*
Laurent, F. 71
Lavergne l'aîné *142, 143*
Lavoisier, A. 15
Law, W. 86, 92, 94
Le Cat, C-N. 5, *5*, 198

Le Dran, H-F. 141
Le Thieullier, L-J. 143
Lees, L. 45
Leibniz, G. W. 198
leisure
   impact on senses of urban 55–9, *57*
Lessing, G.E. 166, 168
letters, letter-writing
   and literature 168
   and medical consultation 140–5, *142, 143*
Lewis, W. 211
libertinism 9, 170
Lieutaud, J. 138
life, public *see* cities; society; towns
lighting, in homes and streets 12, 23, 60
Linebaugh, P. 215
Linnaeus, C. 115, 118–20, *119*
Lister, M. 70
literature
   ability to stir the senses 156–62, *161*, 172–6, *175*
   and cultivation of sensibility 168–72, *171*
   tickletexts 169
   turn to darkness in 162–6
Locke, J. 3, 4, 6, 13, 30, 91, 125, 157, 176, 184–5, 187, 188, 207
Lordat, J. 141–2
Lowood, H. 114
Loyola, I. 96
Luhrmann, T. M. 99, 106

Macartney, G. 123
Machiavelli, N. 28
Maine de Biran, F-P. 175
Malebranche, N. 16–17
McLuhan, M. 205, 206, 212, 216, 218–19
Mann, H. 78
manufactures, 123–30, *130*
magnetism, vital 18, 20, *20*
Marieschi, M. 46, *47*
Marivaux, P. C. de 71

marketization
  of luxury goods 80–2, *81*
materialism, philosophical 4, 6, 17–18, 169, 174, 177, 181, 185
mathematics
  role of senses in understanding of 111–15, *114*
mechanization and automation 127–30, *130*
media
  oral communication 207, 209, 214–15, 221–2 *see also* bells, bellringing; drums, drumming
  print circuits 207–23 *see also type e.g.* news, circulation of; print and printing
medicine
  physician use of perception in diagnosis 135–52, *142, 143, 146, 150*
  role of senses in medical training 15, 134–5
Mendelssohn, M. 87–8
mental disorders
  effects of sensory experience on 13, 195–7
Ménuret de Chambaud, J-J. 197, 199
Mercier, L-S. 30–1, 57
Merleau-Ponty, M. 131
Mesmer, F. A. 20
Methodism 94–7
Meyer, M. 58
mind-body, relationship of *see* body, bodies
Molyneux, W. 4, 125, 184–5
Montagu, J., Earl of Sandwich, 53
Montequieu, C. de S. 31, 35, 63
Montespan, F-A. de 75
Morand, S-F. 141
"morale sensitive" 13–14
Moravianism 98–105, *100, 101*
Morgagni, G. B. 141, 149–51, *150*, 151–2
Moxon, J. 211
Mumford, L. 214

music
  as noise 199–201
  importance and role in Methodism and Moravianism 94–7, 102–5
  role and powers in configuring the senses 194–201
  therapeutic effects of sound 195–8

Nacquart, J-B. 143–4
natural history 113–23, *117, 119*
  Asian versus European 122–3
Necker, J. 32
Nemeitz, J. C. 70–1
nerves 3, 10–11, 92, 141, 159, 163, 165, 168, 197–8
news, circulation of 32–4, 213–23
Newton, I. 5, 111–12, 162, 168, 176
noise 13, 22, 23, 41, 47, 50, 51, 60, 63, 88, 94, 97, 157, 188, 199–201, 209, 219

observation
  in medicine 136–7
  in natural history and science 110, 116–23
odors, bad 5, 11, 23, 120, 159–60, 223
optics, optical instruments 1, 5, 116, 161

Pagin, J-P. 199–200
Paine, T. 53
painting *see* art, visual
parks
  impact on senses in urban areas 55–8
Pepys, S. 74
perception
  consultation by letter 140–5, *142, 143*
  diagnosis (in medicine) 140–53
  pathological anatomy 149–52, *150*
  percussion of the chest 145–9, *146*
Pététin, J-H-D. 20
"philosophy of manufactures"
  role of senses in understanding of 123–30, *130*
physicians, medical practitioners
  use of perception in diagnosis 135–52, *142, 143, 146, 150*

Pietism 86, 88, 96
Pinel, P. 135, 138, 152
plates, fashion
  development as way of marketing new goods 80–2, *81*
poetry and prose
  and concepts of vision 162–7, *167*
  ability to stir the senses 156–62, *161*
  street poetry 12, 215
police, censors, spies 12, 27–8, 209
politics and statecraft
  roles accorded to the senses in structuring of 27–39, *29, 33*
Pompadour, J. A. P. d'E., 183–4
Pope, A. 161–2, 168, 172
populations
  impact on senses, of urban life 41–64, *47–9, 57*
porcelain 23, 186, 190–1
Potter, I. R. 50
Poussin, N. 182
poverty and the poor
  influences of urban areas on senses of 59–60
Prince de Conti (François Louis) 77, 78
Princess Palatine (Princess Elizabeth Charlotte) 83
print and printing 203–23
  see also elements *e.g.* authors; news, circulation of; type and type casting
Procope, F. 68–70
pulse, pulse-taking 134, 137, 138–9, 141, 149, 151
Pyne, W. *89*

Quakers 9, 86, 88, *89*
"quantifying spirit" 111–15, *114*

Rameau, J-P. 195, 200
Rath, R. C. 15–16
reading, reading practices 169, 92–3, 215–22, *217, 220*
Réaumur, R. de 116
Rediker, M. 215

Reiser, S. J. 148
religion and theology
  concept of transgression 97–105
  significance for the senses 90–105, *92, 100, 101*
  see also aesthetics, spiritual; senses, spiritual; sermons; *types e.g.* Methodism; Moravianism; Catholicism, Judaism, Quakers
restaurants and taverns 9, 26, 32, 39, 53–5, 70, 88, 112, 130, 205, 215, 220–1
Reynolds, J. 137, 191
Richardson, S. 168–9, *170*
Roberts, L. 15–16
Rosenthal, A. 193
Rossini, G. 194
Rousseau, J-J. 2, 13–14, 16, 60, 169–70, 171, 172, 194–5, 196
Roussel, P. 16
Rubens, P. P . 182, 183
Rulhiere, C-C. de 200
Rumphius, G. 115–16, *117*
Rush, B. 15, 144

Sade, D. A. F. de 170
satires involving senses 2, 57, 63, 160, *161*, 169, 172, 178
Saunderson, N. 111–12
Sauvages, F. B. de. 136, 137, 138, 149, 151–2
Schmidt, L. E. 18, 88–9
scent, scents 6, 23, 155, 158–9, 165, 170, 172, 176, 177, 223
science
  role of senses in understanding of 111–30, *114, 117, 119, 130*
  see also branches of e.g. natural history
Scientific Revolution 1, 2, 177
secrecy and veiling
  influences on senses and socio-political life 36–9
Senebier, J. 118, 136, 137–8
sensationalism, philosophical 6, 13, 30, 124–7, 169–70, 172, 175, 181, 183

sense(s), inner 6, 15, 18, 20, 96–7, 163, 169, 174, 191, 193–4 *see also* sixth sense
senses, as paths to knowledge 1–6, 9–15, 18, 21, 30, 60, 109–10, 116, 124–7, 131, 138–39, 156, 169, 187–8, 190 *see also* observation; perception; pulse, pulse-taking; sensationalism; science
senses, sensibility
  distrust of 9–11, 15–16, 18, 139, 159 *see also* blindness; perception
senses, ranking of 1–2, 126, 158–63, 198, 206, 209, 218
senses, spiritual 96–7
sensibility, concept and culture of 1–20, 30, 106, 156, 162, 168–72, 177, 191–4
sensitivity
  acute 9–11, 63, 139, 161–2, 168, 170
  cultivation through art and literature 168–72, *171*, 191–4
sensualism, philosophical *see* sensationalism
sensuality 22–7, 44–5, 52, 54–7, 59, 90, 102–3, 156–8, 162–4, 166, 168, 172–8, 182–4, 185, 187, 193–4
sermons 87–90, 103, 106, 205, 207–8
Serres, M. 131
sentimentalism 7, 13, 170, 190, 192–4
Sévigné, M. de 71
sex, sexuality 6, 16–17, 23, 54–6, 104, 168, 170 *see also* eroticism; libertinism; women and gender
Sharpe, W. 58
Shelley, W. B. 176
sight, sense of
  impact of urban development on 41–64, 47–9, 57
  in socio-political life 22–36, *24, 25, 29, 33*, 36–9
  nature of 2, 4–5, 62, 125, 184–85 *see also* art, visual; blindness; medicine; observation

silence 28, 50–1, 88, 164
  silent reading 155, 207
silk 23, 57, 76, 127–9
Simonides 158
Singy, P. 15–16, 118
sixth sense 12, 54, 158, 169, 179, 225
smell, sense of 2, 5, 15, 17, 22–5, 27, 34, 46–7, 50, 53, 54, 96, 102, 106, 120, 122, 134, 135, 158–61, 174, 176, 181, 205, 233 *see also* odors; scents
Smith, A. 169
Smollett, T. 11–12, 41
society
  roles played by senses in structuring 22–7, *24, 25,* 52–3, 41–64, 115, 122–3, 129–31, 190
sound *see* hearing and listening
slaves, slavery 111, 121–2, 129, 131, 191, 214–17
Stamp Act (1765) 218
Sterne, L. 169
Stolberg, M. 10–11
sublime, sublimity
  as aesthetic category 12–13, 159, 164–6, 169, 177, 201
  in religion 96
Swedenborg, E. 18
Swift, J. 159–60, *161*
sympathy 6–7, 168, 169, 192, 197–8

Taricco, S. 28, *29*
Taussig, M. 98
taste, sense of 2, 12, 15, 16, 18, 21, 25, 26–7, 52–5, 60, 65, 67, 77, 89–90, 95, 120–1, 122, 129, 134, 135, 156, 159, 163, 169, 174, 187, 190, 192, 223 *see also* aesthetics
Taylor, W. T. 213
tea, tea-drinking 11, 23, 55, 89–90, 94, 103, 159, 190
textiles
  history of development and tastes in Europe 72–6, *73*
Thomson, J. 162–3, 166

Thunberg, C. P. 122
Tissot, S-A. 10, 133–4, 136, 139, *142*, 144, 145, 146, 153
touch, sense of
  in philosophy 2, 13, 62, 126–7, 184–5
  as metaphor of sensibility 168–9, 170, *171*
  in visual arts 15, 183–7, 191
  role in medical diagnosis 15, 145–9, *146*
  royal 27, 223
  and urban experience 62–3
towns, life in
  impact on senses of development of 41–64, 47–9, *57*
transparency, maximal 22, 30–6, *33*
travel, tourism 3, 32, 45–6, 50, 58, 67, 118, 120–3, 128, 160, 168
Tronchin, T. 141, 144–5
type and typesetting 211–13, *212*

upholstery
  history of development and tastes in Europe 72–6, *73*
  marketization of 80–2, *81*
Ure, A. 129

vapors, vaporous ailments 10–11
Vaucanson, J. D. 127–30
Villiers, P. de 199
Voltaire 2, 26–7, 138
vision *see* sight

voting
  and sensory openness or secrecy 22, 35–9

Walpole, H. 58, 78
Watteau, A. *180*, 181, 182–3, 184, 189, 193, 194
Watts, I. 103, 104, 105
Webb, D. 197–8
Wellek, R. 166
Wesley, C. 51, 89–90, 94, 95, 97, 105
Wesley, J. 91, 92, *93*, 94–5, 96–7, 99, 104
Whewell, W. 124
Whiston, W. 112
Whytt, R. 4
Wilkes, J. 53
Wollstonecraft, M. 60, 170, 172, 177
women and gender 10, 14–17, 26–7, 44–5, 67–8, 71, 72, 74, 83, 90–1, 99, 101, 104, 137, 160, 168, 170–2, 183, 185, 188–9, 192–4
Wordsworth, W. 173–4
work, mechanization of
  role in "philosophy of manufactures" 125–7
Wortley Montagu, M. 44–5
Wren, C. 44

Young, E. 164, 176

Zimmermann, J. G. 136–7, 144
Zinzendorf, Count N. von. 91, 99–100

www.ingramcontent.com/pod-product-compliance
Lightning Source LLC
Chambersburg PA
CBHW080535300426
44111CB00017B/2742